Women, Monstrosity

Women occupy a privileged place in horror film. Horror is a space of entertainment and excitement, of terror and dread, and one that relishes the complexities that arise when boundaries – of taste, of bodies, of reason – are blurred and dismantled. It is also a site of expression and exploration that leverages the narrative and aesthetic horrors of the reproductive, the maternal and the sexual to expose the underpinnings of the social, political and philosophical othering of women.

This book offers an in-depth analysis of women in horror films through an exploration of 'gynaehorror': films concerned with all aspects of female reproductive horror, from reproductive and sexual organs, to virginity, pregnancy, birth, motherhood and finally to menopause. Some of the themes explored include: the intersection of horror, monstrosity and sexual difference; the relationships between normative female (hetero)sexuality and the twin figures of the chaste virgin and the voracious *vagina dentata*; embodiment and subjectivity in horror films about pregnancy and abortion; reproductive technologies, monstrosity and 'mad science'; the discursive construction and interrogation of monstrous motherhood; and the relationships between menopause, menstruation, hagsploitation and 'abject barren' bodies in horror.

The book not only offers a feminist interrogation of gynaehorror, but also a counter-reading of the gynaehorrific, that both accounts for and opens up new spaces of productive, radical and subversive monstrosity within a mode of representation and expression that has often been accused of being misogynistic. It therefore makes a unique contribution to the study of women in horror film specifically, while also providing new insights in the broader area of popular culture, gender and film philosophy.

Erin Harrington is Lecturer in English and Cultural Studies at The University of Canterbury, New Zealand.

Film Philosophy at the Margins

Series editor:
Patricia MacCormack, Anglia Ruskin University, UK

Film Philosophy at the Margins picks up on the burgeoning field of 'film philosophy' – the shift from film analysis and explication to bringing together film with philosophy – and coalesces it with films, genres and spectator theory which have received little critical attention. These films could be defined as marginal due to containing marginalizing representations of violence and marginal invocations of sexuality and queer performativity, showing the margins of bodily modification from disability to performance art, being marginal in their abstraction of representative codes or in reference to their address to the politics of social control, spectatorship and cinematic pleasure as marginal due to its unique status and quality, and many other interpretations of extreme.

The film philosophy which underpins the exploration of these films is primarily Continental philosophy, rather than the more dominant field of cognitive film philosophy, utilizing increasingly attractive philosophers for film theory such as Deleuze, Guattari, Ranciere, Foucault, Irigaray and Kristeva. The series ultimately seeks to establish a refined and sophisticated methodology for re-invigorating issues of alterity both in the films chosen and the means by which Continental philosophers of difference can paradigmatically alter ways of address and representation that lifts this kind of theory beyond analysis and criticism to help rethink the terrain of film theory itself.

Titles in this series

1. Female Masochism in Film
Sexuality, Ethics and Aesthetics
Ruth McPhee

2. Women, Monstrosity and Horror Film
Gynaehorror
Erin Harrington

Women, Monstrosity and Horror Film
Gynaehorror

Erin Harrington

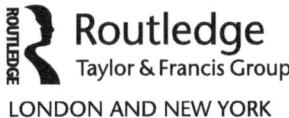

Routledge
Taylor & Francis Group

LONDON AND NEW YORK

First published 2018
by Routledge

2 Park Square, Milton Park, Abingdon, Oxfordshire OX14 4RN
52 Vanderbilt Avenue, New York, NY 10017

Routledge is an imprint of the Taylor & Francis Group, an informa business

First issued in paperback 2018

British Library Cataloguing in Publication Data
A catalogue record for this book is available from the British Library

Library of Congress Cataloging in Publication Data
Names: Harrington, Erin Jean, author.
Title: Women, monstrosity and horror film : gynaehorror / Erin Harrington.
Description: Abingdon, Oxon ; New York : Routledge, 2017. | Series: Film
philosophy at the margins | Includes bibliographical references and index.
Identifiers: LCCN 2017005807 | ISBN 9781472467294 (hardback) |
ISBN 9781315546568 (ebook)
Subjects: LCSH: Horror films--History and criticism. | Women in motion
pictures.
Classification: LCC PN1995.9.H6 H385 2017 | DDC 791.43/6164--dc23
LC record available at https://lccn.loc.gov/2017005807

ISBN: 978-1-4724-6729-4 (hbk)
ISBN: 978-0-367-20806-6 (pbk)

Typeset in Times New Roman
by Taylor & Francis Books

Contents

cannot, then, come from some sort of cool distance, and nor do I think they should. My engagement with expressions of reproductive horror cannot be divorced from the way I respond to cinema in embodied, emotional and psychological ways, which are shaped by things as diverse as my experience of my gendered body, my tastes and distastes, my mood and attention span, my capacity to take some sort of pleasure or interest in suspense and disgust, my life-history of viewing, the environment in which I might encounter a film, and even what I've had for lunch before watching something unexpectedly gory. This book does not attempt to offer a phenomenological account of horror in the vein of recent interesting work by film-philosophers such as Julian Hanich (2010), Dylan Trigg (2014), Anna Powell (2005) and Angela Ndalianis (2012), but it is informed by a mutual interest in the way that films might express complex meanings and provoke complex interactions – interactions that are utterly integral to the way that cinema is experienced and comprehended.

The juxtaposition of Creed and Clover's work, alongside scholars who are exploring new avenues of film-philosophy, highlights a tension that I acknowledge threads throughout this work, but that I hope is provocative instead of problematic. A feminist analysis of female bodies and reproduction in film gestures towards binaries in a manner that can be seen, maybe cynically, as reproducing dualistic modes of representation and interpretation that are often enshrouded in a particularly polar notion of sexual difference and the positioning of woman as dualistic Other. This, arguably, is reinforced through the deployment of feminist theories that are interested in the construction and implications of such difference, let alone their impact upon film and other forms of visual media. This is also related to the insufficient nature of the language often available to us; consider the ocular imperative embedded in the word 'spectatorship', which inherently de-emphasises many of the ways that one might encounter media, and which distils the complex relationship between media entity and individual to the seen and the unseen, the gazer and the gazed-upon. This, perhaps, is a form of linear thinking but it is nonetheless of value. Moya Lloyd (2005) reminds us that "to invoke a stable subject as the active agent of politics is *not* to refer to a subject that precedes discourse or politics... [i]t is to understand the political effects this mode of subjectification generates" (p. 58); that is, this allegedly stable subject is a construct that is politically useful. An emphasis upon the lived, embodied and subjective experience of women, of diverse female subjects, requires an acknowledgement of the very modes of entrenched power that, in the west at least, have created long-standing, deeply felt inequities through the creation and normalisation of asymmetrical relationships between the one (the norm, the centre, the reasoned, the mind, Man) and the Other (the abnormal, the periphery, the uncontained, the body, Woman).

At the same time, such identity politics do not always mesh well with the reappraisals of subjectivity that have emerged in recent decades. These range from posthuman and poststructural accounts of the subject that look to multiplicities, emergences, transformations and provocative teratologies, to accounts of queer and trans* subjectivities and phenomenologies, to the destabilisation of the notion of human-centric subjectivity in Human Animal Studies, Critical Animal Studies and some areas of ecocriticism. This might even extend to more oblique explorations of bodies in the more abstract sense; consider Jean-François Lyotard's offering in *Libidinal Economy* (1993) of a hypothetical, ambiguously sexed body, cut into a flattened band and twisted to form of a Möbius strip across whose singular surface desire circulates, intensifies and dampens, in a transformative figure of ontological playfulness that reframes libidinal impulses within groups and societies outside of gendered hierarchies.

Thus, in the discussions that follow, my identification, articulation and interrogation of such binaries serves to unpick their hierarchical, segmented logic. To draw from the conceptual tools and relationships offered by Gilles Deleuze and Félix Guattari's work on schizoanalysis in *A Thousand Plateaus*, such binaries indicate a mode of fixed, arborescent molar 'being' that operate in a different register to the rhizomatic, multiplicitous 'becoming'; as they suggest, where the tree 'is', in that it "imposes the verb 'to be' ... the fabric of the rhizome is the conjunction, 'and ... and ... and ...'" (Deleuze and Guattari 2004, 27). This ongoing production can be linked to 'desire', a material flow that is the continual production of difference. A becoming isn't an end or even a means to an end, nor is it systematic and linear (Deleuze and Guattari 2004, 24); instead, each 'plateau' of becoming is a change-event, or a snapshot of congruence. As Rosi Braidotti (2002) frames it, "The different stages or levels of becoming trace an itinerary that consists in erasing and recomposing the former boundaries between self and others" (p. 119). This erasure and re-composition makes 'becoming' an ideal way to consider bodily transformations and mutations in horror film, for it reframes 'the body' as an unstable category, not a fixed entity, and these shifts and metamorphoses as something potentially generative rather than negative and threatening. As such, becomings are inherently risky, for they challenge bodily boundaries and can unsettle "a coherent sense of personal self", but they offer the promise of "new forms of living" (Lorraine 1999, 183). After all, any consideration of the reproductive body-in-process cannot take as writ the notion that the body is a fixed, discrete and even hermetic entity.

Although the molar and the molecular coexist, one is not privileged over the other. Their relationship could be categorised as 'both/and', not 'either/or', and Deleuze and Guattari (2004) note that "Every society, and every individual, are thus plied by both segmentarities simultaneously" (p. 235). The "great binary aggregates" such as sex (i.e. man/woman) are not pre-formed independent entities but are made up of smaller molecular assemblages, multiple molecular combinations "bringing into play not only the man in the woman and the woman in the man, but the relation of each to the animal, the plant, etc.: a thousand tiny sexes" (p. 235). The molecular and the molar are not distinguished by their size or shape, but by what they do and by the system of reference within which they are envisioned (p. 239); for example, Claire

Colebrook (2002) gives the example of 'molecular experiences' that "are then organised and extended into 'molar' configurations... Before there is a 'child' that relates to a 'mother' – before there are social selves – there is a pre-personal perception, the connection of mouth and breast" (p. 82). This is the point at which we might re-state the use-value of situating sometimes binary formations of sex and gender that might inform some feminist accounts of identity politics alongside a more expansive, molecular and productive way of considering bodies' capacities and connections.

In this light, I offer the concept of gynaehorror, and the notion of the gynaehorrific, as something that is less linear, more granular, more discursive and more specific than pre-existing configurations of female, feminine and reproductive horror: gynaehorror as a type of signification and content, as an interpretive lens, and finally as a mode of aesthetic, cinematic expression and conceptual representation.

Firstly, gynaehorror, and the gynaehorrific, signals a certain type of specific content, a set of representations, and a matrix of signification that might act as generic markers. The (gynae)horror films I discuss in this book draw from a wide range of gynaehorrific constructions and scenarios, and in this usage I sit most closely to Creed's work on the monstrous-feminine. These films include sacrificial virgins, menstrual monsters and ravenous succubi. They frame the vagina as vulnerable, but also as a site of terror: rotting and dying, or filled with teeth or snakes. They feature a variety of monstrous mothers, who range from the abusive to the psychotic to the vengeful, and who inevitably place their children in the danger from which they then must be rescued. They look to supernatural pregnancies, violent births, and acts of rape and sexual coercion. They interrogate a wide range of reproductive technologies that may victimise and fragment individuals, empower the unborn and attack and dismantle the coherency of the woman's subjectivity, and render biological conception (and even gendered subjectivity, as it is currently framed) irrelevant. They highlight the way ageing women are presented as inherently monstrous – as witches, as demons, as insane, but also as productively transgressive. At the stranger end of the spectrum, they feature aborted foetuses who return to wreak revenge against those who aborted them, houses that detain and rape their occupants, and – as indicated above – ghoulish, improvised emergency caesarean sections. This is gynaehorror as a category that marks women not only as monsters, as with the monstrous-feminine, but also as victims, heroes and subjects in ways explicitly bound with their femininity, their woman-ness and their reproductive capacities, affects and potentials. To interrogate such representations, I often employ what might be thought of as orthodox modes of close reading and textual analysis.

Secondly, I use the concept of gynaehorror to signal a sociocultural, *discursive construction* of female sexuality, subjectivity and reproductive embodiment that marks the female body as always-already monstrous, no matter its age, and that suggests that female embodiment is failure and entrapment. Women and female-ness have been consistently framed historically as inferior to man.

There exists a significant historical conceptual division between the masculine, rational mind and the body-as-feminine, which I outline further in Chapter Three. In addition, women's subjectivities have historically been pushed to the margins of western philosophy, which theorises the male body-and-self as the ideologically-neutral, default subject-position (Battersby 1998; Irigaray 1985a; Irigaray 1985b; Young 1990a), and which in turn marks the body, for women themselves, as a 'problem' (Rich 1996; Young 1990b). In *Volatile Bodies* Elizabeth Grosz (1994) notes that in the West female corporeality is conceptually constructed in terms of viscosity and liquidity, flows and secretions. This ontological structuring of the female body is marked by a sense of uncontrollable 'seepage' that positions women's bodies as both passive and dependent, and unruly and disordered, but ultimately secondary to those of men, even though men's bodies are just as prone to said seepage (pp. 202–3). As Nancy Tuana outlines in *The Less Noble Sex* (1993), the

> conception of the rational person is in complete opposition to all characteristics historically conceived as female and associated with woman – the body, emotion, and passivity. For centuries prior to Descartes and for centuries after, woman was seen as inescapably bound to the concerns of the body by her role in reproduction – her pregnancies, her lactations, and her menses. (p. 63)

These mythic and philosophical assumptions, attitudes and constructions in turn have a profound and insidious effect upon the way that the female body is discursively constructed in medicine, psychology and science. Psychologist and feminist theorist Jane M. Ussher, in remarkable works such as *Managing the Monstrous-Feminine: Regulating the Reproductive Body* (2006) and *The Madness of Women: Myth and Experience* (2011), offers an in-depth, cogent and ultimately unsettling appraisal of how the taken-for-granted notion of female monstrosity operates in medical and psychological discourses, such that the othering of female bodies and experience is normalised, and the construct of woman-as-other is situated as a neutral baseline. It is not that sociocultural, political and biomedical discourses simply accept that women and their bodies are fundamentally unruly, in need of intervention and regulation, and dangerously unstable; indeed, the female reproductive body is specifically *made* monstrous and rendered mad, again and again, in a manner that significantly shapes women's own lived experiences of and knowledge(s) of their bodies and reproductive lives. Such productions of knowledge serve to illustrate a loose circuit whereby difference is expressed, co-opted, and expressed or created again, and the narrative structure of mainstream film, with its looping between order and disorder, is a helpful form through which to explore these relationships.

Throughout this book I look as much to the sociocultural work of scholars such as Ussher, who work to unpick and attack some of the taken-for-grated 'truths' about the nature of the female body, as I do the work of scholars of horror, gender and film. I connect philosophical accounts of the reproductive body, their 'real world' complications, and popular cultural artefacts, such as horror films, so as to demonstrate how they all operate within the same conceptual, yet tangible eco-system. The notion of the gynaehorrific, then, is a way of situating the intersections of female monstrosity (and the misogynistic assumptions from which this springs) in a corporeal sense, through the long-standing dismissal of the relevance of the lived experience of the female body and the alignment of female corporeality with traits that are positioned, structurally, as negative and inferior. This, in itself, is a gynaehorrific construction, for by positing that the heterosexual male body is that which is normal, ordered and ideal, anything other to that takes on the mantle of the other and becomes explicitly gendered not just in and of itself, but in opposition *to*, but identifying and challenging this explicitly is a political act. Gynaehorrific narratives, then, can both interrogate or contribute to the making-horrific of the sexed, reproductive female body.

Thirdly, gynaehorror signals a value-laden mode of aesthetic *expression* and cinematic *representation* that denigrates the female body and defines it foremost by its reproductive capacities in a manner that is negative and damaging, although whether this type of expression is specifically misogynistic, or is a way of exposing misogyny, depends significantly on the film – and, perhaps, the spectator. My use of the term 'expression', in addition to content and representation, is intended to deliberately invoke the notion, which I borrow from Deleuze and Guattari (2004), that expression (or 'enunciation') and content cannot be treated as discrete modes, but instead have a reciprocal relationship (pp. 160–1; see also Shaviro 1993, 3). As Anna Powell demonstrates in *Deleuze and Horror Film*, the 'diagrammatic components' of style such as framing, editing, image or sound – that is, those "regimes of signs or forms of expression" that might combine and interrelate to form assemblages (Deleuze and Guattari 2004, 161) – offer a particular sense of "cohesive force" within horror film (Powell 2005, 6), much as the genre itself is well-disposed to such analysis and experience. For my purposes, the productive interrelationship of gynaehorrific content, representation and expression may operate through imagery, framing and movement; through the use of sound, light and colour; through the fragmentation or the dissolution of the representational image of the body; through the audio-visual expression of a sense of reproductive dread and terror; or through the way that the female body is elided or rendered present-through-absence within the moving image. Of course, the viewer (and their body) is also drawn into these relationships given the experiential, sensory and affective properties of film (see, for instance, Ndalianis 2012; Powell 2005; Powell 2007; Shaviro 1993; Sobchack 2004), although a deep appraisal of such relationships is secondary to my project here beyond its undeniable impact upon the ways that I have engaged with these films.

Many of the films discussed in this book offer images of the female body that are perhaps provocative in their grotesquery, such as in David Cronenberg's body-horror film *The Brood* (1979), the found footage horror *The Taking of*

Deborah Logan (2014), or the *vagina dentata*-themed horror-satire *Teeth* (2007). In many cases, I offer readings of these images that utilise the challenge that they offer as a way of re-thinking, or of thinking through, the body. In some cases, reproductive monstrosity takes on non-human, alien or animal forms, as in the science fiction horror films *Alien* (1979) and *Aliens* (1986), or in the eco-horror *Prophecy* (1979), which features a mother bear and her cub who have been mutated through the effects of industrial pollution. Such non-human monstrosities and their implicit association with a conceptual, constructed female-ness that connects human bodies to non-human ones, offer entry points from which we might think through our nominally molar constructions of the body and self of the woman-in-film. Other films offer scenes or images that are hard to read as doing anything other than exercising outright misogyny for the sake of gross-out shock value, such as a scene in *Contracted* (2013) in which a woman, who has been raped and infected with a type of sexually transmitted virus that makes her die from the inside out, has maggots collect within and then fall from inside her vagina. Such imagery and relations are easy to confidently read as identifiably gynaehorrific. This situates horror, aesthetically and narratively, within and around women's reproductive bodies, even though the interpretations and the effects of these images may vary. Such gynaehorrific bodies are marked by their sexed-ness, their reproductivity, their unruly fecundity and their maternal fleshiness; they 'do' the messy and reproductive, and their relations and capacities connect them in ways that move past categories of strict signification.

However, gynaehorror also expresses itself in less literal terms. It is also apparent in the way that the woman and her body itself is present, absent or fragmented within the frame. I discuss this in depth in Chapters Two and Three, in which I consider how the female body may be visually abstracted and displaced, linking the dissolution or fragmentation of the body-image to a destabilisation of the sense of the woman as coherent subject in a manner that marks such a dissolution as negative and reductive rather than an expansion of capacity and a new mode of being or becoming. This renders the moving image as more than an audiovisual allegory (see Powell 2005, 3), and operates in a manner that articulates (in the sense of making speech, as well as in the sense of joining together disparate parts) abstract meanings, ideas and affects. In the case of a film such as *Triangle*, a time-loop narrative that I discuss in Chapter Two, the temporal plasticity of film as medium becomes a key part of the temporal slippages within the world of the story, which in turn engage with issues of maternal guilt and trauma in a stimulating manner that asks us to think through issues of free will, responsibility and predetermination. The unsettled intersection between linear and non-linear storytelling, as we follow the protagonist Jess through her 'own' time loop and across the loops of other iterations of herself, is a queasy and uncertain exploration of how a person's actions and capacities define who they are more than their articulations of self-definition. Our burgeoning understanding of cause and effect within the loop troubles our ideas about the nature of love and culpability, and the increasing violence of the action gives the impression of wounds that open, close and re-open in a never-ending, fatalistic circuit. What I will make clear, throughout, is that there is violence in the frame. The acts of cutting and editing, especially when done so to specifically deny the female subject-character her personhood or to render her no more than a collection of parts, is itself an insidiously damaging mode of representation and expression that normalises gynaehorrific attitudes and constructions of the body, even as such medium-specific expressions and modes of storytelling also offer nuanced ways of expressing the impossible tensions and contradictions within the discursive construction of woman as (reproductive) subject.

In this context it is worth highlighting that cinematic images of women's reproductive capacity, even in forms that we might think about today as benign, have often been controlled and eliminated. For example, representations of pregnancy and birth in American film were almost non-existent in the first half of the 20th century. This was, in large part, because of the impact of the rules supplied by the Motion Picture Production Code (Hayes 2009) in the United States, an in-house system of regulations adopted by Hollywood studios regarding morally acceptable and unacceptable content that was introduced in 1930 and came to be enforced stringently from 1934, until its post-War weakening and ultimate dissolution in 1967. Until December 1956 the Code decreed that scenes of birth, be they actual representations or even in silhouette, were unacceptable, and after 1957, this was amended to state that such scenes should be shown "treated with discretion and restraint within the careful limits of good taste" (Hayes 2009; see also Oliver 2012, 27–9), much as discussions of pregnancy itself were excluded from public discourse in the 1940s and 1950s (Longhurst 2000, 457).[1] Although the impact of the Code loosened significantly over time, leading to its ultimate dissolution and its replacement in 1968 – incidentally the year *Rosemary's Baby* was released – by a system of 'voluntary' film ratings through the Motion Picture Association of America, the impact of such strictures upon the representation of birth and pregnancy, as well as abortion and issues of 'sexual hygiene', was profound. Such industrial pressures, including the assumptions and attitudes that underpin them, inform gynaehorrific representations and modes of expression throughout the history of cinema. The nature of the taboo, the restricted and the deviant serves to highlight, even through visual absences or sleight-of-hand, what might be deemed challenging, disgusting or dangerous, and also increases the impact of films that breach these boundaries for the first time.

Gynaehorror from virginity to menopause

To account for the shifts in the representation and expression of sexualised, gendered female monstrosity, I offer an account of gynaehorror that follows the trajectory of the normative cisgendered female reproductive lifecycle, from menstruation and first sex, through to pregnancy and birth, to motherhood, and then finally to menopause and post-menopause. In doing so, I offer an account of ageing that highlights shifts in sexual experience, maturation and subjectivity, as well as in corporeal and affective experience. How might gynaehorrific narratives, texts or images chart anxieties about the nature of female subjectivity – of the seeming horror of sexual 'difference'? How might they offer spaces in which to challenge negative constructions of the female body? After all, the experience of one's own sexed, gendered, reproductive body, and the way that gynaehorrific discourses, images and narratives serve to shape our own experiences, provide us with narratives through which we might understand our own bodies and how they operate within the world.

This structural scaffolding is not designed to suggest that this is how all women live their lives or experience their bodies, that all women can or should have children (or even want to), that pregnancy and motherhood are and should be the centre of a woman's life, that all women were assigned female at birth (or vice versa) or identify with binary gender formations, and so on. Instead, I am interested in the bluntly normative – the taken-for-granted sets of norms and ideals about the nature of sex and reproduction that accompany, and perhaps constrain, women as they age. Such a matrix of hegemonic normativity sets parameters of representation, which also act as constraints in terms of the cinematic representation (or lack thereof) of diverse intersections and expressions of ethnicity, class, appearance, sexuality, and gender identity and expression. I also wish to explore how and why, no matter a girl's or woman's age, female sexuality and the sexed female body is rendered monstrous in profoundly insidious and often blatantly contradictory ways. These horror films, then, offer a key site through which to unpack the nature of the gynaehorrific.

I have tried to offer a representative account of this subgenre, but what I have not offered is a representative account of women. Despite its many monsters and its numerous horrors, at present the horror genre is not a site that can be particularly praised for its social and cultural diversity, and it is important to flag that the women who feature in the films I discuss are overwhelmingly heterosexual and cisgendered – something I discuss at the close of Chapter One. More often than not, they are coded as middle class, whether or not they have any further degree of social, political, economic or personal agency. They are also, almost to a woman, white (or 'European'). This lack of racial and ethnic diversity continues to remain pronounced throughout the genre, even in light more inclusive casting of individual titles, such as the 2014 adaptation of *Rosemary's Baby*, a mini-series that cast black actress Zoe Saldana in the role of Rosemary. This is, perhaps, frustrating for the viewer – and certainly this viewer – but I posit that this overarching essentialism is nonetheless helpful from an analytic perspective. It means that as a corpus these collected films offer a degree of enlightenment regarding taken-for-granted assumptions about the nature of femininity and normative female (hetero-) sexuality through their reproduction of a hegemonic bias towards a certain *type* of woman. This is doubly so if we consider the intersection of gynaehorrific attitudes towards sex and bodies with broader cultural and industrial pressures and constraints on the casting of women, including the sorts of structural representations engendered, decision by decision, by filmmakers, producers and distributors. As film theorist Annette Kuhn suggests, if we accept the argument that

> in a sexist society both presences and absences [of women in film] may not be immediately discernible to the ordinary spectator, if only because certain representations appear to be quite ordinary and obvious, then the fundamental project of feminist film analysis can be said to centre on making visible the invisible. (1994, 71)

In keeping with this sentiment I write as a cultural studies scholar, drawing from feminist poststructural and film theories, to interrogate not only apparently "ordinary and obvious" *representations* of women in horror, but to address significant absences alongside *expressions* of gynaehorror, be they aesthetic, thematic or narrative.

To provide a baseline for this discussion, in Chapter One, "Roses and Thorns", I offer an account of normative female sexuality, with an emphasis upon the ways that the horror genre expresses a fascination with the sexuality and sexualisation of women – particularly young women, the construction of virginity, and the act of first sex. It is telling that in his 2012 book *Horror and the Horror Film* Bruce F. Kawin regularly focuses his attention on a trope that, in his index, he calls the 'unconscious woman' or 'the monster and the girl', which features the merging of sex, desire and voyeurism (by both characters and the viewer) with horror. Very early in the book he highlights a scene from the B-movie *Tarantula* (1955) in which the eponymous giant spider voyeuristically spies on the vulnerable, normatively attractive heroine, who is undressing in her bedroom. Despite the almost ridiculous disjunction between arachnid–human relationships, the spider it becomes so excited and agitated that it destroys her house (Kawin 2012, 20–1). This connection between sex, desire and violence is, perhaps, a particularly apt representative account of a gendered power dynamic that recurs throughout the genre, and this is certainly an obvious relationship in the slasher subgenre. Indeed, as Andrew Welsh (2010) demonstrates in his intensive quantitative study of sex and violence in slasher films, women in such films are far more likely to fall prey to eroticised violence than men, and women who engage in sexual behaviour in these films are not only more likely to die than their male and female counterparts, but their death scenes are likely to be longer and more explicit. However, the interplay between female victimhood and the overt display of female sexuality is prominent beyond the monster movie and the slasher, for the sexualised, potentially reproductive woman is present in horror film as hero, villain, victim and monster.

To account for and broaden these constructs, in this first chapter I expand this focus on sex and sexuality to provide a detailed account of the way that taken-for-granted ideas about normative female (hetero)sexuality are articulated, recycled and policed in horror film. While I offer a sociocultural account of such constructions, I also look to Luce Irigaray's critique of the way that female subjectivity is less constructed than it is elided in male-centric psychoanalytic articulations of the male subject, rendered both necessary and invisible. Here I suggest that female sexuality in the horror film is often presented in simplistic, binary terms. One hand, it is both fetishised and contained through the figures of the tenacious virgin-hero and the chaste, feminine sacrificial virgin, each of which shore up the explicit cultural association of virginity with reductive modes of femininity. These archetypes sit in clear contrast to the representation of virginal men, who tend to be presented in feminised terms as weak and emasculated, or as stern ascetics whose self-denial of sexual pleasure and other forms of eroticism or appetite is a measure of their masculine moral strength and thus a repudiation of the femininity that is central to broader understandings of virginity. On the other hand, the unbounded sexual threat of the mythical *vagina dentata*, the toothed vagina, suggests that female sexuality, sensuality and eroticism is dangerous, voracious and monstrous, although this negative framing of such an open, desirous figure bears witness to the way that 'appropriate' (phallocentric, procreative) sexuality is policed. These paradigms serve to constrain and simplify broader cultural conceptualisations of female sexuality while nonetheless turning the body of the woman into an object that is either available for (male, masculine hetero-) sexual consumption, or that is deemed disgusting, terrifying and threatening to phallocentric domination. These constructs co-mingle in the horror-satire *Teeth* (2007), a film in which a chaste young woman discovers that she has a toothed vagina that functions as both a protective mechanism and a form of sexual weaponry. Here, I suggest that the film leverages these archetypes to critique facile, restrictive and often misogynistic understandings of female sexuality and sexual agency, with a sharp emphasis upon those that are propagated through American sexual education programmes that valorise and fetishise virginity, particularly the virginity of young women, and that emphasise abstinence and ignorance over awareness.

   In the following two chapters I move from the area of critical sexualities to theories of subjectivity, an area of profound relevance to horror given the genre's interest in the nature of the boundary between 'self' and 'other'. In Chapter Two, "The Lady Vanishes", I focus on pregnancy, abortion and foetal imagery. There is a key sticking point in the philosophical consideration of female subjectivity that, beyond its own issues of gender and corporeality, has implications for the image of the female body on screen: the historic construction of the ideal subject of western philosophy is that of an in-divisible 'whole' individual who is implicitly male, young, fit and healthy (for whatever 'health' means). Clearly this sits at odds with the state of pregnancy, in which a woman moves from 'one', then 'more-than-one', to a forever changed 'one', if such terminology is even appropriate for a body-in-process. A helpful point of engagement is the work of feminist philosophers Iris Marion Young (1990b), Christine Battersby (1998) and Imogen Tyler (2000), who have each accounted for alternative pregnant subject positions or reconfigured dominant modes of subjectivity.

I had, initially, hoped to find that the fleshy corporeality of the horror genre was a place in which alternative modes of being and subjectivity could be explored and considered, be it through narrative or through the representation of the body and self within the film-image – something that I consider through a discussion of the 'spatiality' of women's bodies, and the long-standing gothic tradition of the conceptual conflation of women's bodies with domestic spaces such as houses. However, I suggest that horror films about pregnancy instead set up a strong oppositional relationship between the pregnant woman and the foetus inside her, both narratively and through cinematic means, such as through framing, editing and the manipulation of off-screen and on-screen space. I argue that this schema has been popularly exacerbated through the ongoing development of foetal imaging technologies, which indicates a provocative intersection between the popular film, medical technology and philosophical models of the self and the subject, especially given the way that pregnancy itself is so often pathologised. For all their medical and social benefits, these technologies allow the foetus *itself* to be considered as an autonomous subject-entity that exists in competition with its mother, sometimes displacing her entirely. Horror films about pregnancy leverage this oppositional, antagonistic relationship to gynaehorrific ends, and demonstrate disquiet about how to best conceptualise, express and explore the uniquely temporal and coextensive embodied relationship between woman and foetus.

Roman Polanksi's 1968 film *Rosemary's Baby* is one of the best examples of the dilemma of the pregnant subject in horror. Its protagonist, Rosemary, is impregnated by a demonic presence after her husband secretly barters her body away to a group of Satanists so that his acting career may prosper. Rosemary acts as the vessel for the Antichrist, and much of the film centres on the tension between the physical and emotional violation of Rosemary-as-subject, her role as unwitting maternal host and the needs of the gestating foetus. *Rosemary's Baby* is, perhaps, the best-known gynaehorror, and certainly a film against which others covering similar territory position themselves and are judged. Throughout this chapter, and this book more widely, I deliberately move beyond this film to consider how issues of pregnancy and subjectivity are expressed elsewhere in the genre. Instead, I interrogate how the pregnant body is positioned and imagined, and the manner in which the pregnant subject herself becomes abstracted, in the technohorror *Demon Seed* (1977), and in religious and ecological horror films such as *The Reaping* (2007) and *Prophecy* (1979) respectively. This oppositional relationship between woman and foetus is made most apparent in the aforementioned French film *Inside/À l'intérieur* (2007), which offers a particularly unusual mode of representation in its inclusion of a computer generated unborn child, who appears as an *in utero* subject.

Stories about pregnancy and birth are well-represented in the genre, but there remains one particularly resonant taboo: abortion, a subject that is conspicuous by its near-absence in Anglophone horror film. I suggest that the dearth of films that feature abortion is indicative of the fraught political nature of the topic, particularly in the United States, in that the heated, some-times violent debate over a woman's right to choose is so deeply embedded within the topic that those few films that choose to include abortion seem compelled to either dance awkwardly around the issue or engage with it head on. A small handful of films about abortion offer a provocative account of the way that the subjectivities of the pregnant woman and the foetus are often pitted against one another. Their political manoeuvring, be it sophisticated or ham-fisted, offers an interesting perspective on the politicisation of gynaehorror. Beyond acknowledging a few exploitation films that leverage the shock value of using aborted foetuses as vengeful entities, I close Chapter Two by comparing the self-proclaimed 'pro-life' American independent horror film *The Life Zone* (2011) to John Carpenter's contribution to the American cable television horror anthology *Masters of Horror*, "Pro-Life" (2007), which is set in an abortion clinic that is under siege by both militant anti-abortion activists and a demonic presence. Both demonstrate how the presentation of abortion in specifically American horror, at least, is irrevocably tied into abortion politics. I also outline how each film explores the subjective power and agency of pregnant women, which differs depending on the text's political position.

In Chapter Three, "Not of Woman Born", I continue my discussion of subjectivity by shifting from the 'embodied' states of pregnancy and abortion to a consideration of 'disembodied' reproduction, that is, the way that the reproductive female body is compromised, elided or eliminated altogether in horror films about reproductive technology – what I term reproductive tech-nohorror. Reproductive technologies such as *in vitro* fertilisation are radical in that they challenge the heteronormative, biologically deterministic procreative imperative that suggests that certain types of families are the 'ideal' family, for they open up new forms of family configuration. They alter the nature of conception and reproductive embodiment itself, by challenging what it means to be an efficient, effective or even necessary reproductive body or participant. They provoke questions about what bodies can and should be able to do, and how flesh and technology might (re)productively co-mingle. They highlight the degree to which we are always-already posthuman, and look to the new modes of being and becoming that might otherwise be engendered through the alliances and symbioses of flesh and technology. And yet, they are inevitably presented as ambivalent: they also inhabit a space marked by corporeal and ethical ambiguity, and as such they are a rich source and site of gynaehorror.

This dis-ease is particularly apparent in 'mad science' narratives, stories like that of Victor Frankenstein and his monster, which explore the creation of life – from conception and sometimes through to gestation – outside the body of the woman and, thus, outside of the so-called 'natural order'. Here I recall Chapter One's discussion of heterosexuality and heteronormativity, for 'mad science' narratives situate reproduction within a molar, dualistic conceptual schema that is structured with regards to the historic association of science to what genre theorist Robin Wood (2003) called the horror film's "disreputable" status (pp. 29–30). Some films have certainly proven themselves to be richer veins of gynaehorror than others, but I have endeavoured not to reinforce explicit and implicit hegemonic hierarchies of taste, nor to cast a distinction between the scholarly value of so-called 'high' and 'low' culture. Films that are well-crafted, thoughtful pieces of cinema-as-art are as valuable here as those that are messy, fragmented and ideologically incoherent; if anything, the latter are more revealing, given their perhaps kneejerk reactions to issues of gender politics, their emphasis upon bottom-of-the-barrel shock tactics, and their sometimes clumsy playfulness with the aesthetics of cinema. As a genre, horror also lends itself well to such a consideration, for as Ian Conrich (2009) remarks in his introduction to *Horror Zone: The Cultural Experience of Contemporary Horror,* "Such is the cross appeal of a core of contemporary horror that it can cater for both a subculture and the mainstream" (p. 3).

I also contextualise these films through an appraisal of other cultural texts and practices; for instance, in Chapter One, I connect horror films about virginity and *vagina dentata* to popular constructions and representations of virginity and female sexuality found in pornography, fine art, American in-school abstinence programmes and urban legends spread by American soldiers. Chapter Three charts some of the connections between the representation of reproductive technologies, including foetal imagery, in horror film, alongside contemporaneous engagements with these issues in the popular and scientific arenas. In this case I demonstrate how these horrific representations take on their own life, mapping lines of flight that dance beyond the interface between film-artefact and viewer, and become an important, populist interpretive lens, within public discourse. These acts of contextualisation are important to my broader analysis because popular films do not exist in a cultural vacuum; much as so-called 'low-brow' and 'high-brow' films can be analysed alongside one another, and indeed often 'do' the same work, it is important that films are considered (and contextualised) against other forms of cultural praxis, and that connections between seemingly heterogeneous media and practices are formed.

I have also deliberately looked beyond films that have achieved 'canonical' status so as to broaden and complicate the discussion of gynaehorror, and in doing so I hope to offer unusual and provocative combinations, intersections and juxtapositions – multifaceted gynaehorrific assemblages. I recognise and sometimes challenge dominant readings of films that are frequently cited or analysed, such as *Rosemary's Baby, The Brood* and *Psycho* (1960), but I also engage with a variety of sometimes idiosyncratic films that have not received in-depth scholarly attention, such as *The Killing Kind, Demon Seed, Prophecy, The Unborn* (1991), *Grace, Triangle, Teeth, The Life Zone* and *Inside.* In some ways my criteria have been very prosaic: is this a film that I, as a fan of the genre, am able to acquire and view? Have I recognised or responded to the sort of exploration or expression of the gynaehorrific? I certainly do not consider myself the 'ideal viewer', but I do wish to acknowledge the breadth of cinema, that is easily available to the enthusiastic English-speaking audience, at the same time as paying heed to the transnational flows that exist within contemporary film viewership (let alone filmmaking itself). Some of these flows, especially regarding the impact of new technologies upon the creation and dissemination of horror films, are considered briefly in Chapter Five.

This issue of transnational context is an important one, and one that recurs throughout this book. It is important to note that the films to which I refer are almost entirely Anglophone and are predominantly made in the United States, although some come from other areas, such as Western Europe.[3] I have not deliberately sought out American films, yet this focus is, perhaps (and, possibly, debatably), unavoidable, especially given horror's position within the history of American film as a staple genre (Hantke 2010, p. vii) and the importance of North American horror films to the development of theory and scholarship surrounding horror as a film genre. However, while the American film industry, particularly the Hollywood system, has been profoundly influential on global and genre cinema, these flows are not one way. There is now a broad range of films that come from complimentary communities of film makers that are no longer – if they have ever truly been – bounded by strict geographical borders. Christina Klein, writing on horror film in 2010, points out the way that genre films are open to transnationali-sation and can be easily localised (pp. 3–4). She also indicates that Hollywood is now a global industry, not just an American one, and its most successful films make more money outside of the United States than they do domestically (p. 4). Klein goes on to argue that:

> the national and cultural identity of many contemporary horror films is increasingly open to question… This question of cultural identity extends, of course, beyond the realm of genre films and into questions about audiences and national culture more generally, all of which are becoming less culturally coherent. (p. 12)

Further, even as Hollywood expands its production and business model into foreign markets, so too do international filmmakers come to Hollywood – as they always have done. One example is French director Alexandre Aja, whose film *Haute Tension* (2003) I discuss at the close of Chapter One. He cites American horror directors Wes Craven, John Carpenter and Tobe Hooper as key influences in his work, indicating that he "grew up with [their] films" (Faraci 2005) in France. His work exhibits a playful, genre-savvy inter-textuality, such as in the way that *Haute Tension* poaches from and reworks an iconic scene in the infamous 'video nasty' *Maniac* (1980) in which the film's killer stalks a woman through a deserted subway station. Pascal Laugier, the director of French horror film *Martyrs* (2008), has argued that French horror cinema lacks legitimacy in its own country (White 2009); it is telling, then, that according to box office reporting service Box Office Mojo, *Haute* through the assemblages and aggregates formed by their personal viewing histories and experiences, and through the way that films might elicit the various affective registers of the 'sensorium': the interplay between a media text and the emotional, cognitive, sensory and physical reactions, engagements and responses effected as one's embodied self interfaces with media.

I belong to a group of horror-loving women who get together regularly to watch horror films, eat, drink, heckle, clutch at each other, debrief and share our love for the genre. We are active, not passive, spectators. In watching gynaehorrific films we think through our own sexual and reproductive lives; we get angry at the often restrictive, reductive nature of representations of women on screen; we celebrate the liberatory and subversive power of the abject and the monstrous; we boo at and denigrate framing that objectifies women and we cheer at female and female-identifying characters (and monsters!) who challenge boundaries and defy the expectations of both genre and society. In our effusive, loving viewing and our sense of community we also refute the idea that we are people first and bodies second, or that perspectives, stories and aesthetics that connect to our own ways of being in the world should be side-lined. Our own experiences with sex, sexuality, gender identity, relationships, pregnancy, birth, menstruation, endometriosis, hysterectomies, menopause and decisions to have children (or not), are undeniably points of fleshy, mucky intersection with our love for and experience with the genre. They provide the emotional, affective and embodied contexts within which we encounter cinema.

Although some of us explicitly intersect with other, similar female-centric fan communities, our own small-scale practices as active spectators, fans and academics are also connected in a broader sense with the emergence in the last ten years of female horror and genre festivals that centralise and promote the work of female and female-identifying filmmakers who are actively working to make horror (as genre, as industry) more diverse. These include the Women's Alliance of Fantastic Film Festivals, American Cinematheque's Etheria Film Night, Tokyo's Scream Queen FilmFest, Australia's Stranger With My Face International Film Festival, and the delightfully vulgarly-named Ax Wound Film Festival, which is organised by international grass-roots organisation Women in Horror Month. I would also argue that the most important piece of feminist horror criticism in recent times comes not from within the academy, but in Canadian writer and film festival programmer Kier-La Jannisse's remarkable autobiographical appraisal of female neuroses in film, *House of Psychotic Women* (2012). Beyond its comprehensive annotated filmography, it highlights the extent to which women, as individuals and as groups, use films as the cultural material through which we might shape and understand our own lives; to invoke the well-worn phrase, they are matter (stuff, material), and they matter (have resonance and importance). All these endeavours work to challenge the notion that horror is a space that is misogynistic and threatening by belligerently reframing the genre as potentially inclusive and positive, working for and not against women.

Horror, then, might also be radical. It is a genre that recycles and rearticulates certain images, but it also destabilises then creates new meaning(s), and fashions a space in which challenges to the status quo and non-normative bodies, identities, expressions and affects are actively centralised. In unpicking the gynaehorrific underpinnings of the representation of women, sex, reproduction and monstrosity in horror – that is, the social, cultural and discursive means by which female gendered monstrosity operates – and in exposing the mechanisms through which horror functions as art, as industrial product, as affect engine and as cultural artefact, we can also untangle molar issues of female monstrosity. After all, we must accept that the nature of the 'monstrous' isn't itself, inherently negative. The monstrous is disobedient, unruly and disrespectful of borders – although this begs the question, 'who is being disobeyed and whose borders disrespected?' The monstrous is generative, rhizomatic and creative, given to proliferation of new modes of unsanctioned, uncontrolled being and expression, and productive lines of flight. Monsters produce and reproduce cultural meaning; as Asa Simon Mittman (2012) attests, "Monsters do a great deal of cultural work, but they do not do it *nicely*" (p. 1). Similarly, Jeffrey Jerome Cohen (1996) suggests that we might try to expel monsters, but when they return "they bring not just a fuller knowledge of our place in history and the history of knowing our place, but they bear self-knowledge … they ask us why we have created them" (p. 20).

The monstrous also signals a body-in-process – and given the cyclical nature of the female reproductive life cycle, and the way that these shifts shape and impact upon women, perhaps leveraging such changes, such malleability and such fleshy corporeality is a distinctly political mode of thinking about and (re-)framing the body. Gynaehorrific films and themes highlight misogyny and fear through their stories, their preoccupations, and the way that they shape and frame the female body through the temporality and spatiality of cinema, but they also offer representational and aesthetic space in which women's bodies and embodied lives insist on being seen and insist on being important. The monstrous expresses dynamic movement across multiple planes; monsters are events. If we are to think of the radical, expansive, productive use of horror, or of monstrosity as a way of breaching boundaries and offering new modes of being, then gynaehorrific narratives and expressions of gynaehorror may also be able to be reconsidered in a manner that emphasises, rather than marginalises the potentialities of the female or feminine body and various expressions of diverse female subjectivities through a celebration of otherness, a way of placing bodies-in-process at the centre of modes of representation, and an attempt to re-centre, not (r)eject, forms of female experience. Thus, my appraisals of gynaehorror throughout this book will dance between and through horror as radical and transformative, and horror as conservative and reductive, not to suggest that these dipoles cannot be resolved, but to highlight productive, rich dissonances, and to celebrate the complexity of a genre that is, too often, written off as low-brow and reactionary.

Notes

1 Similarly, abortion was deemed to be a taboo subject: from 1951 to 1956 the Code explicitly stated that "Abortion, sex hygiene and venereal diseases are not proper subjects for theatrical motion pictures", and prior to this, the topic of abortion was implicitly covered under the regulations regarding "sex perversion" and "sex hygiene". Even after December 1956, the amended code discouraged the subject of abortion, insisting that it should never be discussed, or shown directly or by inference, that stories should never indicate that an abortion had been performed, and that abortion should always be condemned and treated with the utmost seriousness, to the extent that the word itself was disallowed (Hayes 2009).
2 The American Genre Film Archive, for instance, focuses on "exploitation era of independent cinema – the 1960s through the 1980s" (About AGFA 2016).
3 The exclusion of horror films from other territories, such as the burgeoning South East Asian horror industry is both practical and theoretical: it is due to my own ignorance about these film traditions, and the pronounced difference in the history of gender and feminist studies and theories in these areas. This sort of broad transnational study of horror and gender, although a fruitful area, is beyond the scope of this project, although Higbee and Lim (2010) offer a fruitful discussion of some of the potential areas of study and debate within such transnational film studies. In terms of gynaehorror, Sarah Arnold also offers some interesting work in her cogent comparative analysis of Japanese horror films about motherhood and their American remakes (Arnold 2013).
4 A white New Zealander of 'European' descent.

Bibliography

'About AGFA' 2016, *American Genre Film Archive*, accessed March 30, 2016, from <http://americangenrefilm.com/about>.

Aldana Reyes, X & Blake, L 2015, *Digital horror: haunted technologies, network panic and the found footage phenomenon*, London and New York: I. B.Tauris.

Arnold, S 2013, *Maternal horror film: melodrama and motherhood*, Basingstoke, Hampshire and New York, NY: Palgrave Macmillan.

Battersby, C 1998, *The phenomenal woman: feminist metaphysics and the patterns of identity*, Cambridge, UK: Polity Press.

Berenstein, R J 1996, *Attack of the leading ladies: gender, sexuality, and spectatorship in classic horror cinema*, New York: Columbia University Press.

Bordo, S 1987, *The flight to objectivity: essays on cartesianism and culture*, Albany, NY: SUNY Press.

Braidotti, R 2002, *Metamorphoses: towards a materialist theory of becoming*, Cambridge, UK and Malden, MA: Polity Press in association with Blackwell Publishers.

Braidotti, R 2011, *Nomadic theory: the portable Rosi Braidotti*, New York: Columbia University Press.

Carpenter, J 2007, 'Pro-Life', *Masters of Horror*.

Cherry, B 2002a, 'Refusing to refuse to look: female viewers of the horror film', in M Jancovich (ed), *Horror, the film reader*, London and New York: Routledge, pp. 169–178.

Cherry, B 2002b, 'Screaming for release: femininity and horror film fandom in Britain', in S Chibnall & J Petley (eds), *British horror cinema*, London and New York: Routledge, pp. 42–57.

Church, D 2010, 'Afterword: memory, genre and self-narritivization; or, why I should be a more content horror fan', in S Hantke (ed), *American horror film: the genre at the turn of the millennium*, Jackson, MS: University Press of Mississippi, pp. 235–242.

Clover, C J 1992, *Men, women and chain saws: gender in the modern horror film*, Princeton, N.J.: Princeton University Press.

Cohen, J J 1996, 'Monster culture (seven theses)', in J J Cohen (ed), *Monster theory: reading culture*, Minneapolis, MN: University of Minnesota Press, pp. 3–25.

Colebrook, C 2002, *Gilles Deleuze*, London and New York: Routledge.

Conrich, I 2009, 'Introduction', in I Conrich (ed), *Horror zone: the cultural experience of contemporary horror cinema*, London: I. B. Tauris & Co. pp. 1–8, accessed February 17, 2014, from <http://public.eblib.com/EBLPublic/PublicView.do?ptiID= 676670>.

Creed, B 1993, *The monstrous-feminine: film, feminism, psychoanalysis*, London and New York: Routledge.

Deleuze, G & Guattari, F 2004, *A thousand plateaus: capitalism and schizophrenia*, London: Continuum.

Faraci, D 2005, 'Exclusive interview: Alexandre Aja (High Tension)', *CHUD.com*, accessed February 17, 2014, from <http://www.chud.com/3284/exclusive-interview-a lexandre-aja-high-tension/>.

Gamson, J 2011, 'Popular culture constructs sexuality', in S Seidman, N Fischer, & C Meeks (eds), *Introducing the New Sexuality Studies: 2nd Edition*, , Hoboken, NJ: Taylor and Francis, pp. 27–31.

Grosz, E 1994, *Volatile bodies: toward a corporeal feminism*, Bloomington, IN: Indiana University Press.

Hanich, J 2010, *Cinematic emotion in horror films and thrillers: the aesthetic paradox of pleasurable fear*, New York: Routledge.

Hantke, S 2010, 'Introduction: they don't make 'em like they used to', in S Hantke (ed), *American horror film: the genre at the turn of the millennium*, Jackson, MS: University Press of Mississippi, pp. viii–xxxii.

Hawkins, J 2009, 'Culture wars: some new trends in art horror', *Jump Cut*, no. 51, accessed from <http://www.ejumpcut.org/archive/jc51.2009/artHorror/>.

Hayes, D 2009, 'The Production Code of the Motion Picture Industry (1930–1967)', *The Motion Picture Production Code*, accessed December 10, 2013, from <http:// productioncode.dhwritings.com/multipleframes_productioncode.php>.

Heise-von der Lipp, A 2015, 'Hypertext and the Creation of Choice: Making Monsters in the Age of Digital Textual (Re)Production', in L Piatti-Farnell & D L Brien (eds), *New directions in 21st-century gothic: the gothic compass*, New York and London: Routledge, pp. 117–131.

Higbee, W & Lim, S H 2010, 'Concepts of transnational cinema: towards a critical transnationalism in film studies', *Transnational Cinemas*, 1(1), pp. 7–21.

'High Tension (2005) – Box Office Mojo' 2014, *Box Office Mojo*, accessed February 17, 2014, from <http://www.boxofficemojo.com/movies/?id=hightension.htm>.

Irigaray, L 1985a, *Speculum of the other woman*, Ithaca, NY: Cornell University Press.

Irigaray, L 1985b, *This sex which is not one*, Ithaca, NY: Cornell University Press.

Jackson, K 2013, *Technology, monstrosity, and reproduction in twenty-first century horror*, New York, NY: Palgrave Macmillan.

Jancovich, M 2002, 'General introduction', in M Jancovich (ed), *Horror, the film reader*, London and New York: Routledge, pp. 1–19.

Janisse, K-L 2012, *House of psychotic women: an autobiographical topography of female neurosis in horror and exploitation films*, Godalming, UK: Fab Press.

Kaplan, E A 1992, *Motherhood and representation: the mother in popular culture and melodrama*, London and New York: Routledge.

Kawin, B F 2012, *Horror and the horror film*, London and New York: Anthem Press.

Kellner, D 2003, *Media culture: cultural studies, identity and politics between the modern and the post-modern*, London: Routledge, accessed from <http://books.google.co.nz/books?id=DlyKAgAAQBAJ>.

Klein, C 2010, 'The American horror film? Globalization and transnational U.S.-Asian genres', in S Hantke (ed), *American horror film: the genre at the turn of the millennium*, Jackson, MS: University Press of Mississippi, pp. 3–14.

Kleinhans, C 2009, 'Cross-cultural disgust: some problems in the analysis of contemporary horror cinema', *Jump Cut*, no. 51, accessed from <http://www.ejumpcut.org/archive/jc51.2009/crosscultHorror/index.html>.

Kristeva, J 1982, *Powers of horror: an essay on abjection*, New York: Columbia University Press.

Kuhn, A 1994, *Women's pictures: feminism and cinema*, London and New York: Verso.

Lloyd, M 2005, *Beyond identity politics: feminism, power & politics*, London, Thousand Oaks, CA and New Delhi: Sage.

Longhurst, R 2000, '"Corporeographies" of pregnancy: "bikini babes"', *Environment and Planning D: Society and Space*, 18(4), pp. 453–472.

Lorraine, T E 1999, *Irigaray & Deleuze: experiments in visceral philosophy*, Ithaca, NY: Cornell University Press.

Lyotard, J-F 1993, *Libidinal economy*, Bloomington, IN: Indiana University Press.

MacCormack, P 2008, *Cinesexuality*, Aldershot, UK and Burlington, VT: Ashgate.

McPhee, R 2014, *Female masochism in film: sexuality, ethics and aesthetics*, Farnham, Surrey, UK and Burlington, VT: Ashgate.

Mittman, A S 2012, 'Introduction: the impact of monsters and monster studies', in A S Mittman & P Dendle (eds), *The Ashgate research companion to monsters and the monstrous*, Farnham, UK and Burlington, VT: Ashgate, pp. 1–14.

Mulvey, L 1990, 'Afterthoughts of "Visual Pleasure and Narrative Cinema" inspired by *Duel in the Sun*', in E A Kaplan (ed), *Psychoanalysis & Cinema*, London: Routledge, pp. 24–35.

Mulvey, L 2000, 'Visual pleasure and narrative cinema', in E A Kaplan (ed), *Feminism and Film*, Oxford readings in feminism, Oxford and New York: Oxford University Press, pp. 34–47.

Ndalianis, A 2012, *The horror sensorium: media and the senses*, Jefferson, NC: McFarland & Co.

Neale, S 2000, *Genre and Hollywood*, London and New York: Routledge.

Ochoa, G 2011, *Deformed and destructive beings: the purpose of horror films*, Jefferson, NC: McFarland.

Oliver, K 2012, *Knock me up, knock me down: images of pregnancy in Hollywood films*, New York: Columbia University Press.

Perrello, T 2010, 'A Parisian in Hollywood: ocular horror in the films of Alexandre Aja', in S Hantke (ed), *American horror film: the genre at the turn of the millennium*, Jackson, MS: University Press of Mississippi, pp. 15–34.

Pinedo, I C 1997, *Recreational terror: women and the pleasures of horror film viewing*, Albany, NY: SUNY Press.

Powell, A 2005, *Deleuze and horror film*, Edinburgh: Edinburgh University Press.

Powell, A 2007, *Deleuze, altered states and film*, Edinburgh: Edinburgh University Press.

Rich, A 1996, *Of woman born: motherhood as experience and institution*, New York: W W Norton & Co.

Shaviro, S 1993, *The cinematic body*, Minneapolis, MN: University of Minnesota Press.

Shildrick, M 2002, *Embodying the monster: encounters with the vulnerable self*, London: SAGE Publications.

Sobchack, V 2004, *Carnal thoughts: embodiment and moving image culture*, Berkeley, CA: University of California Press.

Trigg, D 2014, *The thing: a phenomenology of horror*, Alresford, UK: Zero Books.

Tuana, N 1993, *The less noble sex: scientific, religious, and philosophical conceptions of woman's nature*, Bloomington, IN: Indiana University Press.

Tyler, I 2000, 'Reframing pregnant embodiment', in S Ahmed, J Kilby, C Lury, M McNeil, & B Skeggs (eds), *Thinking through feminism*, London and New York: Routledge, pp. 288–302.

Ussher, J M 2006, *Managing the monstrous feminine: regulating the reproductive body*, London and New York: Routledge.

Ussher, J M 2011, *The madness of women: myth and experience*, London and New York: Routledge.

Vosper, A J 2014, 'Film, fear and the female: an empirical study of the female horror fan', *Offscreen*, 18(6–7), accessed August 29, 2016, from <http://offscreen.com/view/film-fear-and-the-female>.

Welsh, A 2010, 'On the perils of living dangerously in the slasher horror film: gender differences in the association between sexual activity and survival', *Sex Roles*, 62(11–12), pp. 762–773.

White, J 2009, 'Interview with Pascal Laugier (director of Martyrs)', *Film @ The Digital Fix*, accessed February 21, 2014, from <http://film.thedigitalfix.com/content/id/70486/interview-with-pascal-laugier-director-of-martyrs.html>.

Wood, R 2003, *Hollywood from Vietnam to Reagan – and beyond*, expanded and rev. ed., New York: Columbia University Press.

Young, I M 1990a, *Throwing like a girl and other essays in feminist philosophy and social theory*, Bloomington, IN: Indiana University Press.

Young, I M 1990b, 'Pregnant embodiment: subjectivity and alienation', in *Throwing like a girl and other essays in feminist philosophy and social theory*, Bloomington, IN: Indiana University Press, pp. 160–176.

1 Roses and thorns

Virgins, *vagina dentata* and the monstrosity of female sexuality

Within the world of the horror genre, virginity is of great importance: it is a state, a category, and an expression of femininity that is endowed with power, significance and prestige. In a typically intertextual scene in the post-modern slasher *Scream* (1996), the aptly named virginal, geeky film nerd Randy Meeks outlines the conventions of the horror film to a crowded room of party-goers who are watching director John Carpenter's 1978 slasher *Halloween*: if you want to survive you can never have sex, because sex equals death. You can't drink or do drugs either, because like sex, these are sins, and teen vice is a quick and bloody road to dismemberment and destruction. To prove his point, Randy cites actor Jamie Lee Curtis's roles as a heroic, virginal 'scream queen' in a series of early slasher films: *Halloween, The Fog* (1980), *Terror Train* (1980), *Prom Night* (1980), *Halloween II* (1981) and *Road Games* (1982). When another party-goer announces that he wants to see Curtis's breasts, Randy replies that Curtis didn't show her 'tits' until she hit the mainstream and went 'legit' in her BAFTA-award winning role in the 1983 comedy *Trading Places*. By contrast, in her roles as a horror heroine her virginity and her sexual 'purity' was always assured.[1]

This wry, self-reflexive commentary on the nature of sex and transgression in the horror film, and the way that virginity appears as character trait, expression of sexed and gendered implicitly feminine (or feminised) identity, and, sometimes, plot device within the genre, serve to highlight how widespread and taken-for-granted ideas about male and female (hetero)sexuality come to be represented, expressed and reinforced in popular culture. As sexuality researchers Holland, Ramazanoglu and Thomson argue, "the meanings of virginity and its 'loss', and the acquisition of heterosexual identities, continue to be socially gendered and differently embodied for men and women" (1996, 143), such that virginity is associated more with femininity, passivity and penetrability than it is with masculinity, to the extent that the concept of male virginity is shaped by an association with incompleteness or even outright failure. However, this construction of virginity does not exist in a vacuum; the stereotype of the chaste, virtuous female virgin, who appears in horror film as both victim and hero, is defined explicitly in opposition to unbounded carnal female sexuality. Such sexuality, which is presented as monstrous and voracious, is persistently illustrated in the horror film through allusions to the toothed vagina,[2] or *vagina dentata*. Through its associated iconography and expressions, the toothed vagina is often leveraged to articulate profoundly negative and hostile attitudes towards women's genitalia. And yet, it is also a provocative and expansive expression of embodied sexuality that refutes the suggestion that women's sexualities and desires must be contained, domesticated or positioned as for the use of another.

Within the popular, violent and abject space of the horror genre, myths about virginity are informed by, and in turn contribute to, normative and often very restrictive binary representations of heterosexual sexuality and femininity that deny a breadth of sexual expressions and identities. In this chapter I consider how, at a surface level, horror films engage with and enforce a dualistic socio-cultural construction of heteronormative female sexuality, and assumptions about sexual difference, in a largely uncritical manner. Very often this relies on simplistic tropes such as the feminised yet desexualised sacrificial virgin and the predatory, hypersexual vixen or she-demon, each of whom evoke an archetypal engagement with female sex: one that looks to female sexuality as either docile and contained, or expansive and dangerous. Indeed, even in instances where there may be a greater degree of ambiguity or nuance in the development of character, horror narratives have a tendency to force characters into these strict, sexually demarcated roles, refusing nuance or complexity in the name of generic standardisation. Nonetheless, popular culture is a dynamic site of struggle and contestation of meaning, and the complex richness of these archetypes, images and expressions of female sexuality cannot be easily boxed in. I suggest that thinking through these representations, expressions and relationships as 'gynaehorrific' offers a way of complicating engagements with sex that trouble and expand the aggregation of traits implied through molar binaries such as safe/unsafe, angel/demon and virgin/whore. As I will discuss, the 'danger' of female sexuality, sensuality and desire can certainly be shoehorned into a schema that positions monstrosity simply as the messy dipole of the closed, pure, virgin, to the extent that one becomes the negative image of the other. However, throughout this chapter I also indicate ways that the becomings inherent in the configurations of monstrosity offer a more provocative, proactive way of thinking through expressions of female sexuality. These may serve to trouble the assumptions that are emphasised through the construction of such dualisms, and in doing so challenge the reductive shorthand and the conventions of a genre that has a tendency to fall back on, if not trade upon, sexual essentialism and stereotypes.

Defining virginity

Throughout this chapter I move between sociocultural constructions of virginity and heterosexuality and more conceptual engagements with female sexuality, and as such it is important to consider baseline assumptions and constructions that inform the construction of the figure of the virgin. In popular parlance virginity is spoken about as if its definition – "the state of never having had sex" (Carpenter 2009, 1673) – were natural and ahistorical, but it is a complex cultural construct that amalgamates centuries' worth of ideas about sex, gender, agency and morality, let alone the nature and function of sexual difference. Virginity is important: sociologist Laura M. Carpenter (2009) indicates that "Distinguishing between virgins and non-virgins is an ancient practice" (p. 1673), and virginity has certainly been celebrated in myth and antiquity, such as in the ancient Greek veneration of virgin goddesses. The term is first found in written English near the beginning of the 13th century with specific reference to pious, unmarried women who were celebrated by the Christian church; the first mentions in English of the Virgin Mary are likewise found around this time. The association of the term with chastity and purity – that is, with the presumption of a lack of sexual activity and desire, as separated from its strictly ecclesiastic meaning – is first noted in the late 14th century ("Virgin"). The word 'virgin' comes from Latin root *virgo*, or maiden, and despite a long history of celibate male religious orders, in general the term has been applied almost exclusively to women (Blank 2007, 13).

French post-structuralist philosopher Luce Irigaray's conceptualisation of virginity is helpful at this point, for she connects this historic figure of the virgin to two modalities. In *Speculum of the Other Woman* (1985a), her landmark critique of the construction of the female subject in male-centric (Freudian, Lacanian) psychoanalysis, Irigaray begins by scathingly unpicking Sigmund Freud's masculine bias in his construction of the implicitly male/masculine subject, alongside his positioning of woman as perpetual riddle or enigma (p. 13). Irigaray asserts that the implicitly masculine subject needs – indeed wholly relies upon – the figure of the woman and the feminine so that it may define itself in opposition to it. Toying with the images of both gynaecological tools and the mirror central to Lacan's formulation of the 'mirror stage', in which an infant's recognition of 'his' external, unified self establishes an ideal "I" that he will forever seek to attain, the speculum of the title is the "faithful, polished" mirror (p. 136) that woman becomes in the construction of the male subject. This renders the figure of man/the male subject visible to himself – "wholly in the service of the same subject to whom it would present its surfaces, candid in their self-ignorance" (p. 136) – as she is eclipsed. The woman, here, is therefore necessary to the construction of the masculine subject for the feminine's negativity sustains the masculine's positivity; that is, it is not simply that male subject is inherently, by default, the positive, and the feminine its Other, but rather that the male subject *needs* its other, its *not-*, to define it, even though this need is also a site of extreme vulnerability. The feminine, then, is "a sort of inverted or negative alter ego … like a photographic negative" (p. 22) as opposed to a symmetrical Other. The primacy of the masculine is a construction that thrives on the invisibility of this of this relationship, such that the feminine has "no part of the masculine mastery of power": shaped by and defining the male, she is "Off-stage, off-side, beyond representation, beyond selfhood" (p. 22). The (passive, contained, perpetual) virgin, then, is denied her subjectivity. Irigaray argues that she is a foil to and props up masculine, patriarchal power, agency and phallic primacy through two things: her facilitation of the masculine divine and her exchange value.

Irigaray notes the relationship between the Virgin Mary, the masculine God, and the virgin-born Son of God, in which the figure of the virgin is "the condition for the incarnation of the masculine divine" (1993c, 117): her virginity is "mandatory for the purity of conception" (1985a, 345). The symbolic archetype of the masculine divine, in the figure of the paternal God (as well as his perfect Son), becomes "an identificatory figure for masculine perfection" and an anchor point for masculine identity (Deutscher 1994, 93) that similarly displaces the woman and the feminine into the role of Other. Looking again to the figure of the mirror, Irigaray notes the way that such purity of conception becomes a "polished surface that will not be scratched or pierced, lest the reflection be *exaggerated* or *blurred*" (1985a, 345). Julia Kristeva, in "Stabat Mater", similarly critiques the relationship between the myth and cult of the Virgin Mary, the "*consecrated* (religious or secular) representation of femininity" (1985a, 133), and the way that such mythic femininity is integral to the construction of the motherhood and maternity, for the "Virgin's only pleasure is her child who is not hers alone but everyone's, while her silent sorrow is hers alone" (Oliver 1993, 50). Like Irigaray's suggestion that the role of women in a patriarchal society is to act as the present-yet-absent reference point for the construction of male subjectivity, Kristeva suggests that the patriarchal construction of the cult of the Virgin works to highlight and accommodate femininity while simultaneously controlling it. Instead, the mythic figure of the Virgin mother erases the abject nature of the maternal body and the mother–child relationship, denies the articulation (in terms of the stating as well as the piecing together) of a matrilineal line and disavows the pleasure, enjoyment and eroticism (that is, *jouissance*) that may have accompanied conception and the presence of female subjectivity that this supposes. This last point is important, for as Kristeva suggests, the labelling of Mary as a virgin "was an error of translation: for the Semitic word denoting the social-legal status of an unmarried girl the translator substituted the Greek *parthenos*, which denotes a physiological and psychological fact, virginity" (1985, 135). Kelly Oliver (1993), in her reading of Kristeva, looks to the transgressive, threatening nature of this non-married status, indicating that the *jouissance* associated with the primal scene, then, is a type of 'outlaw *jouissance*', for neither it nor its 'bastard' offspring come under paternal code. Conversely, the mythic figure of the Virgin has no *jouissance*, and is thus recuperated (p. 51).

It is important, then, that it is not simply that Mary was a 'virgin', but that she "remained forever a virgin" (Kristeva 1985, 210). Her mythic, blessed virginity is perpetual, renewing and enduring, seemingly dynamic but locked in its crystalline, circular sameness, such that the son of God is "begotten … without shame of copulation" (1985, 210). The mark of this copulation, the 'blurring' trace of the feminine in the (re)production of both Son and the masculine ideal ego, would serve to destabilise the taken-for-granted phallologocentricism of the masculine divine. The masculine divine, like the aborescent root-tree discussed by Gilles Deleuze and Félix Guattari, *is*, in that it is predicated on and imposes the verb 'to be' (2004, 27), and in this *be*-ing it is rendered always-already present and perfect. "Man is able to exist because God helps him to define his gender" (Irigaray 1993c, 61), but in contrast, the female subject is lost, forgotten: "Providing the basis for the auto-logical speculations, she lives in darkness" (Irigaray 1985a, 345).

Irigaray also emphasises that the value of the virgin stems from the way that she exists and is defined both *for* and *between* men: the virgin has significant exchange-value; she is "a cash-convertible body" (1993b, 87). The mandatory virginity of the divine Virgin becomes the mandatory virginity of the virgin bride, who is passed from father or brother to husband as a means of establishing marriage and thus codifying the transfer of property (Irigaray 1985a, 120–3). The virgin, here, is both possession-object and relationship or vector, and woman's work (her "domestic slavery" (1985a, 122)) keeps her locked within the home, just as the enforcement of her own monogamy (but not that of the man) submits her body and subjectivity to the power and desires of her father-husband. This capture and erasure of feminine subjectivity (let alone sexuality) both assures and privileges a patrilinear bloodline, for she is an invisible matrix – *matrix*, here, drawing from its Latin and Middle English meanings of mother, breeding female, and 'womb' – through which the patriarchal economy structures itself, congratulating itself on its apparently self-sustaining endurance, and erasing the blood-relationship between women (1985a, 125). It is for this reason that Irigaray calls for a reconfiguration of the legal codification of virginity that centralises the subjectivity and autonomy of women. She argues that this might open a pathway to the feminine divine, in which 'virginity' (as a sort of "physical or moral integrity" (1993b, 86)) becomes a part of a woman's identity that is legally protected, just as the women's right to consent (or not consent) to sex is essential for an ethical, mutual relationship that is not predicated on the alienating force of masculine power (1993b 87; see also Irigaray 1993a).

These relationships are echoed in more recent popular usage of the term 'virgin', which moves away from its specifically sexual sense and comes to indicate a novice or someone naïve or uninitiated in something, such as a 'political virgin'; similarly, a 'maiden voyage' refers to a ship's first outing. The term virgin also alludes to possession and alteration: virgin land is that which has not been explored or developed, a virgin city or fortress is one that has not been conquered, virgin forest has not yet been milled or felled, and virgin waters have not been sullied or fished. These terms imply both impending consumption and economic use-value, and given the conflation of virginity with femininity and women, they also signal a denial of female self-possession: Rebecca Whisnant posits that a "woman's body cannot be her sovereign territory precisely because it is the 'virgin' (at first) territory for someone else to conquer and annex" (2010, 161). These metaphors are indicative of the way that, within a patriarchal heterosexual framework, first sex begins with a man's penis entering a woman's vagina and ends with his orgasm. Where sexual debut is the "young man's moment" (Holland, Ramazanoglu and Thomson 1996, 146), virginity is a passive state in which the female body has not (yet) been acted *upon*. The widespread use of the term 'penetration' as a word for sexual intercourse, which marks the penetrator as active and the penetrated (be they male or female) as passive, further evokes this asymmetrical relationship.

To tease out some of this implications of the relationship between the virgin, her feminine passivity, her significance and her exchange-value, I offer here a series of sites of cultural meaning-making – sociosexual practices, invasive acts that impact upon autonomy and self-determination, social and ideological movements, pornography – that each express and explore the cultural impulse to reify the virgin-figure in terms of her use-value. Given the circulation and exchange of meaning within popular culture and cultural practice, each of these expressions casts light upon the way the virgin is structured and repre- sented in horror film; that is, these are all a part of the broader, dynamic cultural ecosystem within which horror and film exist. I work from the sup- position that virginity is a concept that is less concerned with a lack of sexuality per se, but instead indicates a particularly feminine value or potential (untapped, nascent, or otherwise), be that potential sexual, cultural or some- thing else entirely. What is important, though, is that this value is situated as less for the woman herself – that is, that her value is not self-contained nor self-sustaining – and instead acts as a relationship with an-other: she is the material through which an implicitly masculine other, interest or relationship envisages and enacts itself.

Female virginity is, to a large degree, discursively constructed as a state that marries embodiment with morality: it is often popularly defined anatomically with regards to the status of the hymen, the small porous membrane that can cover all or part of the vaginal opening (or not even be present at all). The presence of blood-spotting has long been an (unreliable) indicator of first penetrative sex, but the role of the hymen itself as a *specific* mark of virginity was first posited in the 14th century by the physician Michael Savonarola, who noted its rupture at the time of 'deflowering' (Blank 2007, 45). Although the hymen exists in many terrestrial and aquatic species and is hypothesised to fulfil both reproductive and protective functions (Blackledge 2003, 145), the human hymen – named for the Greek and Latin words for membrane, but also coincidentally sharing the same etymological root as Hymen, the Greek god of marriage – has long acted as a cultural signifier for morality and female virtue. This is well evidenced by some of its colloquial and figurative names, such as 'maidenhead', 'veil of modesty' (Blackledge 2003, 143) and 'knot of virginity' (Blank 2007, 49). As Catherine Blackledge notes, the "hymen has, over the centuries, been invested with more social, moral and even legal significance than any other piece of human flesh" (2003, 142).

Given the strong cultural imperative for women to manage their bodies in a way that is considered normatively (and, usually, heterosexually) desirable, it is unsurprising that the hymen becomes a site of both anxiety and mutability. Women who wish to have their hymens replaced, often for cultural reasons or to 'revirginise' themselves, can undergo hymenorrhaphy, a surgical reconstruction of the hymen. This is an act and a transaction that situates the physical, invasive alteration of the body within a patriarchal economy, (re)creating something that perhaps never existed in its 'ideal' form, only for it to be destroyed by those it serves to placate. There are less invasive means of intervention, too, for artificial hymens filled with small amounts of a substance resembling blood can be purchased for use as a sex aid or to fulfil a man's expectations of what 'should' happen as a part of first penile-vaginal penetration, such as in cultures where there is an expectation that a woman's first such sex act should occur on the wedding night, ensuring the smooth transfer of woman-as-property and woman-as-heir-bearer from family to husband. One well-known Japanese product, with the tongue-in-cheek name 'Joan of Arc Red', advises its users that the "effect will be better if the woman pretend feel pain and shy [sic]" ("Artificial Virginity Hymen (Joan of Arc Red)") so as to increase the alleged authenticity of the experience for the male sexual partner and reinforce the stereotype of the passive, inexperienced feminine virgin. Nonetheless, such products' very existence signifies a complex negotiation with sexuality, power and embodiment, rendering the 'improper' and 'unclean' nature of blood-letting a performative act that slyly expresses feminine agency, suggesting that the masculine codification of sex, property and ownership is precarious and easily manipulated.

Nonetheless, the (non-)existence of the hymen is at best a poor indication of virginity. Hymen inspection, the vulgar making-visible of the metonymic membrane, is an inadequate way of testing for evidence of penetrative sex for the hymen, depending on its size, position and shape, can be easily separated or stretched through medical examination, tampon use, masturbation or vigorous physical activity, and smaller or flexible hymens can stay intact after intercourse. Human rights organisation Amnesty International (2005) considers 'virginity tests', in which a woman's genitals are forcibly inspected for evidence of a hymen, to be a contravention of a woman's human rights due to the reasons for testing, the invasive and undignified methods of testing and the negative and potentially life-threatening ramifications that it has for those who are tested and found wanting. It is of particular significance that similar tests are not and cannot be performed upon men, which further structures virginity as a particularly female or feminine concern, albeit one that is monitored by both men and women alike given the significance of female monogamy within a patriarchal, patrilineal economy of exchange. Indeed, the way a woman's morality, chastity and worth, both physical and moral, can be so tied up in a mucous membrane is also a clear expression of the way in which women's subjectivities are deemed to be more embodied than those of men. Where first heterosexual intercourse may be seen as a deliberate 'act' of doing (and an accomplishment) for a man, critical sexualities scholar Annie Potts (2002) indicates that women come to this experience already in a subjective position of 'being' given the social and cultural constitution of women-as-bodies – something that is exacerbated through women's experiences with menstruation and puberty (p. 198; see also Holland, Ramazanoglu and Thomson 1996, 45). Given these somewhat dubious physiological terms of reference, it follows that although virginity is often spoken about as an agreed-upon term, there is no one medical or diagnostic standard for virginity (Valenti 2009, 19). And yet, as Hanne Blank notes, "By any material reckoning, virginity doesn't exist" (2007, 3): it is a concept that co-mingles absence and presence, a construct, a relationship (between spirit, economies, bodies), and a space through which masculine power is expressed and then written on, even imposed upon, the body of another.

Virginity, then, is a concept that is defined (and redefined) through discourse and practice in keeping with the dominant patriarchal construction of human sexuality, which frames 'normal' (and 'real') sexual behaviour as heterosexual penile-vaginal intercourse (Potts 2002, 198); as sociologist Diane Richardson (1996) wryly suggests, "If we do not engage in such activity we are not recognised as sexual beings, [and] we are still virgins after a lifetime of 'foreplay'" (p. 6). However, although it is ostensibly a straightforward physiological issue, virginity is also associated with a degree of agency and willpower: it may be that your virginity is only gone if you *want* it to be gone. Such a phenomenological, experiential construction of virginity marks it as a state that can also be reclaimed, in a re-inscription of the history of the body by the mind and spirit. Consider the recent practice of 'born-again virginity', which has largely been associated with the evangelical Christian movement and abstinence-only education in the United States (Alexander 2008) and which allows individuals to 'take back' their virginity by pledging abstinence until marriage, even if they have previously engaged in sexual activities. This construct, which I discuss in more detail later in this chapter, frames virginity as a deliberate mind-set and an intentional demonstration of piety, as well as an embodied, empowered act of self-love and self-control (Keller 1999, xiii–xix). The language of such practice explicitly invokes the imperative of heterosexual, monogamous marriage and the use-value of the woman: as one now defunct American pro-abstinence website once framed it, individuals who have "already unwrapped the priceless gift of virginity and given it away" and who "feel like 'second-hand goods' and no longer worthy to be cherished" can "re-wrap it and give it only to [their] future husband or wife" (Pregnancy Support Center: Take2 Renewed Virginity 2013). Despite the seemingly even-handed emphasis upon the virginities of both men and women, these practices, and the onus for compliance, disproportionately falls upon the woman. Thus, virginity is framed as both an actual thing that can be 'lost' or 'given' as well as a process, a rite of passage, a destination and a state of being (Carpenter 2005), but the popular idea that virginity both exists and is 'lost' through penile-vaginal penetrative sex is one based upon a heterosexual, able-bodied bias that ignores the wealth and breadth of possible sexual expression. Virginity is a term, then, that is widely utilised and seemingly agreed upon but rarely adequately defined, and I suggest that it is exactly this nebulousness that makes it a conceptually powerful touchstone in popular media narratives about sex.

What is not in question, though, is the way that female virginity is fetishised and constructed as a mythic ideal – something that is apparent in the number of pornographic websites that play on notions and tropes of youth and purity. These range from sites who claim their models to be 'barely legal' (which plays doubly upon the exchange-value of the woman), to those presenting young women's (alleged) first times on camera, to those that offer scenes of so-called defloration, complete with staged pre-coitus images of the models' hymens and mid- and post-coitus images of blood spotting. The visual grammar of these pornographic sites teeters on the tenuous boundary of the virgin/whore binary, juxtaposing explicit images of women's genitals with signifiers of girlhood. The set dressing features soft toys, child-like costumes and sets that resemble girls' bedrooms, at the same time as eschewing raunchy lingerie and hypersexualised settings. As a representative example, consider the pornographic website Defloration.tv, which markets itself as the first and largest virginity porn website in the world, a veritable clearinghouse for young women's 'virtue'. After outlining the rarity and so-called privilege of seeing such a "fragile object", the pitch on the site's landing page promises "cute virgin girls, hymen photos, juicy teen pussies, real videos, real stories... No scripts! Only real emotions shot on-the-fly!" (Defloration.tv 2016)

The narrative structure of this subgenre of pornography bestows upon the spectator a degree of voyeuristic agency; that is, such sites claim to offer a 'legitimate' *experience* of conquering and consuming a young woman's body in a manner that is mythologised as authentic yet constructed as performative in that it offers the (presumably heterosexual male) viewer an empowering fantasy of domination and the bestowal of sexual education.[3] The act of 'defloration' itself, alongside scenes of alleged seduction and post-coital celebration (or commiseration) is framed as for the exclusive benefit of the consumer-spectator, and marks women's bodies and their virginities as items available for purchase and consumption. The emphasis on "real emotions" evokes the sense of a momentous occasion and acknowledges, even engenders through expectation, a peculiarly affective connection between actress and consumer. However, conquest narratives in virgin porn also serve to venerate and fetishise the "unwilling or faux-unwilling female sexual partner" (North 2010) by framing the penetration of a 'closed' female body as a form of achievement that valorises active male sexuality while treating the virginal body as something to be ruptured, violated, invaded and owned by men (Potts 2002, 198–9; 204). Perhaps more than many other category of mainstream pornography, this positions the actresses on the website as objects of exchange within a patri-archal economy of flesh and fluid, whose performances render them obsolete and presumably unemployable within the same genre.

I highlight these brief but diverse examples of cultural practices that shape and hinge upon virginity to suggest that these sexual dynamics and power imbalances, alongside the sociocultural construction of the 'ideal' virgin and her embodied exchange-value, are widespread and an integral part of the way that women's sexualities are shaped and codified. As I will demonstrate, such constructions and attitudes, which are by no means limited to the practices discussed above, also provide rich material for the horror genre.

Virginity in horror film

When *Scream's* Randy Meeks instructs the drunken teen party-goers on the vagaries of slasher film transgressions, the film's protagonist, Sidney, is upstairs preparing to lose her virginity to her boyfriend Billy, who is later revealed to be one of the killers. The film delights in both critiquing and fulfilling horror film tropes, so although Sidney both loses her virginity and evades death – ready to return for a series of sequels, of course – she nonetheless stands in for the first of two key virginal horror film stereotypes: the female virgin hero, a figure who at first seems to repudiate Irigaray's conceptualisation of the virgin in her assertiveness and self-sufficiency, but whose significance within the genre emphasises the shoring up of a mythic femininity that is predicated on restraint.

The virgin hero is a staple trope in the slasher genre. This mode of representation owes a great debt to the narrative and thematic prominence of both the punishment of sexual activity and the veneration of the virginal heroine in John Carpenter's 1978 film *Halloween,* a film of utmost importance within the genre and that "is the blueprint for all slashers and the model against which all subsequent films are judged" (Rockoff 2002, 55). *Halloween* is also used extensively by Carol J. Clover as she formulates and scaffolds the figure of the victim-hero in her landmark book *Men, Women and Chain Saws* (1992). In particular, Clover demonstrates how Curtis's character, Laurie Strode (a name that is both masculine and dynamic), takes on a more assertive role than women in similar films, such as survivor Sally in the original *The Texas Chain Saw Massacre* (1974). Where Sally ran, screamed and exhibited little agency, Laurie actively fights back, and although Laurie herself is rescued from villain Michael Myers' silent predation by Michael's psychiatrist, who shoots Michael repeatedly in the head and chest in the film's climax, her successors often make the killing blow themselves.

These Final Girls, as Clover terms them, are important because they are set apart from the other women in the films. They are given interests that are coded as masculine (or at least un-feminine), they demonstrate sexual reluctance or disinterest, and they are marked as somehow other to their female peers (p. 48), which is often signalled through their more masculine names such as Joey, Stevie and Max (p. 40). They are watchful, resourceful, responsible and intelligent, and developed in more psychological detail than their peers (p. 44). They look *for* the killer, and instead of running, they ultimately confront the monster face-to-face (p. 44). One of Clover's most important contributions is the assertion that the female victim-hero's expression and experience of abject terror – an emotional state coded as passive and feminine – allows the spectator to share such an experience in a culturally sanctioned manner. This allows space for a slippage in or queering of the gendered identification on the part of the (presumably male[4]) horror audience. Clover suggests that this means that the viewer can dance between identifying with an active villain, whose implicitly masculine point-of-view drives early portions of the film but whose masculinity is in some way compromised (p. 47), and sharing the abject, feminised terror of the heroine. This tension is resolved when the Final Girl 'un-mans' the killer by asserting herself in a manner coded as active and masculine, often through the acquisition and use of phallic weaponry, and then through the disruption or penetration of the killer's body.

By centralising the narrative importance of the virgin-hero, and by having Michael Myers' murderous actions explicitly framed as a form of punishment dealt to his promiscuous teenage victims, *Halloween* correlates sexual activity with death. Although it is by no means the first film to have done so, the connection within the slasher genre has remained resonant, as evidenced by the rules laid out by *Scream*'s Randy Meeks. This association with moral purity may no longer apply in the 'real world': in their exploration of gendered experiences of (hetero)sexual debut, Holland, Ramazanoglu and Thomson (1996) argue that "the acquisition of sexual identities is increasingly detached from moral discourses of purity and sin" (p. 143). Nonetheless, these discourses remain deeply ingrained within horror narratives: a quantitative content analysis of slasher films conducted in 2010 showed that female characters who engaged in sexual behaviour were not only less likely to survive than their non-sexual female peers and their male peers, but that their death scenes were measurably longer (Welsh 2010).

Even as female characters have developed and become more sexually active in horror films, and as the trope is subverted, recycled or parodied in postmodern and millennial horrors, the Final Girls are still presented as different from – both less than and more than – the other female characters. Very often, the Final Girl relinquishes her femininity or avoids the trappings of overt feminine sexuality, either through 'actual' virginity – that is, a lack of sexual, carnal experience, even if she still desires or is desired – or through some other engagement with the implications of cinematic presentations of normative femininity. As an example, consider how literal virginity is increasingly replaced by engagements with virginity in an abstract or metaphorical sense, such as a demonstration of sexual reluctance, temperance or personal moderation. This may articulate itself through a heightened awareness or intelligence: in *It Follows* (2015), a film that draws heavily from the visual language and cinematic legacy of *Halloween,* quiet victim-hero Jay, named for Jamie Lee Curtis, is sexually active but nonetheless presented as 'other' to her female peers, especially as she is the only one of her friends who can see the shape-shifting, sexually-transmitted 'it'-monster that is stalking her.

This sense of 'other-ness' also marks other post-modern Final Girls, to the extent that a degree of creativity regarding the generic expectations surrounding her construction as a mythic figure has become a hallmark of the genre. In Rob Zombie's reimagining of *Halloween* (2007), Laurie is recast as Michael Myers' intelligent, knowing long-lost sister, and the film and its 2009 sequel explore family dysfunction and intergenerational abuse. Laurie appears to defeat Michael at the end of the film, but in the film's sequel, as Michael returns to find her, she is revealed to be perhaps as susceptible to psychopathy as he is. In *Hostel: Part II* (2007) the apparently virginal and innocent Final Girl is shown to be just as bloodthirsty as the film's killers, and she chooses to join them in their 'hunting' of travellers and backpackers rather than succumb to their torture. In the horror-comedy *You're Next* (2011), the Final Girl's resourcefulness acts as a key plot element: Erin was brought up by survivalists in the Australian outback and is more than equipped to fight back violently against the masked home invaders, much to the shock of her boyfriend who had secretly engineered the attack. Horror comedies such as *The Final Girls* (2015) and the American television series *Scream Queens* (2015–), both consider the Final Girl from an intertextual and intergenerational perspective. The Canadian horror series *Slasher* (2016), which explores the tropes of the genre, brings a married Final Girl back to the house where her parents were butchered by a masked killer, who reappears upon her return to the small town. In this instance her acts of revenge against this new incarnation of 'The Executioner' are deliberate, bloody, violent and satisfying. Each of these films and series highlight how Clover's work has, in and of itself, become an important part of the horror corpus, marking a clear articulation of a set of generic markers that have been deliberately, playfully bent and challenged since the publication of *Men, Women and Chain Saws* in 1992.

I suggest that the virgin hero of the horror film can be further contextualised through the lens of radical feminist Andrea Dworkin's provocative account of Joan of Arc, which marks Joan as someone who eschewed the trappings of womanhood – not only her dress and subservience, but her 'to-be-fucked-ness'. For Joan and the virgin saints who appeared to her in divine visions, "virginity was an active element of a self-determined integrity, an existential independence … not a retreat from life but an active engagement with it; dangerous and confrontational because it repudiated rather than endorsed male power over women" (Dworkin 1997, 96). Unlike Irigaray's discussion of virginity, which posits the virgin as both necessary prop to masculine subjectivity and invisible enabler of the masculine divine, Dworkin's interpretation of Joan marks her as able to achieve in the world by specifically *bypassing* male desire through the repudiation of everything that marked her as Woman. Most notably, this included her denial of a woman's dress and appearance and her engagement in activities associated with men and militarisation, to the extent that her gender was called into question (MacLachlan 2007, 11). This is also a powerful disavowal of everything that the concept of Woman inferred, such as property, sexual availability, recalcitrance, submissiveness, accessibility and social inferiority: "she refused to be fucked and she refused civil insignif-icance: and it was one refusal; a rejection of the social meaning of being female in its entirety, no part of the feminine exempted or saved" (Dworkin 1997, 85). This centralises virginity – or 'militant', oppositional, political virginity, at least – as a site of feminine strength and power, which in the case of Joan is linked to her own connection to and communi(cati)on with figures of feminine divinity.

The archetypal virgin hero of the horror film rarely reaches the militant extremes of Joan, but she certainly disavows aspects of her femininity in a manner that may be coded as asexual or masculine, and her refusal of (or inexperience with) sex perhaps acts as both nexus and signifier of her power and difference. And yet, though I acknowledge the sly, subversive power of a certain slippery female-centric perspective of the kind that Carol J. Clover articulates in *Men Women and Chain Saws*, and am certainly interested in the centralisation of female protagonists, I also express a degree of uneasiness about the enduring figure of the virgin-hero, even as she has shifted over time to express more figurative forms of constraint, moderation or recalcitrance. It seems perverse that the way to survive the unknown, to overcome the monster or villain, is to wrap oneself up within expressions of sexual denial as if virginity, here, is a protective mantle. If we accept, even at face value, Laura Mulvey's (2000 [1975]) famous suggestion that the cinematic spectator of mainstream narrative cinema implicitly internalises a specular agency that is coded as masculine, then Clover's argument that the final girl allows this spectator-subject to actively, violently overcome (kill, penetrate) the villain while facilitating the experience of abject (that is, feminised) terror in a sanctioned manner that resolves any gendered dissonance, perhaps reinforces the notion the female subject is both utilised and occluded in the construction of male subjectivity.

In addition, the prominence of the virgin hero – the 'special' girl – indicates that survival comes less from the protections offered by the smooth, closed and untainted mantle of virginity and more from the imperative to be Not Like The Others, where the others are women who have sex, who diverge from traditional expectations of monogamy and domestic exchange, who pursue pleasure and sexual self-expression, or who are otherwise marked as threatening or unworthy. I suggest, then, that it is this compulsive return to the figure of the 'special' girl that is something insidiously problematic. The deaths of trans-gressive, active, often implicitly 'unlikeable' women who assert their agency in threatening ways, in a genre that is often accused of loving to punish women, is not something to celebrate. It is of utmost significance that there is no com-parably consistent model of sex, death and survival for male hero-protagonists in horror film. Perhaps the virgin hero, for all her developments in the last forty years, does not express difference, renewal and progression but instead a perpetual collapse back towards the static figure of the divine, unchanged/unchanging virgin. Her survival, which ensures our own path through the film's narrative and horrors, is predicated on the (re)production of similarity.

As Joan of Arc's martyrdom indicates, the importance of virginity and the ideals implicitly bound up within it are further demonstrated in the second key articulation of female virginity in the horror film: the trope of the sacrificial virgin, whose death offers some sort of transition, offering or exchange. In these instances, the victim is almost invariably an attractive adolescent or young woman, indicating that sexual capital is as important as the state of virginity. Where a child or older virgin could, hypothetically, fulfil the same requirements of virginity, it is the destruction of nascent sexuality that lends itself towards the notion of sacrifice. Hanne Blank (2007) indicates that there are different types of virginity: children have a type of default virginity, and are considered, to borrow from Carl Jung, presexual (p. 13); nuns or other religious celibates are considered vowed virgins (p. 16). However, adolescent virginity can be qualified not as perpetual but as "transitional" virginity, which relies on the assumption that people will enter the "game" of sex and eventually procreate. This marks adolescent virginity (and virginity loss) as a passage that links childhood's end to the beginnings of adulthood (p. 14). It is at this point that "virginity really begins to count for something" (p. 13); that is, the destruction of an attractive, fertile "transitional" virgin is a loss in the present and in the future, for with the death of the virgin comes not only an offering of inviolate purity and sanctity, but the nullification of future children and the perpetuation of the family line. The life and body of the virgin becomes a commodity to be traded for civic protection or success, or to appease or please gods or monsters.

The figure of the sacrificial virgin is most stereotypically (and even comically) articulated in fantasy films, in which female sacrifices are presented as passive, naïve and available to be consumed or destroyed. In both the sword-and-sorcery fantasy epics *Conan the Barbarian* (1982) and *Conan the Destroyer* (1984), which are easily representative of the excesses and campy pleasures of the genre, the titular barbarian saves virgin princesses from the hands of cultists. In the latter film, the virgin-victim is both able to summon the monster by acquiring and using a special and particularly suggestive magic horn, and she is to placate the monster by being devoured.[5] The similarly-themed *Dragonslayer* (1981) features a village that, twice-yearly, must sacrifice a virgin to a nearby dragon so as to save their village. Such representations also draw from myth and legend; in *Clash of the Titans* (1981), which draws from Greek myth, demigod Perseus must rescue Andromeda from being sacrificed to the Kraken, an ancient sea monster. These films all draw from and contribute to the archetypal image of the virgin sacrifice, that is, a young, normatively attractive woman who is bound to rocks or stakes in a way that alludes to fantasies of domination and submission. This is something that is reinforced by the sacrifice's screaming and her ineffectual struggle to break free; there are certainly thematic connections here to the visual grammar of virgin pornography. In each of these instances, the virginal female is a "reservoir of energy … that could serve patriarchy" (MacLachlan 1997, 8) and "a substitute for all the members of the community, offered up by the members themselves" (H. Parker 1997, 75), yet also presented in a manner that conforms to normative constructions of attractiveness, so that the virgin is as much for the visual consumption of the gaze of the ideal (that is, heterosexual male) viewer as she is for the literal consumption of the monster.

Virgins retain this special quality in horror films about black magic and monsters, even in instances where sacrifice itself is less overt than it is implied; for example, in *Sleepwalkers* (1992), the eponymous shapeshifting were-cats need to feed on the life-force of virgin women to stay alive, and they are hunted or seduced instead of sacrificed. Early horror films notably feature unwed young women who discover and are pursued by some sort of monster, and in doing so combine the demands of both an audience who expect thrills and the Hollywood star system's hunger for attractive female starlets. *The Phantom of the Opera* (1925) is perhaps the most explicit narrative featuring a virgin 'taming' (or attempting to tame) a monster, and *King Kong* (1933) and other early RKO and Universal films explore similar material. In Bram Stoker's widely adapted novel *Dracula* (2009 [1897]), which conflates vampirism with sexuality, both newlywed Mina Harker and the ingénue Lucy are virgins; depending on the film adaptation in question, Lucy's transformation into a vampire awakens in her a carnal bloodlust that stands in contrast to her former demure figure.[6]

By framing a woman's virginity in terms of consumption and commodity, it cannot be seen as a private or personal issue; indeed, virginity can be socially constructed as a community concern whereby the body of the girl or woman becomes abstracted and conflated with broader entities or attributes, marking her less as an autonomous individual and more as the material out of which broader civic and civil issues are moulded. This is most famously exemplified by the Vestal virgins of ancient Rome, whose chastity was directly linked to the wellbeing of the Roman state, as their "Feminine virtue was used ... as a sign of the moral health of the commonwealth" (H. Parker 2007, 66). As Vestals were both daughters of and embodiments of Rome, sexual congress with them was considered an incestuous act of treason. The Vestals' punishment for breaking their vow of chastity was to be buried alive with a small amount of food – a necessarily passive-aggressive method of execution, for it was also illegal for a citizen to spill their blood or actively contribute to their death (H. Parker 2007; Dowling 2001).

This sense of collective ownership and exchange-value is bluntly expressed in the wryly named *Cherry Falls* (2000), in which young virgins in the eponymous town are being murdered by an apparently female killer. The high school students decide to protect themselves by staging a school-wide orgy, which is presented a little like a distorted, bacchanalian school prom, in an amalgamation of one adolescent rite of passage with another. The killer, a teacher, is the illegitimate son of a woman who 27 years prior lost her virginity when she was raped by four young men, including the father of the female protagonist, in a 'sins of the fathers' story that echoes other teen horrors such as *A Nightmare on Elm Street* (1984) and *Friday the 13th* (1980) (Falconer

2010, 136). The killer's idiosyncratic revenge for his mother's violation is to dress up as his mother and rob the *parents* of their virginal children – and their children's virginities. The horror, according to the film's logic, is less for the students than it is for the wealthy parents who can do everything for their children except safeguard them, be it their 'innocence' or their role as 'innocents'. Here, the teenagers' collective virginity is a signifier and expression of both good parenting and wholesome small town values, and so long as this social façade is maintained it keeps a bitter historic truth tidily repressed.

Male virginity is generally less visible and of less significance in horror films than the sexual activities, or lack thereof, of their female counterparts. Nonetheless, male virgins are still present in the genre, and their sexual status takes on narrative and thematic import in a manner that differs from women's, but that is just as instructive. Where virginal women have been stereotypically framed as passive victim or victim hero, I suggest that the implied femininity and lack of agency that is inherent in the discursive construction of virginity offers the male virgin only two forms of representation: the effeminate failure, or the noble, monastic ascetic.

The first, negative construction marks male virginity as a form of weakness that draws its (im)potency from the devaluation of the feminine within patriarchal culture. The conceptual conflation of virginity with femininity necessarily renders the male virgin as powerless, for if the virgin exists *for* or *between* men, and as Irigaray suggests disavows her own female subjectivity in her facilitation of the formation of the male subject, then a male body that falls into this role can only be framed as a failure. Given sociocultural associations of masculinity with agency and power and femininity with passivity and subordination, a lack of sexual activity on the part of a men is thus inherently coded as a weakness that must be endured or, preferably, overcome, so that young men can be 'properly' inducted into adult masculinity through their first experience of penetrative heterosex (Holland, Ramazanoglu and Thomson 1997, 144). The situation of heterosex as an essential event in terms of sociosexual development and masculine subject formation is particularly evident in sex comedies such as the *Porky's* (1982) and its sequels, and, more recently, *The 40 Year Old Virgin* (2005), each of which mine the comedic loss-of-virginity trope mercilessly. Consider teen coming-of-age comedy *American Pie* (1999),[7] which centres on four boys' quest to lose their virginities before their senior prom so that they may become 'complete' men before leaving the liminal adolescence of high school and moving out into the adult world. The film, which wryly critiques the myriad insecurities and anxieties that inform the performance of heterosexual, white masculinity, is driven by the boys' horrified realisation that graduating high school without having had penetrative heterosex is an appalling proposition. Everyman protagonist Jim laments that going to college as virgins will mark them as inferior and broken – 'special', in the most derogatory way – even though Jim himself is shown to be an enthusiastic and prodigious masturbator, and his friends are sexually active in various other ways. Where "[female] virginity is in not yet having been subsumed: one's being is still intact, penetrated or not" (Dworkin 1997, 113), male virginity – the act of not having penetrated a woman – is seen as a type of incompletion. Thus, when Jim loses his virginity to a sexually aggressive female peer who was only interested in a one night stand, he expresses delight that he was 'used', for despite lacking agency and being rendered object, not subject, he has nonetheless successfully achieved manhood (Holland, Ramazanoglu and Thomson 1997, 146–152).[8]

When male virginity appears as a plot element or character trait in the horror genre, it is predominantly associated with this sense of impaired or failed masculinity. Carol J. Clover (1992) asserts that traditional masculinity does not do well within the slasher genre (p. 65), but I suggest that when it comes to narratives about sex in the horror film, neither does non-traditional masculinity. Instead, virginity is framed as a dangerous state of ignorance, with the implication being that if a man is not inducted into manhood thorough heterosex, rendered a whole subject through his penetration of a female or feminised other, he remains 'open' for attack; that is, by not asserting himself as a literal penetrator, his own boundaries are insecure. This impending sense of victimhood informs the horror comedy *Once Bitten* (1985): Mark is frustrated because his girlfriend isn't yet ready to have sex, so he starts trawling singles bars where he is picked up by a vampire Countess. She needs his virgin blood to stay youthful, and as Mark's status as possession consolidates as their relationship progresses he begins to express vampiric qualities. However, Mark is eventually rescued by his girlfriend who quickly and uncomfortably 'devirginises' him, in an expedient, eleventh hour act that renders him useless to the Countess. In this case, the loss of virginity is imperative: any notion of romance or love is stripped away from the sex act, and it becomes a way to thwart the Countess's appetite as opposed to a way for Mark and his previously-reticent girlfriend to solidify their relationship. Where virginity loss, at the outset of the film, is framed (for his girlfriend) as something meaningful and worth waiting for, the film ultimately ratifies the idea that men's virginity is shameful, as well as is a valid motivation for cheating on one's partner, and in this instance it is something inherently dangerous that must be hurried and done away with.

However, the effeminacy that is conflated with male virginity is occasionally framed as a virtue as well as a weakness, even if it still results in death or destruction. Without this 'achievement' of normative heterosexual manhood there is also if not an outright rejection of, then at least a deep ambivalence towards the negative and harmful aspects of the socially and culturally dominant construction of what it means to be a 'real man', such as the association of normative masculinity with violence, domination and sexism. Consider *Borderland* (2009), in which college student Phil is nearly goaded by his boorish friends into losing his virginity to a prostitute in a brothel on the Mexican-American border. He reneges, but is then abducted and used as a human sacrifice by a group of drug smuggling cultists. Phil is an apt sacrifice and exchange-object because he is presented as specifically *less* masculine than his friends: he is feminised through what is framed as his care for the wellbeing of 'his' prostitute and her child, as well as for the way that he 'values' his virginity enough to not want to have his first penetrative sexual experience with a sex worker, and as such he is presented as a 'good' guy. In this instance, the trope of the sacrificial virgin is upheld, but the nature of the sacrifice speaks more to the precarious or contested nature of masculinity, rather than an allegedly inherent, feminine vulnerability that takes the form of implicit sexual availability and consumability.[9]

This association between a lack of sexual experience and degree of empathy and emotional maturity is also present in *Decoys* (2004), in which two male college students who are desperate to lose their virginity discover that many of the beautiful women on campus are refugee aliens who are seeking hosts for their offspring. The aliens impregnate their male hosts by penetrating them, using tentacles that sprout from their chests, in a violent and deadly process that freezes the men from the inside out. Wiseacre Roger discovers that he has a 'sensitive side' and takes on a stereotypically feminine, hesitant role when he tries to convince his alien love interest, the ironically named Constance, to wait until the right moment before she takes his virginity. Even though Constance has developed feelings for Roger and tries to 'go easy' on him, he barely survives the impregnation process and dies shortly thereafter.[10] Both Roger and his friend Phil are presented much more caring and respectful than their friends and classmates, and therefore 'better' people, but for them both sex and virginity are dangerous – a double bind that indicates a great deal of anxiety about both the nature and performance of normative masculinity.

Although these films associate male virginity with an impaired sense of normative masculinity and a sense of physical weakness, the deliberate act of (sexual) self-denial can be coded as a sign of strength. As such, the second, more assertive construction of male virginity, posits that male chastity or celibacy, vis-à-vis 'virginity' in its broader sense, can be express(ive)ly masculine if it is associated with a militant and ascetic intentional *disavowal* of (heterosexual) desire altogether, for removing the celibate from the sexual economy does not impugn his status as subject, and nor does it challenge masculine power. As an example, Pete Falconer (2010) helpfully suggests that although the titular vampire-human hybrid hero of action-horror *Blade* (1998) and its two sequels is not presented as a sexual virgin *per se*, his disinterest in sex, and his active repression of his need for human blood, give the image of a man who is militantly and successfully denying his baser needs (pp. 128–130), thus allowing his will to triumph over his body.

This denial is also present in religious representations of abstinence in the horror film, such as in *The Wicker Man* (1973), where celibacy is a sign of moral and spiritual fortitude. A young, religious and celibate Police Sergeant Neil Howie is lured to the Hebridean island of Summerisle by the community's inhabitants by way of a bogus missing person case, where he is to be sacrificed on May Day in a giant, burning wicker man to the island's pagan gods so as to restore the island's ailing orchards. Howie represents the perfect sacrifice, according to the Lord of the island, as he came willingly, as a virgin, as a representative of the king (as a policeman representing the Crown) and as a fool (that is, a naïve idiot). The film ends with the islanders joyfully singing an old English hymn as the Howie shouts Psalm 23 from his burning wicker cage. However, Howie's presence is indicative of more things that just his virginity: he is active, strong and a representative of the law and authority. His devout religious beliefs stand in contrast to those of the islanders, and we are asked to compare their actions and beliefs: where they are sexual, fecund and permissive, he is guarded and physically aloof; where they place their beliefs in old gods, sexual energies and supernatural rituals, he has an unwavering faith in paternalistic, conservative Christianity. Howie is no passive feminised sacrifice for his virginity and his faith gives him strength, and his solid Christian 'goodness' serves to increase the horror of his demise at the hands of the pagans, leaving viewers to watch as the moral and spiritual corner-stones of British society are undermined and cast away, only to embolden the unruly gods and practices that Christianity itself suppressed. Howie dies as a martyr, not a victim – and notably, it is rare to find filmic accounts of female virginal martyrdom in the horror genre that evoke such ideas of strength.[11]

These virginal categories – the female sacrificial victim, the victim-hero, the deficient man and the masculine ascetic – have come to be fixed generic types, although they are increasingly acknowledged in a knowing, ironic and media-literate manner. However, even in critiquing and playing with these tropes, postmodern horror films nonetheless seem compelled to fulfil them. This is overtly apparent in *The Cabin in the Woods* (2012), which like *Scream* is interested in exposing and deconstructing horror film tropes, but which, like many other self-referential horror films, can only become the thing that it is seeking to critique through its repetitive (re)production of similarity. The film posits that five American horror film archetypes – the jock, the scholar, the slut, the fool and the virgin – must be sacrificed every year to appease a Lovecraftian elder god. This sacrifice is an international endeavour, and each participating country's own contributing sacrifice plays out in a manner that fits within their own horror traditions; in the United States this is achieved through a ritual that plays out much like a stereotypical slasher film, which is posited to be simply the latest incarnation of an ancient practice. The people orchestrating the sacrifice point out that the virgin must be the last alive, to live or die as fate sees fit, but that what matters is that she visibly suffers for the benefit of the watching gods and, by proxy, the spectator, who is impli-cated in perpetuating the film's violence and voyeurism. Here, the five college students 'inadvertently' unleash a specific monster by mucking about with one of many archetypal horror artefacts found in the cabin's dim, crowded base-ment, and they are then terrorised and killed one by one. In this instance, the group are attacked by a family of redneck zombies who are summoned when Dana, the 'virgin', reads aloud from a young girl's mouldering diary. As such, Dana is at once set up as transgressor, virgin hero and sacrificial victim, offered agency yet defined as object.

The parameters of the American slasher genre are quickly enforced: the friends, who begin as relatively diverse and well-rounded individuals (within the parameters of mainstream film), are shoehorned into their archetypal roles through drugs, tricks and environmental conditioning. Dana is certainly not sexually inexperienced, and it's made clear in the opening minutes that she's been having an affair with one of her college professors; instead, we are told drolly that under modern conditions the ritual's overseers must make do with the insufficient material they are presented with. On one hand, the film bluntly questions the appeal and narrative necessity of the youthful, attractive Final Girl and her experience of abject terror. At the film's close Dana and Marty, the pot-smoking comic relief, decide not to fulfil the ritual if such a brutal practice is what it takes to keep the world alive, thus expressing agency by ironically doing nothing. Joss Whedon, one of the film's creators, describes the film as a "very loving hate letter" to the sorts of horror films that they consider have "sung [sic] a little too far in [the] direction" of sadistic so-called torture porn (Joss Whedon talks The Cabin in the Woods 2012). Nonetheless, the film – perhaps necessarily – fulfils exactly the parameters that it sets out to critique, especially in a scenes in which Dana, dripping wet, is savagely mauled by one of the zombies, and Jules, the slut, is attacked while half-undressed and in the process of having sex with jock Curt. The audience member's recognition of their own bloodlust is reflected back to them, particularly as the white-collar puppet masters take bets on the outcome and celebrate what they initially believe to be the successful completion of the ritual, but this is not necessarily tempered by the film's ironic distance. Instead, I suggest that one comes to knowingly shrug off the other. The production and distribution of this critically and financially successful horror film succeeds, in part, through its objectification and punishment of attractive young women, as well as through its playful perpetuation of the widely understood 'terms of engagement' that come with such a film – a case, perhaps, of having things both ways, and succeeding because of it.

The virgin's other: *vagina dentata*

The chaste sacrificial virgin is only one side of the dyadic form of the sexed woman in horror: the converse is the articulation and visual expression of what occurs when the female virgin's nascent sexuality is released. Take, for example, the playful exploration of a ritual gone wrong in *Jennifer's Body* (2009), in which a struggling and fairly unmemorable band of indie rock musicians decide to advance their fortunes by making a deal with the devil and sealing it with the sacrifice of a virgin. At a small town gig they set their sights on Jennifer, a stereotypically attractive and hyper-sexualised cheerleader from the local high school. Jennifer lies about her sexual experience, initially to appear coquettish to the lead singer and again, later, when she is taken away by the band and begins to fear that she has been abducted so that they can have sex with her. However, she has been sexually active since middle school and is not even a 'back door' virgin, as she puts it, and as such the sacrifice goes terribly wrong. The band receives their boon and head towards stardom, but Jennifer comes back from death: her body absorbs the summoned demon and she becomes a succubus. She must devour men approximately once a month to satisfy her hunger and maintain her appearance, which moves after feeding from supernaturally radiant and beautiful to lack-lustre, wan and spotty over the course of a few weeks. The needs of her inner demon are freely equated with the ways in which women's bodies can be affected by their menstrual cycle, her 'withdrawal symptoms' mimic those of a drug addict, and her hunger is a source of pain as well as pleasure. When Jennifer seduces and feasts on her male schoolmate victims she adopts her demon form: she has an enormous snake-like articulated jaw that is lined with sharp teeth with which she tears off the genitals of her victims. This image of her dangerous, gaping maw, framed by bright red lipstick, is a symbolic representation of the other, more dangerous and unruly side of female sexuality: *vagina dentata*, or the toothed vagina. If the virgin can be considered a hermetic or closed system of contained sexuality, *vagina dentata* plays on anxieties surrounding unbounded female sexual power and desire, the interiority of the female genitals, the origins of life, and the mechanics of birth. It also acts as a cautionary tale to men about the hypothetical dangers of sex with unknown women, and expresses rapacious, unbounded desire in a manner that is coded as threatening and transgressive.

Vagina dentata is a primal and ancient construct of femininity. Erich Neumann, in his work on the archetypes of the Great Mother, indicates that this "destructive side of the Feminine ... appears most frequently in the archetypal form of a mouth bristling with teeth" (Rees 2013, 222). Literary and cultural theorists have linked this monstrous conceptualisation of female embodiment and desire with broader issues, such as the spiritual and mythic interconnection between birth and dying, for as mythologist Joseph Campbell (1993) highlights, "The universal goddess makes her appearance to men under a multitude of guises ... The mother of life is at the same time the mother of death" (pp. 302–303). Feminist philosopher Elizabeth Grosz (1994), in turn, aligns the destructive horror of the mythic *vagina dentata* with the abject fear of being consumed, submerged and absorbed into something that is boundary-less; here, horror is evoked not because of the thing itself, but because of the way that this sense of fluidity and viscosity troubles fixity and the laws sur-rounding the clean and proper (pp. 194–195). As such, the vaginal opening, as the transitional space between the interior of the woman's body and the exterior world, takes on a conceptual indeterminacy that turns on its head the notion of penetrator and penetrated; instead, the vagina is capable of sub-suming the penis, of taking it, actively, inside the depths woman's body, as well as acting as the passage through which the newborn enters the world.

As with stories about virgins, purity and sacrifice, motifs expressing variations on the *vagina dentata* are prevalent in myths and stories from around the world (Caputi 2004, 28). In Māori legend, Hine-nui-te-pō – the 'great woman of night' and ruler of the underworld – has gnashing teeth of obsidian in her vagina. Trickster-hero Māui attempts to make humankind immortal by climbing up inside her vagina as she sleeps, reversing birth; however, she is awoken by a bird laughing at how ridiculous Māui looks and she crushes him with her thighs, bringing death into the world (Kahukiwa and Grace 1984, 58). Related myths feature women with snakes, eels, carnivorous fish or dragons in their vaginas, or stories of women or goddesses who, like the Lamia, look like beautiful women from the waist up, but from the waist down resemble monstrous beasts (Blackledge 2003, 168). The fairy tale Briar Rose – more commonly known as Sleeping Beauty – portrays a beautiful maiden surrounded by a seemingly impassable forest of thorns; by conquering these teeth and breaking through the dangerous entrance, the hero is rewarded with the young woman, whose name references the long-standing association of the images of roses with female genitalia and sexuality (Bernau 2008, 74–77).

Barbara Creed's account of the resonance of *vagina dentata* imagery in horror in *The Monstrous-Feminine* (1993, 105–121) connects such issues with psychoanalytic accounts of personal and sexual anxiety. Creed argues that the vicious, aggressive image of the head of the Medusa is a visual expression of the threat of castration that is evoked in the male child by the adult female genitals, rather than acting as a symbol of castrated female genitals, as Freud argued. Within this schema, Medusa's hair of phallic serpents and her 'stiffening' (that is, erection-causing) gaze are not a comforting, consoling, fetishistic image of the imaginary phallus; instead, her tusks, tongue, enormous mouth and hair of twisting, hissing snakes are an image of the castrating *vagina dentata* (p. 111), and as such allude to both a literal castration and a symbolic one, such as one that results in the child's loss of the mother's body or his loss of identity (p. 107). Creed also asserts that the castrating function of the *vagina denata* plays into fears of orality – firstly, the oral sadistic mother who is feared by her children, who imagine that as much as they gain pleasure from feeding from her, she will gain pleasure in feeding on them, and secondly the dyadic, pre-Oedipal mother who threatens symbolically to engulf the infant, thus obliterating them (p. 109).

The impact and resonance of these stories is apparent in the way that *vagina dentata* appears in modern day myths and urban legends that frame women's sexed bodies and desires as dangerous, if not fatal to men.[12] A clear example comes in cultural anthropologist Karen L. Pliskin's account of the ways that the figure of the monstrous, toothed vagina is invoked as a metaphor for predatory female sexuality in World War Two propaganda about ways to halt the transmission of sexually transmitted infections, particularly those that may be asymptomatic for the carrier, such as genital herpes. Pliskin cites imagery in posters that identified women as the source of venereal disease and men as their unsuspecting victims, such as a well-known poster aimed at soldiers which depicted Mussolini and Hitler walking, arms linked, with a tall woman with a skeletal face:

at the top of the poster, in big letters flanking the woman's head, is 'V.D.' The woman, holding her head back defiantly ... wears a sleeveless clinging dress and high heels. [...] Written at the bottom of the poster is, 'Worst of the three' – referring to the VD woman. (1995, 491)

Other Allied wartime posters framed women and their sexed bodies as weapons of war, and featured catch phrases such as "Fool the axis! Use prophylaxis!", "Juke joint sniper: syphilis and gonorrhea", and "'Innocent looks' and medical 'certificates' may be booby traps that cover up V. D. mines. Don't take chances" (Williams 2013). The dangers of sex, as well as the negative outcomes of casual sex or infidelity, are situated explicitly in terms of the sexualised bodies of women, who act as knowing, untrustworthy 'honey traps' ready to fool unsuspecting men and undermine the war effort, and whose predations might result in the infection of 'innocent' parties such as women and children – that is, soldiers' present or future families. Similarly, folk tales about dangerous vaginas proliferated among soldiers who fought in the Viet Nam war, who recounted urban legends of Vietnamese women, predominantly prostitutes, putting razorblades, sand, ground glass or even grenades in their vaginas; one active serviceman stated "I always put my finger in first. If I pulled back a bloody nub I knew not to stick anything else in there" (Gulzow and Mitchell 1980, 308). The ur-story of these 'real life' horror stories involves the removal or taming of the teeth or dangerous items by the hero, which neutralises the active danger of the female body. The man can then be rewarded with his prize: docile female sexuality (Beit-Hallahmi 1985, 355).

What is important throughout these accounts of *vagina dentata* is not that she/ it signals a symmetrical other to the figure of the virgin, even though popular notions such as the Madonna/whore dualism might suggest or trade upon such a fixed binary relationship. I wish to stress that where the mythic construction of the Virgin might be seen as a contained category, circular in its perpetual purity, such that virginity and women come to operate for and between men within a patriarchal society, *vagina dentata* expresses something open and unbounded: the infinite matrix-womb as juxtaposed with the hard, decisive finality of teeth. It is this, not simply the interiority of the vagina itself nor the mechanics of menstruation, conception and birth that threatens the patriarchal order. Instead, I suggest that *vagina dentata* speaks of a body (and here I speak not of literal bodies, but of bodies in the more abstract sense) as well as a mode of feminine agency that has power for it and does not need the masculine to sustain or justify it. It pleases and pleasures itself, and it chooses what enters into it. Its (auto)eroticism is complex. It does not centralise male pleasure, nor does its potency necessarily submit to male power. Where the 'closed' falls in upon itself, allowing nothing in or out, the 'open' flows forth, expanding and multi-plying in the persistent making-different that similarly marks the notion of the monstrous not inherently negative but as productive and generative.

Where Barbara Creed recalls Freud's invocation of Medusa as signifying the threat of castration and women's status as metaphorically castrated, and reframes her image as an expression of the agency of the castrator (the *femme castratrice*), it is also worth remembering that French post-structuralist philosopher Hélène Cixous likewise looks to Medusa as a misinterpreted symbol. In "Laugh of the Medusa" (2010 [1975]), Cixous argues that we must look for new ways to think about how women might counter the masculine bias of phallo(go)centric modes of language and power that have historically denied women the ability to write their own language, tell their own stories, and stake claim to their own representations and identities. As she advocates for a feminine writing (*écriture féminine*), a writing of the self and the body that acts as a way of "breaking the codes that negate" women (p. 31), she suggests that Medusa is "not deadly. She's beautiful and she's laughing" (p. 38). In this vein of re-interpretation, I put forward that the *vagina dentata*, then, forecloses the idea of the one Woman who is Other, a necessary and invisible condition of male subjectivity. Instead it unfolds into a kaleidoscopic constellation of erotic, sensual possibilities and becomings that recalls, firstly, Irigaray's description of embodied female autoeroticism ("Woman 'touches herself' all the time, and moreover no one can forbid her to do so, for her genitals are formed of two lips in continuous contact" (1985b, 24)), and secondly the destabilisation of binary aggregates inherent in the molecular nature of becoming (Deleuze and Guattari 2004, 235). This situates sex (i.e. coitus) involving the penis or phallic signifier and the openness of *vagina dentata* not as an interaction between the active and that which is acted upon, nor a coupling, but one of a multiplicity of potential conjugations, none of which inherently centralise male power or pleasure. Therefore, when the *vagina dentata* is rendered as misogynist iconography, it is to specifically *displace* these transgressive attributes, reframing the woman's body as a site of horror and co-opting it into a binary scheme, and denying self-sustaining possibility.

Imag(in)ing the vagina

From a sociocultural perspective, the combined myths surrounding *vagina dentata* indicate a deep dis-ease about women's sexuality and reflect broader negative attitudes towards the vagina in contemporary culture that are put to work to actively repudiate any power inherent in the feminine. There is good evidence within some of the earliest recorded art, religious artefacts and history that the vagina, and vaginal iconography, may have been worshipped as sacred (Wolf 2012, 166–171), but more recent images and discussions of the vagina have been eradicated through ignorance and in the name of so-called 'respectability' (Rees 2013, 1–5). The meanings and connotations of the vagina and the vaginal are now conflicted and paradoxical. As psychologists Virginia Braun and Sue Wilkinson (2001) indicate in their nuanced and often openly frustrated accounts of trying to map the sociocultural construction of the vagina, it "is, among other things, the toothed and dangerous *vagina dentata*; the (symbolic) absence of a penis; the core of womanhood; and a symbol of reproduction" (p. 17). However, more often than not, the vagina is portrayed as inferior: as lesser than the penis; as a passive receptacle for the penis; as sexually inadequate, vulnerable and abused; as smelly, dangerous to both men and infants, and ultimately disgusting – a depressing portrayal that "needs to be challenged in order to promote women's sexual and reproductive health" (p. 25). Such negative and normalised portrayals of the vagina – indeed, of the female reproductive and sexual body as a whole – are recognised and ratified in the horror film, which offers very little in the way of positive or affirmative representation. Instead, the horror genre looks to the vagina as a place of disgust: it is a fleshy and conceptual site of monsters, of dread and of dangerously unbridled sexuality that marries terror with obscenity.

The image of the flaccid penis is usually unremarkable within Western artistic contexts, reflecting the reality that the phallus itself is the privileged signifier of masculine power within Western patriarchy, central to the construction of phallo(go)centric language and reason through an asymmetrical account of sexual difference that subordinates the feminine to prop up the masculine. Conversely, the image of the vagina is largely considered to be taboo and pornographic. This is highlighted in the vocal response to the work of Australian artist Greg Taylor, whose 2009 exhibition *CUNTS... and other conversations* featured 141 'porcelain portraits' – sculptures made by taking casts of the genitals of women ranging in age from 18 to 78. The exhibition came under heavy criticism for its allegedly offensive and pornographic content. Postcards advertising the exhibition were considered so vulgar that Australia Post banned them and warned Taylor that he was in breach of Commonwealth law, although – as with artist Jamie McCartney's similarly themed large-scale polyptych *The Great Wall of Vagina* (2008–2012) – the smooth, impersonal whiteness of the porcelain undoubtedly serves to render even Taylor's sculptures less potentially confrontational than they could have been.[13]

The life-sized sculptures and their marketing material were even argued to be degrading to women themselves. The conservative Australian Family Association's spokeswoman Gabrielle Walsh condemned the exhibition, saying that there was no excuse for the "c-word" to be used in public, and that Taylor "shouldn't be allowed to force these images and words upon us in public for all to view, including children... It's an abuse of public space and women, in particular, would find them deeply offensive" (Nankervis 2009). The tenor of these responses stands in direct contrast to the attitudes of Taylor's models with one, Xanya Mamunya, stating that it was:

> empowering because I am from a generation that never even looked down there. I wasn't even told about the menstrual cycle until I thought I was bleeding to death. Modelling for the exhibition made me feel that I was part of something that I think is very important – for everyone. (The O: Cunts ... And Other Conversations)

Taylor, in turn, notes that "All of them want one thing; for young women to be free of growing up with fear, ignorance and loathing of their bodies and sexuality" (New Greg Taylor Exhibition 2009). More pointedly, he states "It's all about the word," asking "why is it that in our culture the most vile and disgusting thing is perceived to be a cunt?" (Kizilos 2009).

These issues are certainly not new, for the controversy echoes the criticisms levelled at American artist Judy Chicago's iconic and monumental 1979 installation *The Dinner Party*, which features 39 beautifully presented ceramic vulvar sculptures placed at 'settings' around a large triangular table. The 39 'guests', accompanied by 999 tiles representing 'women of achievement', are dedicated to historical and mythical female figures, ranging from Hindu goddess Kali, Babylonian goddess Ishtar and the pre-historic primordial goddess, to modern feminist icons such as novelist Virginia Woolf, abbess and polymath St Hildegarde of Bingen, and artist Georgia O'Keeffe.[14] The work utilises forms of arts and crafts traditionally associated with women and domesticity, and that are thus considered 'less-than' other forms of artistic expression due to their quotidian, feminine and often quite practical nature. It aims to counter the often invisible place of women in historical accounts by giving them a 'seat at the table' and undermining phallocentric, patriarchal narratives of power and influence. The *New York Times* review of the 1980 Brooklyn showing described the work as having

> an insistence and vulgarity more appropriate, perhaps, to an advertising campaign than to a work of art. Yet what ad campaign, even in these 'liberated' times, would dare to vulgarize and exploit the imagery of female sexuality on this scale and with such abysmal taste? (Kramer 1980, p. C1)

When the piece was initially gifted to the University of the District of Colombia in 1990, it was described as "ceramic 3-D pornography" by Californian Republican representative, evangelist Pat Robertson, who accused Chicago of blasphemy (Levin 2007, 91), and Republican congressmen threatened to cut funding to the National Endowment for the Arts, which had initially funded the work's creation (Through the Flower – The Dinner Party 2016), using the indignation over the work as fuel for a broader assault on federal arts funding.

Despite *The Dinner Party*'s celebration of women's (often invisible) achievements, it is telling that the inclusion and promotion of the imagery that alludes to, as well as directly represents, female genitalia led many of the work's detractors to label it exploitative or pornographic. Here, the designation of work as 'pornography' means far more than material that is sexually explicit; instead, the implication is that women's bodies are being simultaneously victimised and displayed in a manner that inherently invites or provokes sexual arousal, although the question of who is being aroused, why, and whether or not they wanted to be turned on in the first place is rarely touched upon. The barely-veiled implication here is that although women may be shown and celebrated, it is only if there is a consequent disavowal of female sexuality and biology, which is perhaps deemed a limitation, an obscenity or a distraction. Likewise, the assumption that it is somehow essentialist or reductionist to emphasise vulvar iconography in a making-visible of the work and place of women works to further eradicate forms of expression that emphasise the feminine (Rees 2013, 125). In this case, the denouncement of images and more abstract forms of expression referencing women's sex organs works to argue that a display of women's bodies and positive sexual embodiment is not only inappropriate, but actually bad for women themselves, rendering the ethical obscene (Rees 2013, 141–142). The criticism suggests that women are trapped within or inhibited by their bodies, and as with the mythic figure of the Virgin, only by disavowing their genitals – and, presumably the 'limitations' that come with female embodment and sexuality – will they be free from objectification or debasement.

This is a perversely limiting supposition, especially when one considers the way a diverse, immense and deeply spiritual work such as *The Dinner Party* serves to illustrate and express what might be thought of as aspects of the feminine divine, rather than the masculine divine. This operates figuratively (in the relationship between mothers, daughters and sisters; the recognition of female power; relationships built upon equality and respect; and even in the collective, collaborative process of its creation) as well as literally, as in its inclusion of goddesses, abbesses, saints and other such figures. In her discussion of feminine forms and modes of beauty, Luce Irigaray argues that women have been restricted by the forms and visual image-languages made available to them, and that in order to exist these must be dismantled. Drawing from the image of the flower as representative of a woman's virginity, as something that evokes the perpetual re-flowering that marks productive becomings, she posits that in

> destroying already coded forms, women rediscover their nature, their identity, and are able to find their forms, to blossom out in accordance with what they are. Furthermore, these female forms are always incomplete, in perpetual growth, blossoms, and fertilizes (herself) within her own body. But she cannot be reduced to a single flower, as in the male image of virginity. In line with her own virginity, she is never completed in a single form. She is ceaselessly becoming, she 'flowers' again and again, if she stays close to herself and the living world. (1993b, 111)

The 'flowering', then, in *The Dinner Party* is doubly provocative, for it draws from iconography that has historically been used to limit, simplify or constrain women, as in the abstract representation of the Virgin and her contained, perpetual divinity. Instead, it speaks to an immensity of difference, refusing homogeneity through a powerful leveraging of the essentialist imagery made available through patriarchal systems of representation.

The discursive construction of the vagina as ugly or obscene extends well beyond art and into social practices around sex and medicine. In particular, the notion that the vagina is inherently deformed, vulgar and shameful is echoed in the rapidly expanding field of female genital cosmetic surgery (Stark 2010; Prime 2013; Rabin 2016), a term that first entered the public consciousness in the late 1990s (Rodrigues 2012, 778). Unlike invasive cultural practices such as female genital mutilation or clitoral excision, or reconstructive procedures that may occur in the treatment of disease, or procedures such as sexual reassignment surgeries, female genital cosmetic surgeries are specifically marketed to cisgendered women with 'healthy' vaginas with the alleged intention of enhancing the woman's sexual pleasure, thereby allowing women to proactively engage with their own (hetero)sexuality. However, despite these apparently self-affirming aspects, much of the emphasis is on making genitalia 'pretty', 'youthful', more 'inviting' or more 'feminine' – that is, that changes are made for aesthetic instead of functional or medical reasons. The language surrounding such procedures and the hunt for the perfect 'designer vagina', and the other procedures generally offered – such as the aforementioned hymen replacement, as well as vulval liposuction, clitoral hood repositioning, labia reductions and augmentations[15] and vaginal tightening – frame women's bodies as both imperfect or impeded (Braun 2005, 410). Here, the female genitals are framed as for the appraisal and consumption by another, usually posited as a heterosexual male, with 'optimal' aesthetics serving as a means of disciplinary control (Rodrigues 2012, 779; 784–785).

Although such medical interventions can perhaps be considered an extension of other sexual-aesthetic body modification practices, such as pubic waxing and labial dye products such as My New Pink Button[16] (Braun 2005, 408), it is important to note that the demand and supply of female genital cosmetic surgery points to the reality that most heterosexual women are most likely to have seen the genitals of other women within the context of pornographic media, and that it is the images of airbrushed vulvas in softcore pornography[17] and the highly exposed genitals of hardcore pornography, that set an aesthetic standard.[18] It would be overly simplistic to suggest that these anxieties about sex and body image are being articulated in such a way purely *because* of pornography and its emphasis upon genital visibility, but it is certainly significant that these contemporary fictive vaginas (for want of any other broadly 'available' alternative) are posited as both 'ideal' and 'normal' and thus the most attractive to the heterosexual men who, presumably, respond to them sexually in mainstream pornography (Braun 2005, 413). Such discursive positioning marks the vagina as a controlled space for (heterosexual male) erotic pleasure, as opposed to a liminal or abject space of "ambiguity and indefiniteness" (Rodrigues 2012, 782), or one that exists for the benefit and experience of the woman herself.[19] These anxieties, be they personal or more broadly sociocultural, serve to inform the sorts of narratives about unruly vaginas that play out within the horror genre.

Vagina dentata in horror

Given the myriad expressions of such cultural disgust and dis-ease concerning the vagina, alongside deeply misogynist fears about the power of female sexuality, interiority and pleasure, it is unsurprising that *vagina dentata* is a popular and resonant motif in horror, albeit one can be thought about as ambivalent, even radical in its broader implications. Allusions to the toothed, dangerous vagina are present in the bloodied, fanged maw of the vampire, the mouth of the shark in *Jaws* (1975) and the burrowing monsters in *Tremors* (1990), the writhing, tentacled chests of the female aliens in *Decoys*, the mouths of the alien squid-monsters in *Grabbers* (2012), the insatiable alien-plant Audrey II in *Little Shop of Horrors* (1986), the face of the *Predator* (1987), who is dubbed "pussyface" in *Predator 2* (1990), and the mouths of snake-worshipper Lady Sylvia Marsh and her serpent-deity in the campy *The Lair of the White Worm* (1988). Human mouths, too, evoke the allure of *vagina dentata* – the blood red lips of the disembodied singing mouth during the opening number of *The Rocky Horror Picture Show* (1975) juxtapose sexual invitation with impending sexual danger, prefiguring the film's own radical and joyous repudiation of heteronormativity.

The threat of *vagina dentata* is also present in more abstract or metaphorical senses. In her account of the monstrous-feminine, Barbara Creed (1993) connects the recurring presence of creatures with large, toothed, devouring mouths to films involving castration, as in the 1978 rape-revenge film *I Spit on Your Grave*, alongside films that feature 'castrating', emasculating mothers, such as *Psycho* (1960). The toothed vagina also appears throughout films' mise-en-scène, framing and décor. Creed suggests that allusions to the monstrous vagina are present in the genre's fascination with long dark hallways or corridors, with dangerous doors and thresholds (p. 109), and with stories that, like that of Māui and Hine-nui-te-pō, or of Heracles' trial in the underworld in Greek legend, involve a hero travelling into deep, subterranean spaces of interiority and death to conquer toothed or monstrous creatures. Swiss artist H. R. Giger's strategically and deliberately sexualised designs for the film *Alien* (1979) best evoke abject genital horror and a playful ambivalence about the nature of the unbounded feminine: the large, vaginal caverns of the derelict alien spacecraft and the horrific mouth of the parthenogenetic alien creature are coupled with the film's extensive and canny use of visual and thematic signifiers of the sexual monstrosity to create a film that exudes a deep dis-ease surrounding the power and danger of female sexuality.

These expressions of *vagina dentata* are predominantly metaphorical, but there are more specific, nasty and quite literally explicit examples of monstrous vaginas in horror films. In body horror *Contracted* (2013), a woman is infected with a sexually transmitted virus that renders her dying from the inside out; at various points she bleeds profusely from her vagina and, in one particularly abject scene, maggots fall from her vagina – much to the horror of the man with whom she has just been having penetrative sex. The similarly-themed *Thanatomorphose* (2012) takes the metaphor of feeling 'dead inside' and makes it literal: isolated, emotionally blunted protagonist Laura begins to slowly decay after a sexual encounter. Her dissolution is visually echoed in a leaking, dripping tear in the ceiling, which resembles a vaginal opening and connects her inner rot with that of her dark, oppressive apartment. The mute undead woman at the centre of the cynical *Deadgirl* (2008) is repeatedly raped by a group of young men who discover her naked and bound to a table in the basement of an abandoned psychiatric hospital. When one of the teenage boys forces her to perform oral sex on him she bites his penis and infects him with the same disease that rendered her a zombie, linking sexually transmitted infection to plague, and conflating the explicit danger of her mouth with the implicit danger of her vagina and her undead interiority. Even more explicitly, the Japanese schlock-horror *Sexual Parasite: Killer Pussy* (2004), which draws from a history of Japanese porn-and-gore films, features a woman who has a long, snake-like Amazonian parasite living in her vagina, which makes her insatiably aroused, but which also eats the penises of those who come near it as she reaches orgasm. The misogynistic and often incoherent low-budget British horror *Penetration Angst* (2003) treats *vagina dentata* as a metaphor for sexual dysfunction. Helen, who is coded as both girlishly reticent and sexually available, is repulsed by her body. She has a history of sexual abuse and her hungry vagina demands to be fed, and when men have sex with Helen against her will – which happens with disturbing frequency – the man is devoured, leaving only his clothes behind. Inexplicably, Helen falls in love with a man who has been stalking her, and this resolves her 'penetration angst' and silences her ravenous vagina.

This is not to say that all such representations of monstrous vaginas are similarly negative. *Bad Biology* (2009) engages more playfully with the potential for new modes of sexuality and desire. Jennifer considers her personal mutation – a dripping, cave-like vagina with multiple clitorises which renders her permanently aroused – to be an evolutionary leap.[20] She decides that her God-given insatiable appetite for violent, murderous sex must be a sign that she is destined to be 'screwed' by God and give birth to his holy child. Jennifer sees her vagina as both divine and apocalyptic, a nexus of life and death; she compares her sexual, desirous interiority to the Garden of Eden, to Sodom and Gomorrah, and the equivalent of having the Armageddon and all the Biblical disciples inside her all at once. Her sexual appetite is insatiable and her multiple sexual partners leave her unsatisfied; indeed, sex usually ends with the death of her partner and the swift creation (and disposal) of mutant babies. Her counterpart is a horrified, put-upon man who has an enormous sentient penis, which regularly becomes fed up with its owner's sexual difficulties and insufficiencies and detaches itself so as to go looking for more ways to please itself. The film ends with an explosive sexual encounter in which one outsized, insatiable sexual and reproductive system meets the other. This enthusiastic representation of monstrous sex and desire reflects director Frank Henenlotter's overall corpus of exploitation films, which ironically and humorously revel in the excesses of the body, offering a gleefully gross-out and abject account of transgressive pleasure and corporeality.

In a more humorous vein, it is worth highlighting the idiosyncratic yet surprisingly non-explicit sex comedy *Chatterbox!* (1977), which casts a vagina as its wisecracking comic relief. In this one-of-a-kind film a young beautician's vagina (dubbed 'Virginia') inexplicably starts to talk and sing, often spouting smutty jokes or butting into conversations. Virginia and her 'owner', Penelope, embark upon an ill-fated career on variety shows and eventually find true love (and, presumably, rewarding sex) in a man whose penis also speaks its mind. The film's moral centres on learning to love and live with your body, flaws and all, and in celebrating sex as a part of women's embodied, sexual lives. The connection between Virginia and Penelope is emphasised throughout the film; between being threatened with exorcism by an angry priest, and being challenged by high profile feminists including Gloria Steinem and Betty Friedan, Virginia maintains that she, with Penelope in tow, will show them all up (see also Rees 2013, 229–234). Nonetheless, in each of these examples, whether the film is horrific or humorous, the relationship between the woman and her vagina is synecdochic – that is, the vagina represents the woman herself, so that the woman becomes entirely conflated with her genitalia and its (independent) desires or its trauma, much as the penis is often framed as an entity with a mind of its own (see Potts 2002, 102–133).

How, then, might these conflicting and complicated engagements with female sexuality, from the demure, sacrificial virgin to the voracious, expansive *vagina dentata* combine within the horror genre? So-called 'low brow' films are rich sites of inquiry, given their effusive and largely uncritical poaching of a wide variety of images, myths and allusions, and this is certainly the case in the religious horror *The Unholy* (1988). The film combines myths about female virginity, male chastity and voracious, demonic sexuality in an overwrought, less-than-coherent melange that nonetheless reveals a great deal about the shifting vagaries of sociocultural myths about women, virginity and sex and the way that reductive conceptual binaries are shored up. The film centres on a young priest, Father Michael, who is sent to take over a church in which the previous priests were viciously sacrificed by an unknown force. Father Michael befriends a troubled young woman, Millie, who is involved with a goth fetish club tellingly named 'The Threshold', which, apart from its allusions to the entrance to the vagina, points to the space between sexual immaturity and sexual knowledge. It is not long before Father Michael becomes tangled within the supernatural occurrences. He is haunted by dreams of a naked woman dancing outside his window, as well as images of snakes, and the escalation of the violent, supernatural activity surrounding the church results in the grisly sacrifice of the resident dog by an unknown offender. The convoluted underlying mythology is one of temptation and punishment. Father Michael learns that these events are related to the predations of a demon called The Unholy which attempts to tempt a priest; should the priest succumb then the demon butchers him, meaning that the sinner is killed in the act of sinning and his soul sent to hell. Father Michael, in a confrontation in the church over Easter weekend, is tempted by sex, but he manages to keep his lust for the demon's female form, and for Millie, at bay. He eventually defeats the demon, but he loses his sight in the process.

Within this fairly standard religious horror narrative, *The Unholy* indicates how conflicting and often contradictory representations of sexuality can coexist within narratives that fetishise and (in this case literally) demonise female sexual agency, all while positing that women, in whatever form, are a threat to men. The 'seductress' form of the demon is that of a naked woman who sports exaggerated signifiers of hypersexuality and hyperfemininity: large breasts, long painted nails, long curly red hair and heavy makeup. She never speaks, only beckons and teases. She is often draped in a flimsy gauzy material that looks better suited to boudoir lingerie, as is filmed in a diffuse soft focus effect that draws from the iconography of late night 1980s erotica. She is associated with the image of serpents, which suggest numerous allusions, from Medusa's hair to Eve's temptation in the Garden of Eden, to transformation, and to the devil (Stutesman 2005, 65–66). This ophidian imagery is elsewhere, too: the goth club owner, a stage magician called Luke who performs black magic, has a picture of a woman and a large python in his bedroom, and Father Michael has a nightmare in which his crotch is covered in small snakes. During the attempted temptation of Father Michael we see the image of the demon flicking between that of the enticing succubus and that of its true form: it is a gnarled, scarred, four-legged creature with an enormous fanged mouth and a long, prehensile tongue. The film invites us to be both aroused and repulsed in the knowledge that the previous priests of the church were killed for their spiritual and sexual transgressions by a creature that both conforms to and is completely opposed to normative notions of female hypersexuality and sexual acceptability.

Where the demon is presented as both salacious and serpentine, the film offers up a number of conflicting representations of virginity. Father Michael's virginity is presented as both strength and weakness. It is something from which he draws spiritual and physical fortitude, but it is also the means through which he can be corrupted, especially given his obviously erotic and inappropriate feelings for the troubled runaway Millie. She, in turn, is presented in a sexualised but girlish and naïve manner that, like the pornography that fetishises 'deflowering', asks the viewer to regard her as both coquettish virgin and sexually available object of desire. Millie steals a book of black magic from Luke and is distraught to discover that the demon thrives on purity, and kills virgins who succumb to temptation, so she presents herself to Father Michael, undresses, and asks him to have sex with her so as to protect her. Ironically, both the film's ingénue and the Satanic emissary are shown to be offering exactly the same 'wares' and both promise Father Michael's downfall – for the demon, in taking his soul to hell, and for Millie, by undermining the sanctity of his holy vows.

In keeping with narrative expectations, Father Michael prevails against the evil forces, and he comes through the ordeal having lost his sight – apt, given the visual titillation of the demon – but having also replenished his waning faith.[21] He also establishes a more 'appropriate' relationship with Millie, in effect replacing the abusive relationships she had with both her father and boyfriend Luke with a more prescribed, paternalistic one. His virginity and piety remain firm, the monstrous vaginal monster is defeated, and Millie is sexually rehabilitated, placed back within a submissive role better fitting the stereotypical role of the virgin. Although the film's internal logic is convoluted, its containment of female sexuality and its celebration of the docile re-educated virgin blatantly typify the way that female sexuality is forced into reductive binary categories, so that female sex is both for the benefit of and dangerous to men. It is a threatening horror but one that can be vanquished, even if it is at first enjoyed.

A different sort of *Teeth*: reframing *vagina dentata*

The chaste virgin and the toothed vagina are often paired together to form a problematic dyad, with each standing for a simplistic and reductive representation of women and normative femininity that defines each by their sexuality and sexual availability, and that denies the potential of multiple forms of desire, sexuality and eroticism. The evocations of the toothed vagina discussed above have been predominantly negative and serve to shut down transgressive (that is, non-phallocentric) female desire by inspiring fear, disgust and loathing. However, *vagina dentata* can also be reframed as emancipatory: if the virgin body is to be forcibly annexed, as Rebecca Whisnant (2010, 161) suggests, then perhaps *vagina dentata*'s inherent agency and implicit violence can be leveraged as a deterrent or a line of defence. Instead, *vagina dentata* can be reframed as a discursive strategy through which women can reclaim their bodies, resist corporeal colonisation, or retaliate against a conceptual framing of masculine sexual prowess that serves to denigrate, objectify and subjugate women (Potts 2002, 213).

Vagina dentata is deployed in this sense as a metaphor for sexual self-awareness and self-defence, as well as a means of potentially positive sexual embodiment, in the 2007 American black horror-comedy *Teeth*. The film situates adolescence in suburban America as "a socio-sexual battleground" (Craig and Fradley 2010, 90) that pits young men and women against each other in a social environment shaped by insidious structural misogyny. However, although the film undeniably offers a liberal and progressive attitude towards women's sexuality and self-fulfilment, it nonetheless resolves itself in a troublesome and almost contradictory manner that suggests that, perhaps, one form of sexual violence and victimhood can only be countered by another.

The film draws from popular myths and constructions about female sexuality, specifically the figures of the chaste virgin and the voracious *vagina dentata*, in a strategic, knowing, and often humorous manner. The narrative centres on Dawn O'Keefe, a wholesome and naïve teenager who is an enthusiastic participant in her school's chastity club, even though she is undermined and mocked by her schoolmates for her firmly-held beliefs on abstinence and moral fortitude. Dawn and her first real crush, a scruffily attractive 'born-again virgin' named Tobey, enjoy a flirtatious relationship, and they start to act, hesitantly, on their desires for one another. They go to a local make-out point, a secluded reservoir, but when Dawn tries to halt Tobey's increasingly impassioned advances he rapes her. However, Dawn has a defence mechanism: as Tobey tries to muffle Dawn's cries, her vagina castrates him. Tobey, bleeding profusely from his wound, collapses into the reservoir's waters and disappears.

Dawn is horrified and traumatised, and upon returning home she tries to gain some sort of understanding as to what her body is and does – a difficult task, given her ignorance of her own anatomy and her own previous disavowal of female sexual impulses. She visits a gynaecologist but he, too, assaults her. When he gives her an invasive internal examination using glove-free hands Dawn's toothed vagina again retaliates, and the doctor loses some of his fingers. Dawn looks to her high school anatomy textbooks, which she had previously considered to be immodest, and researches *vagina dentata* on the internet. Distraught, alone and frightened, and panicking about the response to Tobey's disappearance, she turns to a classmate, Ryan, who had previously shown interest in her. He plies her with alcohol and anti-anxiety medication and they have sex – an act that proceeds without his mutilation given, perhaps, his attention towards Dawn's own sexual pleasure and orgasm, even though the dubious circumstances undermine the nature of Dawn's consent. However, even though he proclaims himself to be the 'hero' who will remove her metaphorical thorns, he is more interested in making Dawn break her virginity pledge than in genuinely helping her. When Dawn realises she has been the subject of a wager she is able, for the first time, to consciously exercise her newfound agency, and Ryan becomes one of Dawn's casualties.

As Dawn is coming to terms with her sexuality and her body's abilities, her aggressive and misogynistic stepbrother Brad is implicated in the death of Dawn's terminally ill mother: he fails to hear her shouts for help over the sound of the loud music he is listening to as he has aggressive and demeaning sex with his girlfriend. In an act of vengeance, Dawn decides to take advantage of the quasi-incestuous feelings Brad has had for her since they were infants. She dresses up in a pristine white sundress, seduces him, and then castrates him with her vagina, then hitchhikes out of town. In the film's final moments she is offered a ride up by a man who indicates that he wants sexual favours in turn for his assistance. Dawn rolls her eyes in unsurprised exasperation but then turns to him invitingly, indicating that her toothed vagina is now as much a targeted weapon as it is a defence mechanism.

Teeth's wry and pointed engagement with teenage sexuality and female sexual agency is a part of a larger millennial preoccupation with virginity that is particularly evident in American social and political discourses (Farrimond 2013, 48), including popular feminist work such as Jessica Valenti's 2009 book *The Purity Myth* and Cassie Jaye's documentary *Daddy I Do* (2010), which looks to the culture of so-called purity balls, in which girls and young women make public vows to stay chaste until marriage. Alongside teen-centric films such as the witty rom-com *Easy A* (2010), a modern retelling of Nathanial Hawthorne's book *The Scarlet Letter*, and the tongue-in-cheek religious satire *Saved!* (2004), which centres on the intersection of evangelical faith, homosexuality and first sex, *Teeth* provides a pop cultural response to the discursive construction of virginity that centralises teenage girls' perspectives on the contradictory and messy constructions of teen sex, morality and female sexual identity that are so often imposed upon them. In particular, *Teeth* explicitly addresses with the most pronounced engagement with virginity and sexual education in the contemporary United States: the cultural and political impact of abstinence-only-until-marriage education and its association with the 'purity movement'.

Federal support for American abstinence-only sexual education officially began in a limited capacity in 1982 under the Adolescent Family Life Act, which promoted "chastity and self-discipline" (Kelly 2016), but it was extended significantly in 1996 during welfare reforms. These reforms saw the creation of targeted funding streams – initially US$50 million dollars per year in 1998, which later blew out to US$176 million per year in 2006 and 2007 – that were tied to the promotion of abstinence-only-until-marriage programmes that fulfilled the parameters of a strict eight-point schedule (SIECUS 2010). The provisions for such funding stated that "a mutually faithful monogamous relationship in the context of marriage is the *expected standard* of human sexual activity" (Howell and Keefe 2007, emphasis mine), and that completely abstaining from sexual activity before marriage is the only way to avoid pregnancy, sexually transmitted infections, and a whole slew of (alleged) associated health, social and psychological problems, centring on the notion that any "sexual activity outside the context of marriage is likely to have harmful psychological and physical effects" (Howell and Keefe 2007). This marked a significant ideological shift away from programmes that emphasised the prevention of unwanted pregnancy and sexually transmitted infections and into a more stringent set of guidelines designed to promote an ideal, moral, docile heterosexual citizen who behaves in an ideologically-complicit manner – one who conforms with American 'family values' (Beh and Diamond 2006). Indeed, Casey Ryan Kelly (2016) argues persuasively that this was a way of instrumentalising bodily desire, rather than suppressing or censuring it, and in doing so taking open public discourse surrounding sexuality and re-routing it into a national project of heteronormative, familial (re)productivity. More importantly, the programmes restricted or eliminated information about safer sex practices, including the use of contraception and other safer sex aids such as dental dams, suggesting that this knowledge would *promote* adolescent sexual activity, instead of empowering teenagers to make informed choices.

Targeted funding for abstinence-based sexual education in schools in the United States was introduced by conservative lawmakers under the Clinton administration, and remained present in varying forms until it was removed from the 2017 federal budget, the final budget under the Obama administration, which also increased funding for pregnancy prevention programmes.

However, the 'purity movement' is inextricably linked with the evangelical Christian values that were supported and encouraged under the presidency of Republican George W Bush from 2000 to 2008. The value-driven message of abstinence-only education is not simply that pre-marital sex should be avoided. It actively demonises pre-marital sexual activity, "capitalising on the danger and extreme consequences of knowing and/or acting on sexual desire" (Burns and Torre 2004, 130–131) by presenting "horror-filled images and portrayals of dire life outcomes [that] have a lasting impact" (Burns and Torre 2004, 131) that deny that pre-marital or adolescent sex can be anything other than a negative and damaging experience. This message was reiterated through social and political discourses too; Eric Keroack, who was from 2006–2007 the Deputy Assistant Secretary of the federal Office of Population Affairs, which oversees the United States' government's reproductive health efforts, even proclaimed that "pre-marital sex is really modern germ warfare" and that "sexual activity is a warzone" (Valenti 2009, 54). Such statements equate pre-martital sex with literal pollution as well as moral pollution, much as the anti-VD posters mentioned earlier in this chapter align sex (and the sexual bodies of women) with violence and acts of war. The emphasis on abstinence over comprehensive sexual education also paints contraception as ineffective and dirty.[22] This model has been widely derided as being misleading and generally ineffective in delaying first penetrative intercourse and stopping the transmission of sexually transmitted infections, as well as ignoring the needs of youth of sexual minorities (Beh and Diamond 2006), although there are indications that abstinence can be an effective means of delaying penetrative sex if couched within identity politics – that is, when "chastity functions essentially as a youth counterculture" (Lancaster 2003, 331).

The overwhelming heterosexism of this sexual discourse also draws from very gender-specific and conservative attitudes towards what 'proper' behaviour for young men and women should be. As an example, this sociosexual model puts the onus for avoidance of sex and arousal (and, implicitly, sexual assault) predominantly upon young women, by arguing that they have better sexual self-control than their male peers because they are allegedly less easily aroused and less visually oriented, which in turn places emphasis upon women's bodies as a locus of desire and temptation. Where the figures of the virgin and the whore come to typify a dualistic gynaehorrific construction of female sexuality, the framing of teenage sexual desire within discourses of abstinence similarly posits that women are both sexually threatening yet have the responsibility to actively, even militantly, withhold sex. Under such frameworks, young women must take on responsibility for both male and female arousal by policing sexual behaviour (Valenti 2009, 107), such as by avoiding clothes deemed too tempting and by being trained to forcefully rebuff unwanted sexual advances.

At first, Dawn takes this essentialist construction of sex, and her role within it, as inherently natural and normal. At the film's outset, Dawn gives an impassioned talk to her chastity club on how one's virginity is a precious gift and not a handout. She defends the district school board's decision to place large stickers over diagrams of the vulva in biology textbooks, but not the penis, by arguing that girls have an inherent modesty. When she fantasises about Tobey she frames her desire 'properly' by imagining their wedding night – as erotic a dream as she will allow herself. Desire is framed as dangerous, and chastity worth being vigilant about, and initially Dawn and Tobey avoid spending time alone together outside of the relative sexual and moral safety of their social circle. However, when they finally meet for an illicit swim at the reservoir, Tobey uses his mounting sexual frustration to legitimise his actions: when he rapes Dawn he shouts at her, self-pityingly, that he hasn't masturbated since Easter. Again, virginity is less a set of actions than a state of mind: he tells her that if she just lies still and lets him do what he wants then she will still be pure in the eyes of the Lord, marrying his sexual entitlement and his objectification of Dawn with the assertion that her subjective 'presence' isn't mandatory and that her victimhood and sacrifice somehow protects her morally.

However, although *Teeth* is certainly a strident critique of the misinformation offered by the purity movement, conservative evangelical cultural ideologies regarding sexuality and gender, and the widespread move away from compre-hensive sexual education in large areas of the United States, the film generally alludes to religion instead of engaging with it directly. Even though Dawn's abstinence group clearly plays with stereotypes of American evangelical Christian youth groups, and born-again virgin Tobey refers to being a virgin in 'His' eyes, the only point at which religious language or iconography is explicitly referenced – other than a brief exchange about evolution during biology class in which the teacher is obviously frustrated with talk of so-called 'intelligent design' – is when Dawn gives a presentation to the purity club the day after Tobey has raped her. Unlike the first meeting, in which Dawn warmly promoted 'purity', this one takes on a woozy, almost hallucinatory quality. The assembled crowd of children and adolescents respond to Dawn's hesitant, increasingly horrified articulation of her own experience of the lethal 'thing' inside of her in a manner of call and response that explicitly mimics that of evangelical worship. Dawn's dialogue with the crowd – the de facto congregation – becomes increasingly strained, desperate and fragmented as she stumbles her way through an account of her own femininity as tainted. Dawn struggles to find her place herself within a cultural and moral framework that, on one hand, requires chastity and piety of young women, and that on the other hand marks women as inherently flawed, equating sexuality and (carnal) knowledge with temptation and original sin through the vilification of Eve. Dawn's story, instead, is the discovery that the 'something' inside of her – both her burgeoning desire and her literal *vagina dentata* – isn't wicked or foreign at all. Importantly, the film doesn't ask the viewer to mock Dawn for her beliefs; instead, it asks us to have sympathy for her and to understand that she's been grossly misled and miscast. Dawn is doubly victimised – once by the men who assault her, but also by the movement that professed to have her best interests at heart.

Teeth's satirical project, then, is to take the rhetorical gynaehorrific configuration of sex, as it is presented in an educational, political and religious
framework that demonises female sexuality and considers even the basic
mechanics of sex too raunchy for the classroom, and then make it literally
monstrous. However, the film emphasises that it is not sex *itself* that is dangerous,
but abusive sexual practices, sexual ignorance and misogynistic discourses of
sexuality. Instead, sex is presented as an alluring unknown. When Tobey and
Dawn finally meet at the reservoir after weeks of awkward courtship and
sexual avoidance, they swim across to the local make-out spot, a site that
invokes vaginal iconography and mythology to the point of po-faced parody.
The cave is dark, mysterious, wet and inviting. Set across the lake, it is a place
that the two must actively travel to and climb up within, and its dripping,
verdant opening sits in contrast to the parched desert-like surroundings. The
cave is a place of secrecy and fertility – as evidenced by the blankets left
behind by previous couples – but also a place of danger, not because of sex
itself but because of Tobey. When she returns home, after Tobey has been
castrated and has disappeared into the water, she showers and washes away
the muck from the pond, cleansing herself of the rape, then tears the girlish
posters and photos from her wall, throwing away the trappings of childhood
and naïveté. The wet, vaginal cave was the site of trauma, but it certainly
wasn't the cause of it.

The implication is that abstinence-only education isn't simply misleading,
that it is fundamentally harmful; as legal scholars Hazel Glenn Beh and Milton
Diamond (2006) suggest, it "is anything but educational. At best, it deprives
students of the knowledge necessary to manage their own sexual health. At
worst, it is dangerous to minors and to the public health" (p. 15). This is
made apparent when Dawn realises that she has no real knowledge about her
body and how it is meant to look and function, and that she is hopelessly ill-
equipped to deal with her questions about sex. Dawn manages to remove the
sticker covering the anatomical images of female genitalia in her biology
textbook by lowering the page into water and gently sliding the sticky metallic circle away, in a gesture that seems like a caress. The image of the vulva is
a revelation. Dawn is both relieved and entranced, although she has no idea
what she is looking at, and after studying the image she comically looks down
to her crotch, and then back at the diagram. During her subsequent research
she reads about the myth of the *vagina dentata*, learning that a hero must do
battle with the woman and her toothed, monstrous inner creature and defeat
her power. She also reads that the myth symbolises sexual dread and a journey
back to the womb: the vagina is a 'crucible', a place of origin and end.

Of course, these myths are as little about female empowerment as her
school's sexual education, and it is only after she experiences pleasurable sex
with her classmate Ryan that she comes to be in control of her inner teeth.
When she discovers that she's been the subject of a virginity-breaking wager
and that her seduction was an act of coercion she summarily castrates him, swears,
and mutters about his lack of heroism. In this moment she dismissively

discounts the mythic accounts that she had read; after all, she is her own hero, and her power most certainly does not need to be defeated or dismantled for her to achieve self-sufficiency. As such, her *vagina dentata* isn't necessarily the evocation of an aggressive, primal and hostile female sexuality. It is a necessary protection against a world full of predators and misogynists who try to deny Dawn her bodily and sexual autonomy and a way of exercising agency. So, it is through this self-awareness and practical, embodied knowledge, and sexual praxis, not through moral isolationism, that Dawn comes to be equipped to deal with and confront the pleasures and perils of the sexual world.

While *Teeth* is a serious engagement with female sexual autonomy, it is presented in a knowing and tongue-in-cheek manner that lightens some of the more horrific aspects of its content. It highlights the absurdity of dominant myths of female sexuality through the steady build-up of ironic visual juxta-positions, in particular in its articulation and subversion of a distinction between light and dark, and purity and danger. Most obviously, Dawn's name recalls associations of light and dawn with virginity, much as her last name, O'Keefe, references American modernist artist Georgia O'Keeffe, whose soft, luminescent flower-like paintings evoke images of female genitalia. This juxta-position between light and dark informs the film's climactic sexual conflict. It begins when blonde, radiant Dawn prepares herself for sexual 'combat' by turning herself into a virginal fetish object, by donning a white girlish dress, doing her hair, and carefully applying soft, dewy makeup, before offering herself as a honey-trap to her dark-haired black-clad stepbrother Brad.

Dawn is initially presented as a wholesome cliché, and Brad is her stereo-typical opposite: he is a violent, anti-social, heavily tattooed chain smoker and drug user whose tastes in media tend towards hardcore pornography and death metal. His most fulfilling relationship is with his Rottweiler, Mother, a canine replacement for his own mother, who he believes had been maliciously displaced by Dawn's mother when he was very young, even though the reason for the dissolution of his parents' relationship is never mentioned. (In a comically macabre touch, once Brad has been castrated by Dawn, Mother eats the severed penis.) However, Brad's darkness also stems from his dysfunctional relationship with sex. He refuses to have vaginal sex with his girlfriends and instead insists upon rough, demeaning sex and anal penetration. His perva-sively misogynistic attitude towards women is tied to a half-remembered incident from early childhood, the inciting incident of the film: when he and Dawn were playing in a paddling pool he tried to insert his finger into Dawn's vagina, but the tip of his finger was snipped off. It is Brad who is most afraid of the vagina, not because it is inherently dangerous but because his unwanted probing triggered a defensive mechanism and *made* it dangerous.

This sense of sexual dread is accentuated through the film's self-conscious intertextuality, especially in its playful deployment of tropes and imagery associated with pulpy monster movies. As she watches late-night television, Dawn is horrified by the enormous mandibles of the eponymous stop-motion animated monster of *The Black Scorpion* (1957). Later, asleep and dreaming of a wedding with Tobey, she is clearly aroused, but a flash of the scorpion's head intrudes upon her fantasy just as her hand nears her crotch, her self-policing equating her nascent sexuality with monstrosity. Likewise, at one point the Hammer horror film *The Gorgon* (1964) plays on a television in the background, and Dawn, when researching *vagina dentata*, is startled by images of Medusa. It is notable that once Dawn has taken control of her 'gift', her predatory gaze is accompanied by the sound of a snake's rattle. The soundtrack and cinematography is likewise extremely tongue-in-cheek: for example, Tobey's admission that he has previously had sex is accompanied by heavy, foreboding music and faux-primal drumming as Dawn stares at him with horror. Similarly, other revelations, such as Dawn's discovery of the myth of *vagina dentata*, are accompanied by musical stings that are so overly dramatic as to be rendered camp. Although there are a few brief explicit shots of severed penises and bloody crotches, horror is usually implied through laboured, exaggerated reaction shots that recall those of 1950s scream queens in B-grade creature features.

The threat of taint also looms large over Dawn's home. Close behind the family's house sits a nuclear power plant whose cooling towers spew clouds of unnaturally smoky steam against the blue sky and above the trees of the comically idyllic small town. The film's opening shot pans across the stacks before tilting down to reveal an aerial wide-shot of Dawn's suburban (nuclear!) family home on the day of the film's inciting childhood incident, the small round paddling pool juxtaposed against the parched, patchy lawn. An early scene in Dawn's biology class hints that her toothed vagina may be a beneficial mutation caused by the proximity of the power station; however, the image of it looming over her house indicates the ever-present threat to purity and family by pollution, both literal and spiritual.

Teeth is clearly a film made with a distinct feminist sensibility, and it positions itself as a satirical fable about the dangers of sexual ignorance and the attainment of female self-sufficiency and autonomy. Writer-director Mitchell Lichtenstein acknowledges that he is freely referencing attitudes to women and the perceived threat of female sexuality, but argues that he engages with these issues and images critically, noting that the metaphor of the toothed vagina has little to do with the actual qualities of women, but the attitudes of men (Billington 2008). He also indicates that the monsters of the film are more insidious and quotidian than Dawn and her 'unique anatomy', positioning Dawn away from past representations of monstrous women, such as telekinetic, destructive high school student Carrie in the eponymous 1976 film, whose monstrosity is similarly connected with her sexuality. Carrie's power, he says, is destructive,

> but aimed toward people who, within the context of the movie, deserve it. [...] Carrie is destroyed in the end and Dawn will never be destroyed because she is not a monster. Carrie was a sympathetic monster but in this movie it's really not Dawn who is the monster. (Billington 2008)

Instead, Lichtenstein frames Dawn's journey within the film as an origin story that gives her immense strength and privilege: "it's really about the birth of a superhero" (Interview with Mitchell Lichtenstein 2008). However, the film's resolution, whereby Dawn decides to use her *vagina dentata* punitively as a sexual vigilante – not just against Brad but against the lecherous old man who she hitchhikes with and, presumably, others who fall foul of her – will for some cast doubt over the film's overall success as an empowerment narrative.

This ambivalent resolution, as with the climax of *The Cabin in the Woods,* is indicative of the way that such knowing, postmodern texts engage with issues surrounding women's bodies, in that they both critique patriarchal, heterosexist and often overtly misogynistic material while simultaneously reinforcing the status quo. Katherine Farrimond (2013) suggests that (post) feminist texts – that is, contemporary texts she sees as both taking into account and repudiating selected forms of feminism – are selective, even ambivalent in their approach to feminist issues such that they exhibit "neither a clearly defined progressive response nor a straightforwardly con-servative reaction to ideas around sexuality and empowerment" (p. 44). *Teeth*'s resolution is potentially problematic because it suggests that the misogynistic world that Dawn lives in won't change, and as such she will need to continue to deal with matters in a manner that conforms to and reinforces hostile repre-sentations of female sexuality. Where Jennifer in *Jennifer's Body* becomes a succubus, seducing men to devour them, Dawn is not so far divorced from the American infantrymen's legends of Viet Cong women with grenades in their vaginas invoked in the accounts collected by folklorists Monte Gulzow and Carol Mitchell (1980).

On one hand, *Teeth* critiques conservative identity politics through its rebuttal and handling of conservative evangelical Christian sexual politics. On the other, it nonetheless ironically reinforces other forms of conservative identity politics through its invocation of the lone vigilante, a figure who "actualizes signature themes of U.S. conservatism: strong individualism, distrust of the state, [a] focus on the rights of crime victims, advocacy of the death penalty, and the right to bear arms" (Stringer 2011, 270–271) – or, in this case, bear teeth. This is further actualised by the lack of support that Dawn receives, for although her parents are nominally supportive, she is largely isolated, and her only female ally – her terminally ill mother – dies in part because of Brad's indifference towards her, thus denying her of her female, matrilineal genealogy and the mode of female-centric identification that these engender.

Teeth is not alone in its presentation of such a vigilante figure; indeed, Martin Fradley (2013) asserts that teen horror films as a matter of course deal with "young women's everyday gendered discontent" (p. 209), and recycle and rearticulate a key trope in postfeminist cinema: "women who embrace violence as a refusal of victimhood" (p. 214). This victimhood-to-violence narrative is a staple of the rape-revenge subgenre, in which "Rape and sexual objectifica-tion serve … as a catalyst for an expressionistic violence which offers a way of talking about the violent (re-)emergence of a feminist political consciousness" (p. 217). Such narratives suggest that specific, targeted revenge is the best (or, at least, most satisfying) remedy for sexual abuse and violence. Spectacularly visceral and punishing action is emphasised in films where the crimes against women, as well as their punishment, exist outside of both rationality and the law, as in the case of *I Spit on Your Grave* (1978) and *The Last House On The Left* (1972), although *Teeth* takes significantly less glee in the presentation of sexual violence against women than a film like *I Spit On Your Grave,* where the extended, unflinching presentation of rape and violence is as important, visually, as the bloody revenge. The female vigilante, then, recalls the figure of the *femme castratrice*, or 'castrating woman'. This castration may be presented metaphorically, as in the closing credits of *Jennifer's Body*, where Needy wreaks bloody vengeance on the indie rock band who sacrificed Jennifer (Fradley 2013, 213–214). In *Teeth*, like other rape-revenge films, the castration is literal, and the narrative marks the shift from reactive or defensive murder and violence, to proactive, intentional punitive action (Clover 1992, 141).

As satisfying as this vengeance may be, it elides what has historically been an important part of feminist struggle: collectivity and community. This sort of revenge is, by its very nature, deeply individualistic, both in terms of the way that it is enacted and the highly personal wrongs it addresses. In this vein, Rebecca Stringer (2011) asks how successful the figure of the vigilante is in terms of overall feminist work to challenge male violence against women (p. 280). In her discussion of the female vigilante films *The Brave One* (2007) and *Hard Candy* (2005) Stringer suggests that where these stories emphasise agency rather than victimhood, there is nonetheless a misrepresentation of feminism that finds its "rightful conclusion in violent vigilantism", as opposed to that the sorts of activities and strategies usually emphasised in feminist efforts against violence, "which have primarily assumed the form of collective political struggle and non-violent direct action" (p. 280). Although I do not argue at all that the individualism itself that is expressed in *Teeth* is inherently wrong or anti-feminist – and nor do I agree with Stringer than the only way to address violence is through idealised collectivism – it is important to note that the film's vigilante ending most certainly reflects a broader attitude towards women, victimhood and violence in millennial American film-making that puts the onus on the individual, be that an emphasis on the nature of victimhood or the evocation of punishment that exists necessarily outside the law.

Such a reading complicates *Teeth*'s ostensibly straightforward coming-of-(sexual-)age narrative arc, and its exploration of female sexual self-actualisation. The film positions itself as a rhetorical interrogation of misogynistic and reductionist modes of constructing female sexuality, but it does so by ultimately rearticulating (or, at least, co-opting) another set of negative female constructs and stereotypes. The lone, vigilante *femme castratrice* with her fearsome toothed vagina is a figure that is not necessarily compatible with constructive and hard-won feminist battles about the nature of and responses to violence, both at community and individual levels. Thus, *Teeth* offers a conflicted and troublesome gynaehorrific moral: that, perhaps, only by embodying and deploying masculine fears of voracious female carnality can women best protect themselves and exert an active subjectivity that refuses to be co-opted or constrained. Clearly, this does nothing to challenge a framework wherein women are defined by their sexuality and their relationship towards men's heterosexuality, specifically insofar as women's sexuality relates to such heterosexual narratives of consumption, containment and desire.

Heteronormative horrors

In this chapter I have outlined the way that the mythic construction of the passive, docile virgin and the transgressive figure of the open, unbounded *vagina dentata* are expressed within the gynaehorrific modalities of horror film. These, in turn, inform and reflect broader social and cultural processes of meaning-making within a patriarchal culture that situate women's sexual, erotic and reproductive lives largely in the context of their relationships with and between men, and in service of the ongoing construction of male subjectivity. As a coda: what, then, of the lesbian in horror film? Harry M. Benshoff (1997) offers an illuminating account of the relationship between the horror genre, its monsters and queerness, in particular the way that the genre frames homosexual, queer or non-conforming desire as monstrous, by suggesting that "American culture has generally constructed its ideas about and fears of homosexuality within a framework of male homosexuality", but not really female homosexuality (p. 7). The lesbian monster, in comparison, is perhaps conspicuous by her absence, much as the figure of the lesbian has historically been absent or disregarded in other discourses. Killers and monsters in horror, especially the slasher subgenre, may certainly be associated with some sort of 'impaired' or transgressive masculinity (Clover 1992, 26–29), but there is little overt lesbian presence in the horror film.

   For those interested in diversity in horror, it is dispiritingly easy to formulate a representative roll call of lesbian (or faux-lesbian) figures within the genre. The erotic thriller *Basic Instinct* (1992) is widely touted as featuring a lesbian killer, but this ignores the fact that Catherine, the film's femme fatale, is bisexual and the majority of her on-screen sex scenes are with a male protagonist. Bisexuality, and more fluid forms of sexuality and female-centric sensuality, are also present in *Jennifer's Body*, the dark horror comedy *May* (2002) and the erotic vampire film *The Hunger* (1983); these forms of sexuality might certainly connect to the generative nature of the monstrous, in that they express forms of desire and pleasure that deny a phallocentric authority. Indeed, vampire films have opened up more space for lesbian desire and same-sex eroticism than other areas of the horror genre, such as in camp 1970s films like those in Hammer Studios' Karnstein Trilogy (*The Vampire Lovers* (1970), *Lust for a Vampire* (1971) and *Twins of Evil* (1972)), which reflects, perhaps, the centrality of female same-sex desire in one of the earliest pieces of vampire fiction – Sheridan le Fanu's 1872 novella *Carmilla*. Similarly, other films with a camp sensibility, such as Troma Films' *Chopper Chicks in Zombie-town* (1990) allow much more space for characters who challenge norms and boundaries, especially those predicated on taste and respectability. That said, in many of these instances I would argue that such queer erotic relationships are in large part present to satisfy an implicitly voyeuristic heterosexual male gaze, rather than to adequately express or embody lesbian identity or otherwise queer desire – British horror comedy *Lesbian Vampire Killers* (2009) is a sterling example of this, in its tongue-in-cheek presentation of its Sapphic killers as vampiric Girls Gone Wild – although of course the same cannot readily be said for the reception of such relationships, images and expressions of sex and desire.

More recently, characters who are gay 'on their own terms' have emerged, such as Sarah, the lesbian daughter of the titular character in *The Taking of Deborah Logan* (2014), whose sexuality isn't treated as a novelty or a plot point, nor as a means of objectification. Allusions, too are present: in the torture-centric *Hostel: Part II* it is often implied but never explicitly stated that Final Girl Beth is gay (Wester 2012, 397–398), although this suggestion is treated as something of a punchline. The core female relationship in *Grace* (2009) is strongly implied to have been if not sexual then at least deeply erotic and loving, offering a different mode of connection and affect than the rather bland heterosexual coupling that conceives the baby of the film's title. There is also a very small handful of by-lesbians-for-lesbians films; one such instance is the low budget slasher *Make A Wish* (2002), in which a woman brings together all her ex-girlfriends for a camping trip on her birthday, each of whom represent a clearly defined lesbian stereotype, and each are butchered one by one in what is ultimately revealed to be an elaborate revenge fantasy.

More often than not, though, lesbian characters, like their other non-heterosexual counterparts in horror (as well as further afield), are punished or killed, as in the pregnancy horror *Proxy* (2013), in which lesbian desire is framed as murderous and unhinged, and the revelation that a character is lesbian is marked as a violent plot twist. The protagonist of aforementioned body horror *Contracted* is similarly maligned: Samantha is a lesbian woman who contracts her horrific, body-altering sexually transmitted disease after she is raped by a man whilst intoxicated. Through the rape and the subsequent dissolution and decay of her body she is viscerally punished for her non-conforming sexuality and her past transgressions involving drugs and alcohol. Here, the monstrous disintegration of her body does not offer a new, generative mode of being, but instead signals that without use-value in an oppressive, patriarchal economy of exchange she is not even worth the sum of her parts. There is nothing to hold her together; she kills her former lover, she collapses in upon herself, and she finally becomes a member of the rotting, walking dead.

A rare and troublesome, yet instructive, example of lesbian desire in the horror film is in the French horror film *Haute Tension (High Tension)* (2003). The protagonist, Marie, travels to the countryside with her friend Alex to stay with Alex's family. However, in the night a hulking, filthy and brooding man in a boiler suit, identified in the credits only as *le tueur* (the killer), arrives at the country house and butchers Alex's family before capturing Alex and taking her away in his truck. Marie pursues them to try to rescue Alex and confront the villain – only it is revealed that Marie *is* the killer, and that the immensity of her unrequited lesbian desire for her heterosexual friend has triggered a psychotic break. This is initially expressed through shots in which Marie moves in and out of shadow, through the strategic use of mirrors and the presentation of security footage, and through the symbolic, uncanny cracks that form along the face of a child's doll. The tilt in the film's focus involves a woozy, unsettling looping back that exposes previously innocent events as fictions, for what we see from the perspective of the police exposes Marie's own perspective as unreliable; this is further emphasised through the use of a shifting colour palette that asks us to question not only what is happening, when, and to whom, but from whose point of view (Cameron 2012, 93). The film's climax recalls *The Texas Chain Saw Massacre*: where that film's antagonist, the oddly asexual Leatherface, chases after Sally with a phallic chainsaw, Marie pursues Alex while brandishing a circular saw, a canny choice that alludes to *vagina dentata* and the seeming circularity of her monstrous female desire.

Although Barry Keith Grant (2011) suggests that a reading of lesbian-as-monster in *Haute Tension* is facile, it is nonetheless both cynical and significant to point out that the revelation of Marie's murderous psychopathy is explicitly co-dependent on the revelation of her (closeted, covert) lesbian sexuality. This is to say that the film's narrative success is entirely predicated on the assumption that the audience will believe Marie to be heterosexual, and that the emotional connection between Marie and Alex will be read as nothing more than the platonic love that exists between close female friends. Intertextual elements assist in this deception: *le tueur* is played by actor Philippe Nahon who is best known for playing violent and unpleasant characters in French thrillers, in particular a nameless butcher in a series of films by Argentine provocateur Gaspar Noé. This casting choice explicitly codes Marie's lesbian desire as inherently masculine (or non-feminine), dirty and aggressive. This is exemplified in a presumably fictitious and metaphorical scene early in the film where we see *le tueur* fellating himself with a woman's decapitated head before throwing it out the window of his truck, a feint that seems to situate sexual degeneracy, predation and violence outside of Marie herself. Marie initially fulfils the criteria for the virginal Final Girl[23] – she is watchful, intelligent, androgynous and sexually aloof, and she seems to actively stalk and confront the killer – but these generic features are used to mask her psychopathic desire, to play upon the presumed heteronormative bias of the viewer, and to lay the foundations for the film's twist ending.[24]

These examples point clearly to what Adrienne Rich (1980) termed "compulsory heterosexuality": the bias through which lesbian experience is marked as deviant, abhorrent or simply invisible (p. 632), and through which heterosexuality is deemed innate, natural, a social and economic imperative (p. 634), and actively enforced through social and political means (p. 640). Rich asserts that "the institution of heterosexuality itself [is] a beachhead of male dominance" (p. 633), and it is significant that *Haute Tension* reinforces such dominance through the leveraging of an implicitly heterosexual subjective viewing position. The film's teasing exploration of the initially coincident relationship between the viewer's perspective and that of its apparent Final Girl comes undone at the end, when our point of view is (re-)aligned with that of (heterosexual) survivor Alex, who views the now captive Marie with revulsion and fear. Marie, the murderer, is physically contained although her monstrous, transgressive desire remains dangerous, for she seems to be able to sense Alex's presence even through one-way glass.

To draw from French radical lesbian theorist Monique Wittig (1992), *Haute Tension*, like other films discussed throughout this chapter, are predicated upon the 'heterosexual contract'. Like Jean-Jacques Rousseau's social contract, Wittig outlines that this heterosexual contract is an institution that silently underpins the construction of the body politic, claiming truth and shaping subjectivity (such as through the heterosexual, masculine bias of psychoanalysis) (p. 24). She argues that discourses of heterosexuality oppress heterosexual women, lesbians and homosexual men by "prevent[ing] us from speaking unless we speak in their terms" (p. 25), ensuring that any discussion of difference hinges upon the reification of Man as default, neutral and ideal, such that any other ontological category can only be different-to (pp. 29–30). For this reason Wittig argues that we must change our language and do away with or abstract the terms 'men' and 'women' in favour of other expressions and categories, for the heterosexist language we have only buttresses the status quo (p. 11). Heterosexuality, of course, is itself a social construct; after all, the term 'heterosexual' as a descriptor of sexual behaviour has only been in existence since 1868, when both 'heterosexual' and 'homosexual' were coined by Austro-Hungarian journalist Károly Mária Kertbeny in response to punitive laws that looked to ban sodomy; Kertbeny hoped that such terms might offer a way of describing identities predicated on differing sexual preferences with a degree of equality instead of privileging one sex act over the other (Blank 2012, 16; 33). It was not until the 1880s that the term heterosexual was co-opted by the legal and medical professions, which used the term to define the 'normal', procreative mode of sexuality against which the abnormal could be measured and pathologised.

To connect Rich and Wittig's discussion of the primacy of the heterosexual imperative to my broader discussion of gynaehorror, I suggest that this is also exemplified in the way that at a surface level female sexuality in the horror film is forcibly categorised into dual extremities, even though such a binary relationship belies the more provocative relationship that exists between the 'closed' and the 'open'. At one end, it is horrific and all-engulfing – the toothed vagina, or *vagina dentata* – and at the other it is contained and controlled in the form of the chaste, sacrificial virgin or the virgin hero. Even when playing with or against the gynaehorrific conventions of the genre, horror films have a tendency to actively perform and naturalise normative heterosexuality by framing the woman's body and sexuality as either *for* or *against* man in a looping, circular generic compulsion through which female subjectivity almost always acquiesces to the masculine. This is not to say that such films may not be read against the grain, so to speak, nor that there is no space within these, or any other texts, for different expressions of desire and pleasure, but instead that the dominant, preferred reading of such films is clear. I remain hopeful that embracing a more rhizomatic, generative view of monstrosity might allow for a better account of non-conforming bodies, pleasures and radical horrors that is not implicitly negative but might instead express different articulations of female or feminine desire – especially desire that is for (her)self, and that refutes a phallocentric economy of exchange, bodies or ideas.

Notes

1 When Randy escapes murder in *Scream*, he proclaims that he never thought he'd be so happy to be a virgin. However, he is killed in *Scream 2* (1997), and in *Scream 3* (2000) – through a taped video diary he'd left behind – he states sheepishly that should he have been killed, then having lost his virginity to a woman at a video store was probably not the best idea.

2 To reflect popular usage, throughout this chapter I predominantly use the word vagina to describe the female genitalia, even though the word vulva is the anatomically correct term for the outer genitalia. Sara Rodrigues (2012) suggests that using popular terminology also helps to "release the vagina from anatomical language and, by extension, from the space and gaze of the clinic" (p. 779) so as to incorporate both medical descriptions and cultural conceptions and perceptions of the entire female genitalia, which may serve to "promote a discursive politics that encourages women to employ the terms that best enable them to speak about their genitalia honestly and without shame" (p. 779).

3 This is not to imply that men are the only consumers of pornography; instead, it can be readily assumed that given these narrative descriptions on the site, and the emphasis upon inspecting a woman's genitals before, during and after penetrative penile-vaginal sex, that the site at least intends to portray a heterosexual male viewpoint. Whether or not the viewers of the website engage with or take pleasure in the material in this prescribed manner is another matter altogether.

4 It is important to note that Clover discusses a predominantly male audience, despite declaring her own fandom, a perspective that draws from the gendered nature of subjectivity and spectatorship offered in work such as that of Laura Mulvey's early discussions of pleasure and narrative (2000 [1975]). This specific alignment of gender and spectatorship can, perhaps, be extended in more abstract terms given the much broader distribution of gendered viewing.

5 The visual style of each film is heavily influenced by the work of illustrator Frank Frazetta, who produced covers for *Conan* books in the later 1960s. Frazetta's lush, richly detailed and hyperbolic artwork has had a profound influence on the style and iconography of contemporary fantasy, including its highly sexualised representation of female characters, whether warriors or victims.

6 Andrea Dworkin also offers an in-depth radical feminist reading of the virginities of Mina and Lucy in her book *Intercourse* (1997, 170–9).

7   The film's suggestive tagline is "There's something special about your first piece".
8   Despite this inauspicious beginning – which, had the genders been switched, would have perhaps read as explicitly rather than implicitly abusive (Gavey 2005, 201) – Jim and Michelle pursue a relationship in *American Pie 2* (2001) and then get married in the third film, *American Wedding* (2003), thus conforming to the trajectory of a normative heterosexual relationship. Nonetheless, the emphasis on male sexual 'prowess' and the imperative to lose one's virginity at any cost continue through the franchise's direct-to-video spin-off titles, of which there are four at time of writing. This conservatism is also present in other ways: the first film expresses a strong and quite progressive interest in the personal and sexual agency of its female characters – who, like the young men, represent a diverse range of viewpoints with regards to teenage sex and sexuality – but the latter films, especially the spin-offs, are increasingly predicated on illicit voyeurism, a hazy attitude towards consent, and the sexual objectification of the young women involved, which perhaps link them more clearly to the tradition of films such as *Porky's*.
9   The remarkably charming and good-natured Canadian horror comedy *Teen Lust* (2014) turns this trope on its head: 17-year-old Neil realises that his boring, embarrassing, Satan-worshipping parents have taken a close interest in his ongoing 'good behaviour' as they wish to use him as a virgin sacrifice on his 18th birthday, this invoking the devil and preventing a millennium of peace on earth. With the help of a friend Neil absconds and tries to lose his virginity while being pursued by his parents and their sect, but he discovers that having sex is a lot easier said, or fantasised about, than done.
10 *Decoys*, like *American Pie*, does not address the notion of rape. The female aliens have, effectively, killed their male victims by forcibly penetrating them, but each act is framed in a way that shifts responsibility from the aggressor to the victim. In each case the male victim is sexually active and forward, and the overwhelming feeling is that the men who are killed by the aliens were in part complicit in their deaths due to their sexual activity and their leering objectification of the aliens, perhaps in the same way that young women are often unfairly labelled as partially responsible for sexual assaults if they are, for instance, provocatively dressed or sexually active. Further, it is made clear that up until the point of impregnation the male victims were enjoying themselves, playing on the erroneous assumption that men 'can't' be raped. It is for this reason that Roger is not immediately killed: because of his sexual reticence, he is deemed to be 'different' to (and less aggressively masculine than) the other men, who are considered boorish and lustful, and therefore disposable. Nicola Gavey (2005), in a much broader discussion of how women's sexual coercion of men is culturally and socially framed, suggests that dominant understandings of the rape of men by women are framed by discursive constructions of male sex drive and sexuality that centralise sexual impulse. Alongside the cultural positioning of women as objects of desire and the reification of a binary that situates male as active and female as passive, this suggests that consent is presumed to be the default response to any form of (hetero)sexual engagement (pp.193–213).
11 A rare example of this can be found in the French horror film *Martyrs* (2008), in which a mysterious cult posits that the best way to try to understand what exists beyond life is through the creation of martyrs – literally, witnesses. These martyrs are young women who are subjected to extreme, long-term and systematic torture, and who might glimpse something through the mind-altering effects of transcendent pain. The cult leader, Mademoiselle, notes that for reasons unknown young women, including children, seem to be the best candidates.
12 F. K. Taylor (1979) offers a medical consideration of this myth, and suggests that some instances of these stories could be loosely connected to "penis captivus", a

situation where the penis is 'captured' by the vagina mid-coitus, and its relationship to vaginismus, a painful spasm or contraction of the vagina that can make penetrative intercourse difficult or impossible.

13 The Museum of Old and New Art (MONA) in Hobart, Australia, which currently houses Taylor's exhibition, also sells a series of fragrant, handcrafted 'cunt soaps' designed by the artist, each named for their model.

14 The Brooklyn Museum offers a comprehensive account of the installation, including searchable lists of all of the work's components, including the settings, the 999 tiles on Heritage Floor, the interpretive material on the Heritage Panels, the six large entry banners, and the acknowledgement panels, which depict the 129 people who worked on *The Dinner Party* (Brooklyn Museum: Components of the Dinner Party).

15 Anna North (2010), reporting on a screening of the documentary *After Porn Ends* (also known as *Exxxit: Life After Porn*, 2010), highlights a scene in which "ex-porn star Houston says she became so used to marketing her celebrity status that when she got a labiaplasty, it was a no-brainer to encase her labia 'trimmings' in lucite and sell them" – a move that continues to commodify the female body, even when its constituent parts are no longer attached.

16 The product's website describes it as "a simple to use Genital Cosmetic Colourant that restores the 'Pink' Back to a Woman's Genitals" [sic] (My New Pink Button).

17 A particularly illuminating appraisal of this comes from the Australian news and entertainment show *Hungry Beast*, which in a 2010 segment on labiaplasty suggested that the idealised 'single crease' vulva that was requested most frequently in cosmetic surgery clinics had become popular as the indirect result of the way that softcore pornographic magazines were regulated. In the segment, an anonymous graphic designer who works with pornography explains that the presentation of labia minora in unrestricted pornography, such as *Penthouse* magazine, is deemed unacceptable and vulgar by classification boards, and that his job is to alter the pictures of women's genitalia to fit these prescribed standards of "discrete genital detail" (Labiaplasty 2010).

18 The impact of such airbrushing and manipulation is evident in the 'self help'(!) website labiaenhancement.com, which proclaims that "It's every little girl's dream to have perfect vaginal [sic] and pretty vaginal lips. Women who are not blessed with pretty vaginas (genitals) feel inadequate and deformed in their most intimate body part…"

19 There are a number of initiatives that seek to counter this sense of shame and ugliness. Australian sexual health website The Labia Library offers information on vaginal health and offers a photo gallery that features a diverse range of female genitalia: "Whatever you call them, it's worth knowing that labia are all different" (Victoria Women's Health). Another, the Beautiful Cervix Project, "provides accessible information about women's fertility and menstrual cycles and showcases photographs documenting changes in the cervix and cervical fluid throughout the cycle" and has "Empowering Self-Exam Kits" that allow women to take photos of their own cervix and, if they feel like it, send them in to be featured on the website (Beautiful Cervix Project).

20 The description of the toothed vagina as a favourable evolutionary step is also alluded to in *Teeth*, which is discussed later in this chapter.

21 This happens much in the same way as Father Karras regains his faith in *The Exorcist* (1973), a film that *The Unholy* blatantly pays homage to or rips off, depending on how generous you are being.

22 As an example, in 2009 the (now defunct) abstinence resource website *The Facts Project* claimed that:

> based on typical condom use (and that includes using a condom EVERY time you have sex), a 15 year old teen has a greater than 50% chance of getting

pregnant (or getting a girl pregnant) by the time they are 20. These are the same odds as flipping a coin.

(Common Myths About Sex 2009)

Compare this to figures published in medical resource manual *Contraceptive Technology*, which publishes efficacy rates for all forms of contraception; the authors predict that a typical woman who uses a combination of reversible methods of contraception continuously from age 15 to age 45 would experience 1.8 contraceptive failures (Hatcher et al. 2007, 29).

23 David Greven offers a provocative, in-depth discussion of queerness and the Final Girl in his 2011 book *Representations of Femininity in American Genre Cinema*. In considering queer spectatorship and the viewer's subjective alignment with on-screen characters, he asks "are we the Final Girl, or the monster she destroys?" (p. 8).

24 The extensive online database of pop culture tropes and idioms TV Tropes describes the figure of the "psycho lesbian" in this tongue-in-cheek manner: "This trope can sometimes carry uncomfortable subtext: go straight or go crazy. Or *at least* have the decency of being bisexual so you can be of proper use for men" (Psycho Lesbian, emphasis original).

Bibliography

Alexander, B 2008, 'Born-again virgins claim to rewrite the past', *msnbc.com*, accessed November 7, 2013, from <http://www.nbcnews.com/id/23254178/ns/health-sexual_health/t/born-again-virgins-claim-rewrite-past/>.

Amnesty International 2005, *Women, violence and health*, accessed February 24, 2014, from <http://www.amnesty.org/en/library/asset/ACT77/001/2005/en/f6925f5e-d53a-11dd-8a23-d58a49c0d652/act770012005en.pdf>.

'Artificial virginity hymen (Joan of Arc red)' 2014, *Hong Kong Alito Trade Co., Ltd.*, accessed February 24, 2014, from <http://www.alitonghk.com/ProductShow.asp?ID=422>.

'Beautiful Cervix Project – Love Thy Cervix!' 2014, *Beautiful Cervix Project*, accessed February 24, 2014, from <http://www.beautifulcervix.com/>.

Beh, H G & Diamond, M 2006, 'The failure of abstinence-only education: minors have a right to honest talk about sex', *Columbia Journal of Gender and Law*, 15, pp. 12–62.

Beit-Hallahmi, B 1985, 'Dangers of the vagina', *British Journal of Medical Psychology*, 58(4), pp. 351–356.

Benshoff, H M 1997, *Monsters in the closet: homosexuality and the horror film*, Manchester: Manchester University Press.

Bernau, A 2008, *Virgins: a cultural history*, London: Granta.

Billington, A 2008, 'Sundance Interview with Teeth Director Mitchell Lichtenstein', *FirstShowing.net*, accessed February 24, 2014, from <http://www.firstshowing.net/2008/sundance-interview-with-teeth-director-mitchell-lichtenstein/>.

Blackledge, C 2003, *The story of V: opening Pandora's box*, London: Weidenfeld & Nicolson.

Blank, H 2007, *Virgin: the untouched history*, New York: Bloomsbury USA.

Blank, H 2012, *Straight: the surprisingly short history of heterosexuality*, Boston, MA: Beacon Press.

Braun, V 2005, 'In search of (better) sexual pleasure: female genital "cosmetic" surgery', *Sexualities*, 8(4), pp. 407–424.

Braun, V & Wilkinson, S 2001, 'Socio-cultural representations of the vagina', *Journal of Reproductive and Infant Psychology*, 19(1), pp. 17–32.

'Brooklyn Museum: components of the Dinner Party' 2016, *Brooklyn Museum*, accessed September 4, 2016, from <https://www.brooklynmuseum.org/eascfa/dinner_party/home/>.

Burns, A & Torre, M E 2004, 'Shifting desires: discourses of accountability in abstinence-only education in the United States', in A Harris (ed), *All about the girl: culture, power, and identity*, New York: Routledge, pp. 127–137.

Cameron, A 2012, 'Colour, embodiment and dread in *High Tension* and *A Tale of Two Sisters*', *Horror Studies*, 3(1), pp. 87–103.

Campbell, J 1993, *The hero with a thousand faces*, London: Fontana.

Caputi, J 2004, *Goddesses and monsters: women, myth, power, and popular culture*, Madison, WI: University of Wisconsin Press/Popular Press.

Carpenter, L M 2005, *Virginity lost: an intimate portrait of first sexual experiences*, New York: New York University, accessed February 24, 2014, from <http://site.ebrary.com/id/10137144>.

Carpenter, L M 2009, 'Virginity and virginity loss', in H T Reis & S Sprecher (eds), *Encyclopedia of human relationships*, Thousand Oaks, CA: SAGE Publications, pp. 1673–1675, accessed November 10, 2013, from <http://site.ebrary.com/id/10372803>.

Cixous, H 2010, *The portable Cixous*, M Segarra (ed), New York: Columbia University Press.

Clover, C J 1992, *Men, women and chain saws: gender in the modern horror film*, Princeton, NJ: Princeton University Press.

'Common myths about sex' 2009, *The Facts Project – Abstinence Until Marriage Education*, accessed from <http://web.archive.org/web/20091126063105/http://www.thefactsproject.org/myths.shtml>.

Craig, P & Fradley, M 2010, 'Youth, affective politics, and the contemporary American horror film', in S Hantke (ed), *American horror film: the genre at the turn of the millennium*, Jackson, MS: University Press of Mississippi, pp. 77–102.

Creed, B 1993, *The monstrous-feminine: film, feminism, psychoanalysis*, London and New York: Routledge.

'Defloration.tv' 2016, accessed August 29, 2016, from <http://www.defloration.tv/>.

Deleuze, G & Guattari, F 2004, *A thousand plateaus: capitalism and schizophrenia*, London: Continuum.

Deutscher, P 1994, '"The only diabolical thing about women...": Luce Irigaray on divinity', *Hypatia*, 9(4), pp. 88–111.

Dowling, M B 2001, 'Vestal virgins: chaste keepers of the flame', The BAS Library – Biblical Archaeology Society, accessed February 24, 2014, from <http://members.bib-arch.org/publication.asp?PubID=BSAO&Volume=4&Issue=1&ArticleID=14>.

Dworkin, A 1997, *Intercourse*, New York: Simon & Schuster.

Falconer, P 2010, 'Fresh meat? Dissecting the horror movie virgin', in T J McDonald (ed), *Virgin territory: representing sexual inexperience in film*, Detroit, MI: Wayne State University Press, pp. 123–137.

Farrimond, K 2013, 'The slut that wasn't: virginity, (post)feminism and representation in "Easy A"', in J Gwynne & N Müller (eds), *Postfeminism and contemporary Hollywood cinema*, New York: Palgrave Macmillan, pp. 44–59, accessed November 5, 2013, from <http://www.palgraveconnect.com/doifinder/10.1057/9781137306845>.

Fradley, M 2013, '"Hell is a teenage girl"?: postfeminism and contemporary teen horror', in J Gwynne & N Müller (eds), *Postfeminism and contemporary Hollywood cinema*, New York: Palgrave Macmillan, pp. 204–221, accessed November 5, 2013, from <http://www.palgraveconnect.com/doifinder/10.1057/9781137306845>.

Gavey, N 2005, *Just sex?: the cultural scaffolding of rape*, London and New York: Routledge.

Grant, B K 2011, '"When the woman looks": *High Tension* (2003) and the horrors of heteronormativity', in H Radner & R Stringer (eds), *Feminism at the movies: understanding gender in contemporary popular cinema*, Abingdon and New York: Routledge, pp. 283–295.

Greven, D 2011, *Representations of femininity in American genre cinema: the woman's film, film noir, and modern horror*, New York: Palgrave Macmillan.

Grosz, E 1994, *Volatile bodies: toward a corporeal feminism*, Bloomington, IN: Indiana University Press.

Gulzow, M & Mitchell, C 1980, '"Vagina dentata" and "incurable venereal disease": legends from the Viet Nam War', *Western Folklore*, 39(4), pp. 306–316.

Hatcher, R A, CatesJr., W, Trussell, J, Nelson, A, Kowal, D & Policar, M 2007, *Contraceptive technology*, 19th edn, New York: Ardent Media.

Holland, J, Ramazanoglu, C & Thomson, R 1996, 'In the same boat? The gendered (in)experience of first heterosex', in D Richardson (ed), *Theorising heterosexuality: telling it straight*, Buckingham, UK and Philadelphia, PA: Open University Press, pp. 141–160.

Howell, M & Keefe, M 2007, *The history of federal abstinence-only funding*, Advocates for Youth, accessed February 24, 2014, from <http://www.advocatesforyouth.org/publications/publications-a-z/429-the-history-of-federal-abstinence-only-funding>.

'Interview with Mitchell Lichtenstein, writer/director of "Teeth"' 2008, *The NYC Movie Guru*, accessed February 24, 2014, from <http://www.nycmovieguru.com/mitchelllichtenstein.html>.

Irigaray, L 1985a, *Speculum of the other woman*, Ithaca, NY: Cornell University Press.

Irigaray, L 1985b, *This sex which is not one*, Ithaca, NY: Cornell University Press.

Irigaray, L 1993a, *An ethics of sexual difference*, Ithaca, NY: Cornell University Press.

Irigaray, L 1993b, *Je, tu, nous: toward a culture of difference*, New York: Routledge.

Irigaray, L 1993c, *Sexes and genealogies*, New York: Columbia University Press.

'Joss Whedon talks The Cabin In The Woods' 2012, *Total Film: the modern guide to movies*, accessed November 17, 2013, from <http://www.totalfilm.com/news/joss-whedon-talks-the-cabin-in-the-woods>.

Kahukiwa, R & Grace, P 1984, *Wahine toa: women of Maori myth*, Auckland, New Zealand: Collins.

Keller, W 1999, *The cult of the born again virgin: how single women can reclaim their sexual power*, Deerfield Beach, FL: Health Communications, Inc.

Kelly, C R 2016, 'Chastity for democracy: surplus repression and the rhetoric of sex education', *Quarterly Journal of Speech*, 102(4), pp. 353–375.

Kizilos, K 2009, 'Private matters', *theage.com.au*, accessed February 24, 2014, from <http://www.theage.com.au/news/arts/private-matters/2008/02/26/1203788346904.html>.

Kramer, H 1980, 'Judy Chicago's "Dinner Party" comes to Brooklyn Museum: review', *New York Times*, pp. C1, C18.

Kristeva, J 1985, 'Stabat Mater', *Poetics Today*, 6 (1/2), pp. 133–152.

'Labia Enhancement' 2006, *Labia Enhancement*, accessed February 24, 2014, from <http://labiaenhancement.com/>.

'Labiaplasty' 2010, *Hungry Beast*, accessed November 18, 2013, from <http://vimeo.com/9924049>.

Lancaster, R N 2003, *The trouble with nature: sex in science and popular culture*, Berkeley, CA: University of California Press.

Le Fanu, J S & Tracy, R 2008, *In a glass darkly*, Oxford and New York: Oxford University Press.

Levin, G 2007, 'Art meets politics: How Judy Chicago's Dinner Party came to Brooklyn', *Dissent*, 54 (2), pp. 87–92.

MacLachlan, B 2007, 'Introduction', in B MacLachlan & J Fletcher (eds), *Virginity revisited: configurations of the unpossessed body*, Toronto: University of Toronto Press, pp. 3–12.

Mulvey, L 2000, 'Visual pleasure and narrative cinema', in E A Kaplan (ed), *Feminism and film*, Oxford readings in feminism, Oxford and New York: Oxford University Press, pp. 34–47.

'My New Pink Button' 2016, *My New Pink Button*, accessed February 24, 2014, from <https://web.archive.org/web/20160430015038/http://www.mynewpinkbutton.com/>.

Nankervis, D 2009, 'Genital posters "degrade women"', *The Advertiser*, accessed February 24, 2014, from <http://www.adelaidenow.com.au/news/fringe-display-uproar/story-e6freo8c-1111118996889>.

'New Greg Taylor exhibition: Cunts and other conversations' 2009, *Cunts the Movie*, accessed February 24, 2014, from <http://cuntsthemovie.com/2009/02/new-greg-taylor-exhibition-cunts-and-other-conversations/>.

North, A 2010, 'Exxxit: lust, labia trimmings, and the lasting stigma of porn', *Jezebel*, accessed February 24, 2014, from <http://jezebel.com/5561141/exxxit-lust-labia-trimmings-and-the-lasting-stigma-of-porn>.

Oliver, K 1993, *Reading Kristeva: unraveling the double-bind*, Bloomington, IN: Indiana University Press.

Parker, H N 2007, 'Why were the Vestals virgins? Or the chastity of women and the safety of the Roman state', in B MacLachlan & J Fletcher (eds), *Virginity revisited: configurations of the unpossessed body*, Toronto: University of Toronto Press, pp. 66–99.

Pliskin, K L 1995, '*Vagina dentata* revisited: gender and asymptomatic shedding of genital herpes', *Culture, Medicine and Psychiatry*, 19(4), pp. 479–501.

Potts, A 2002, *The science/fiction of sex: feminist deconstruction and the vocabularies of heterosex*, London and New York: Routledge.

'Pregnancy Support Center: take2 renewed virginity' 2009, *PSC Stark*, accessed November 7, 2013, from <https://web.archive.org/web/20090105161106/http://www.pscstark.com/42>.

Prime, L 2013, 'Genital surgery in NHS rises fivefold in a decade', *OnMedica*, accessed February 24, 2014, from <http://www.onmedica.com/newsarticle.aspx?id=070acb77-1fe4-4a9d-ae35-8670e79a9136>.

'Psycho lesbian – television tropes & idioms' 2014, *tvtropes.org – Television Tropes & Idioms*, accessed February 24, 2014, from <http://tvtropes.org/pmwiki/pmwiki.php/Main/PsychoLesbian>.

Rabin, R C 2016, 'More teenage girls seeking genital cosmetic surgery', *Well*, accessed September 4, 2016, from <http://well.blogs.nytimes.com/2016/04/25/increase-in-teenage-genital-surgery-prompts-guidelines-for-doctors/>.

Rees, E L E 2013, *The vagina: a literary and cultural history*, London and New York: Bloomsbury Academic.

Rich, A 1980, 'Compulsory heterosexuality and lesbian existence', *Signs*, 5 (4), pp. 631–660.

Richardson, D 1996, 'Heterosexuality and social theory', in D Richardson (ed), *Theorising heterosexuality: telling it straight*, Buckingham, UK and Philadelphia, PA: Open University Press, pp. 1–20.

Rockoff, A 2002, *Going to pieces: the rise and fall of the slasher film, 1978–1986*, Jefferson, NC: McFarland.

Rodrigues, S 2012, 'From vaginal exception to exceptional vagina: the biopolitics of female genital cosmetic surgery', *Sexualities*, 15(7), pp. 778–794.

SIECUS 2010, 'A history of federal abstinence-only-until-marriage funding', *SIECUS: Sexuality Information and Education Council of the United States*, accessed September 4, 2016, from <http://www.siecus.org/index.cfm?fuseaction=page.viewpage&pageid=1340&nodeid=1>.

Stark, J 2010, 'Psychiatric help required after vaginal surgery', *The Age*, accessed September 4, 2016, from <http://www.theage.com.au/victoria/psychiatric-help-required-after-vaginal-surgery-20101113-17rx0.html>.

Stoker, B 2009, *Dracula*, Camberwell, Vic.: Penguin.

Stringer, R 2011, 'From victim to vigilante: gender, violence, and revenge in *The Brave One* (2007) and *Hard Candy* (2005)', in H Radner & R Stringer (eds), *Feminism at the movies: understanding gender in contemporary popular cinema*, Abingdon, UK and New York: Routledge, pp. 267–282.

Stutesman, D 2005, *Snake*, London: Reaktion.

Taylor, F K 1979, 'Penis captivus – did it occur?', *British Medical Journal*, 2(6196), pp. 977–978.

'The O: Cunts… And Other Conversations' 2016, *The O*, accessed September 4, 2016, from <https://theo.artpro.net.au/exhibit/720/#exhibit>.

'Through the Flower – The Dinner Party' 2016, accessed September 4, 2016, from <http://www.throughtheflower.org/projects/the_dinner_party>.

Valenti, J 2009, *The purity myth: how America's obsession with virginity is hurting young women*, Berkeley, CA: Seal Press.

'Virgin' *OED Online*, accessed November 7, 2013, from <http://www.oed.com.ezproxy.canterbury.ac.nz/view/Entry/223735>.

Welsh, A 2010, 'On the perils of living dangerously in the slasher horror film: gender differences in the association between sexual activity and survival', *Sex Roles*, 62 (11–12), pp. 762–773.

Wester, M 2012, 'Torture porn and uneasy feminisms: re-thinking (wo)men in Eli Roth's Hostel films', *Quarterly Review of Film and Video*, 29(5), pp. 387–400.

Whisnant, R 2010, '"A woman's body is like a foreign country": thinking about national and bodily sovereignty', in R Whisnant & P DesAutels (eds), *Global feminist ethics*, Lanham: Rowman & Littlefield, pp. 155–176.

Williams, O 2013, '"Say NO to prostitutes": vintage collection of health adverts warning against the dangers of STDs', *Daily Mail Online*, accessed December 5, 2013, from <http://www.dailymail.co.uk/news/article-2345107/Vintage-collection-health-adverts-warning-dangers-STDs.html>.

Wittig, M 1992, *The straight mind and other essays*, Boston, MA: Beacon Press.

Wolf, N 2012, *Vagina: a new biography*, London: Virago.

Women's Health Victoria 2016, 'Labia Library', *The Labia Library*, accessed February 24, 2014, from <http://labialibrary.org.au/>.

2 The lady vanishes
Pregnancy, abortion and subjectivity

The horror genre deals in visceral, often brutal narratives that concern them-selves with the untidy nature of bodily boundaries and the integrity (or lack thereof) of the self. This is especially true of horror films about pregnancies and pregnant protagonists – films that feature demonic conceptions, super-natural gestations, bloody births, and myriad terrified women, who are coded as doubly vulnerable, placed in situations of extreme peril. Gynaehorror films about pregnancy offer a rich vein of material through which to consider the uncanny and the abject (Arnold 2013; Creed 1993; Oliver 2012), and patri-archal fears about the nature of women's ability to reproduce (Berenstein 1990) alongside sociocultural issues such as the intersection of gothic allegory and personal experiences of pregnancy (Fischer 1992) and the cultural idea-tion of pregnancy (Valerius 2005). They are also a fleshy, liminal, conceptual space that explores the nature of the physical, embodied and conceptual struggle between one's 'own self' (should there be such a stable thing) and a mutable body that shifts from one, to more-than-one, to one, although 'one' that is irrevocably changed. This struggle highlights a philosophical tension – a horror of its own: the dominant ontological framework of the self, which is predicated on autonomous implicitly masculine individuality that is presumed to be a fixed state of being, is incompatible with the subjective and lived state of pregnancy, which draws attention to mutability and modes of becoming.

Horror films about pregnancy, then, act as a site of inquiry and exploration, for they bring the question of subjectivity violently to the fore. Narratively, they frequently pit pregnant women not only against external antagonists, but also against their own changing, perhaps unruly bodies, vividly portraying the fluid nature of gestation itself and very often articulating a complicated, sometimes dichotomous relationship between the pregnant-self and the foetal-other. I suggest that this narrative struggle is coupled with a conceptual struggle. Mainstream narrative films must contend with the creation of a believable, knowable protagonist; we expect, perhaps implicitly, that characters are presented in and behave in certain ways, and that they exhibit a coherent sort of 'self-hood'. The fraught conceptual relationship between the pregnant woman and the foetus or unborn child places the women in such narrative films in a peculiar place. As characters, the women exhibit agency and subjectivity: they may drive the narrative forward, be our locus of perception or connection, or become the centre of the film's action, even if the foetus or unborn is framed as more 'important' than she is. At the same time, the aesthetic capacities of cinema offer competing expressions of female subjectivity that explore corporeal malleability in interesting, monstrous, and even productive ways – although, as I will demonstrate, within gynaehorror narratives this very often results in the dislocation or elimination of the woman 'herself' (that is, as a relatively stable or coherent category). This may be through the elision of the woman's image, agency or experience (if we are thinking of the 'character' of woman in a molar or traditional sense). It may also be through acts of framing, editing or audio-visual design that manipulate expressions of body and subject, or that fragment the female body within the *mise-en-scène* in a manner that is reductive or destructive. After all, Roman Polanski's landmark 1968 film is titled *Rosemary's Baby*, even though Rosemary herself is the protagonist.

In this chapter I consider the exploration of pregnancy, abortion and foetal subjectivity in horror film, be they in explicitly narrative or more abstract aesthetic modes, alongside philosophical encounters with pregnant subjectivity. There is a dual purpose to this: firstly, I chart the key concerns of and patterns within gynaehorror narratives about pregnancies and pregnant women to provide a robust account of this thematic sub-strain. Secondly, I explore how the horror genre responds to, expresses and problematises dominant constructions of the relationship between the pregnant woman and her foetus or unborn child through cinematic means. This means that I am less concerned with the implications or potential of the subjective camera, and look more to the interrelationship between narrative and character, the aesthetics of cinema, and 'monstrosity' as a mode of expression, representation and interpretation. Linda Williams' discussion of horror (alongside melodrama and the pornographic film) as a type of 'body genre' in her article "Film Bodies: Gender, Genre and Excess" (1991) is particularly instructive here. She categorises such films by the spectacle of corporeal excess through "the gross display of the human body" (p. 3). This body is often a "sexually saturated" female body (p. 6) that is "caught in the grip of intense sensation or emotion" (p. 4), such that its display in turn effects a pronounced physiological affective response in the viewer such as arousal, tears or horror. My interest here is what such a body genre might reveal about the limitations of our dominant understandings of the body (representationally, as well as how we might experience through the body), especially given that pregnant bodies can most certainly be considered both sensational and sexually saturated, and that the representation of pregnancy itself was historically hidden away, and deemed excessive, taboo or unsightly. The particularly abject and monstrous qualities of the horror genre also offer the possibility of troubling, or moving through, dominant notions of the autonomous, individual, indivisible subject, just as the aesthetic capacities of film offer a valuable way of thinking about how subjectivity might be expressed through sound, movement, imagery, and the manipulation of time and space, as well as dialogue and characterisation. Yet, the visual and narrative languages of the films discussed in this chapter also highlight how deeply entrenched some ideas about the nature of the self are by emphasising asymmetric and hostile relationships, rather than co-extensive corporeal relationships that might function as a dialectic or as blocks of becoming instead of a clean splitting in half (see Young 1990, 167).

A note, firstly, on terminology: throughout this discussion I use terms such as 'foetus', 'unborn child', 'embryo', 'pregnant woman' and 'mother' in very specific ways. This is not to straddle a political fence or to give a sense of political ambiguity, but to reflect the perceived attitudes (or preferred reading) of each film towards both the pregnancy itself and the ontological positioning of the woman throughout the pregnancy in question, be they explicitly or implicitly stated. Beyond issues of medicine and anatomy, politically, and particularly with regards to debates surrounding abortion, the term 'foetus' is favoured by those speaking from a so-called 'pro-choice' perspective – that is, one that favours access to abortion and emphasises a woman's right to bodily self-determination – as it clarifies the position that although the pregnant woman is a subject and a citizen with rights, her foetus is not. This choice of terminology is a political act of depersonalisation that refutes the idea that an embryo or foetus is a human being and a legal subject and that, therefore, abortion is not necessarily the death of a human being. The term 'unborn child' is favoured by those arguing from a so-called 'pro-life' position – that is, one that opposes abortion entirely – as it emphasises a sense of foetal subjectivity. It positions the unborn as inherently human and therefore subject to the same ethical considerations as a born human being, although in doing so it often elides or challenges whatever rights the pregnant woman may have, as well as failing to consider what may happen to the child after birth. The terms 'pro-life' and 'pro-choice' are themselves acts of political framing or agenda-setting (Chamberlain and Hardisty 2000), even though the terms 'pro-abortion rights' and 'anti-abortion rights' are perhaps a more accurate representation of the political positioning of the groups. However, they are the terms widely adopted for themselves by those engaged in debates surrounding termination, and it is not helpful to challenge them within the context of this discussion (see Shepard 2010).

Framing pregnant subjectivity

Philosophical accounts of subjectivity in/and pregnancy are instrumental in understanding how pregnant women are represented in horror films, for taken-for-granted understandings about the nature of the subject and the relationship between the person and their body are an intrinsic part of the visual grammar of cinema, let alone the structure of its narratives and the construction of its characters. Nick Mansfield's (2000) lucid survey of theories of subjectivity is a helpful lens through which to consider these issues. He establishes that 'the subject' can be thought of as a construct that posits the self as "not a separate and isolated entity, but one that operates at the intersection of general truths and shared principles" (p. 3), although what exactly those 'truths' *are* is highly problematic. Subjectivity is of integral importance to the feminist project (see, for instance, Gavey 2005, pp.92–4) although the notion of subjectivity is itself historically and culturally fraught. For example, ethnocentric and feminist interrogations of the autonomous subject have shown how western patriarchal culture and discourse restricts those people whose rights, thoughts, actions and subjectivities are privileged: "Women, as well as, for example, gays and lesbians and the working classes, are categorically excluded from such a definition of the subject; simply put, they do not matter" (Kilby and Lury 2000, 253). Beyond issues of gendered embodiment, such as the framing of pregnant subjectivity, such exclusions also have significant ramifications for the nature of representation and agency in narrative cinema.

Although he notes that in recent decades the notion of the completely self-contained subject has been contested and rejected (2000, 13), Mansfield identifies four broad types of subjectivity, or ways of separating ourselves into distinct selves, and I offer this as a helpful starting point from which to depart. The first is the "subject of grammar", the seemingly discrete "I", who at once seems to originate action but who is inherently tangled up within "a huge and volatile, even infinite, transhistorical network of meaning-making" (p. 3). The second is the politico-legal subject – an individual who is an actor within fixed "codes and powers" (p.4) such as the law and the State. This is a reciprocal obligation, wherein we agree to what Jean-Jacques Rousseau "first called a 'social contract' which asks certain responsibilities of us, and guarantees us certain freedoms in return" (p. 4). The third subject is the free and autonomous philosophical subject of the Enlightenment. This reasoning subject is in part "defined by the rational faculties it can use to order the world" (p. 15); that is, the thinking self, and one's active ability to perceive and be aware of the world (p. 18), sit at the centre of "truth, morality and meaning" (p. 4). Finally, Mansfield identifies the fourth subject as the subject as human person: the 'self' or personality who experiences and perceives (and exists *within*) the world.

Tellingly, the first three of these basic definitions of subjectivity are challenged, or at least made problematic, by pregnancy. These are definitions that are predicated on the notion that we *are* – that we are be-ings, and that although we may move through the world (and through time), our subjectivity remains a fixed coherent point of reference. Further, Western philosophical models of the self, although allegedly gender-neutral, are inherently androcentric: they treat a body that does *not* have the potential to become pregnant as the neutral body-self. Consider the term 'individual', which implies one that may not be divided, but the pregnant body starts as one, becomes more-than-one, then becomes one again.[1] This is a process of mutability and becoming that sits at odds to the indivisible, autonomous subject of the Enlightenment. Instead, the pregnant subject comes to be complicated and decentred in two key ways: through actual lived experience, which is perhaps shaped by the implicit terms of reference with which we conceptualise our bodies, and in the way that the medical profession frames pregnancy as a condition or a disorder that requires intervention, as opposed to a normal way of being in which the woman is an authority on her own body (Young 1990).

One particular feminist challenge to androcentric accounts of subjectivity is to seek to disrupt this sense of internal division between self and other, while critiquing the pathologisation and conceptual sequestering of pregnancy, and here I offer three accounts of the potential philosophical construction of the pregnant subject that each reflect some of the issues that bear in the cinematic expression of pregnancy and subjectivity. Iris Marion Young (1990), for instance, opens her argument in "Pregnant Embodiment: Subjectivity and Alienation" by taking umbrage with the way that subjectivity has been omitted from discourses on pregnancy, which has instead been discursively constructed as a medical condition. She praises the work of 20th-century existential phenomenologists such as Maurice Merleau-Ponty and Erwin Straus for the way that they have advocated for the lived body as a site of knowledge, perception and experience, which challenges the primacy of the 'thinking' self of Descartes' *cogito*. Nonetheless, she highlights that such thinkers continue to rely on dualistic language in the articulation of their anti-dualist claims: there is an inherent supposition that the *subject* (I) is a unified self as distinct from an *object* (not-I), and that this unified self is a condition of experience – even though the very notion of the experiencing-self challenges the suggestion that a division can even be drawn between subject and object (p. 162). Given that there is a tacit assumption in such conceptualisations that the (young, productive, healthy) male body is the neutral, default way of experiencing the world, Young rightly asserts that women's experiences have been absent from cultural discourse surrounding human experience, let alone the narratives of history (p. 161), just as the maternal body and its shifts have traditionally been absent from spaces of philosophy (Tyler 2000, 290–1).

Both Young and feminist philosopher Imogen Tyler (2000) offer interesting challenges to this historic essentialism through their exploration of the embodied experiences of their own pregnancies – their own reproductive becomings. Young highlights the changing shape and sensation of her body, and then how her first awareness of foetal movement – the 'quickening'[2] – produces a sense of split subjectivity (p. 163). For Young, pregnancy is a specific, unique type of temporality in which the subject can "experience herself as split between past and future" (p. 160). The intimate, interior relationship between pregnant woman and foetus is "not unlike that which I have to my dreams and thoughts" (p. 163), but is undermined by the medicalisation of pregnancy, which privileges instrumentation, medical imaging and physical intervention over the knowledge imparted by a woman's own senses. This interventionism takes as natural the idea that there must be mediation between the woman (as self and subject) and her 'disobedient', fecund body, presenting scientific 'rationality' as a way of containing, controlling and rationalising the body.

Similarly, Tyler asks whether philosophical bodies can account for, explain, contain or even comprehend a body or a subject that *literally* reproduces others (p. 289), outside of the figurative (re)production of the male subject at the expense of the female subject that is highlighted in the work of post-structural feminists such as Luce Irigaray (1985a; Irigaray 1985b), Hélène Cixous (2010 [1975]) and Julia Kristeva (1982; Kristeva 1985). To address this she considers her own experience as a heavily pregnant subject, attending an academic seminar, utterly fed up with the indifference of many of her philosopher colleagues towards the importance of sexual difference, stating her desire to go to the front of the room and present her heavily pregnant body *itself* as a question to the visiting philosopher (p. 290). Estranged and frustrated by the disjunction between her academic practice, her lived experience and her mutable pregnant subjectivity, she concludes that philosophically she is a "freak" (p .290). This is delivered with a strong sense of irony for, as she later points out, pregnancy is among the most common, conventional and controlled modes of embodiment that most women can and do encounter (p. 291). Thus, pregnancy exposes an enormous problem at the heart of philosophical models of self and subjectivity (p. 293), for through its shifting, transitional nature and its disruption of fixed frames of reference, pregnant embodiment is ontologically challenging and uncertain (p. 292).

The problems with the formulation of split subjectivity are likewise confronted by feminist phenomenologist Christine Battersby (1998), whose work takes issue with the fact that Western philosophers have largely ignored the ontological significance that we are all born selves (p. 3) and instead have considered birth as "something that simply happened before man 'is'" (p. 18) – even though all 'individuals' have at some stage been in a state of foetal or childhood dependency. Battersby argues that to adequately account for sexual difference, we must do five things: we must recognise "the *conceptual* link between the paradigm 'woman' and the body that births" (p. 7, emphasis original) as an abstract component of embodiment; address the "ontological dependence of the foetus on the mother" (p. 8); acknowledge that philosophically and practically "for the (normalized) 'female' there is no sharp division between 'self' and 'other'" (p. 8); accept that "in our culture, at least, female [cf. feminine] identities are fleshy identities" (p. 9); and consider that the "'experience' of the female human in our culture has direct links with the anomalous, the monstrous, the inconsistent and the paradoxical" (p. 11), in such a way that allows for a re-contextualisation, or an opening up, of embodied identity.

Instead of treating women as a deviation from the (presumably male, individuated) norm, Battersby requires that, in our acknowledgement that we are all born subjects, we position the female body as the starting point for a new fleshy metaphysics. To be flippant, this literally requires some navel-gazing. This would mean that the act of birth is no longer framed (philosophically) as an abnormal state (p. 2) underpinned by the assumption that "the sense of discontinuity and alienation experienced by the male in reproduction is attributed to both genders" (Blaetz 1992, 17). As such, Battersby's project considers the ramifications of what might happen if the potential for pregnancy as "as central to the notion of personhood and self" (Battersby 1998, 17) so as to conceptualise identity in a way that is founded on a "metaphysics of fluidity and mobile relationships" (p. 7) – an identity that privileges becoming over static being, and that acknowledges that all born subjects have, at one stage, been more-than-one. Battersby suggests, somewhat contentiously, that if there is a 'sameness' to women, it originates from a shared metaphysical position: that "Whether or not a woman is lesbian, infertile, post-menopausal or childless, in modern western cultures she will be assigned a subject position that has *perceived* potentialities for birth" (p. 16, my emphasis), and that this "female predicament" (p. 22) must no longer go unconsidered, given its implication for both classical and postmodern understandings of subjectivity and personhood.[3] Thus, in Battersby's framework, the female body and the resultant malleability of embodied experience and subject position become the norm, and not the deviation.

However, these accounts are not without their problems. For example, Young's exploration of pregnant embodiment both challenges yet inadvertently demonstrates the limitations of how we consider female embodied experience. Despite her call for an embodied understanding of pregnant subjectivity, Young nonetheless recycles the dualist language that she critiques: she considers the dissonance between what she terms her "aesthetic interest" in and awareness of her pregnant body *vis-à-vis* her philosophical and personal "aims and projects" (Young 1990, 165), a schism that distances her (as a philosopher) from her embodied experience (as a woman). Her description of a 'split' subjectivity creates an implicit disjuncture between her embodied subject-self and her thinking subject-self, for each mode of 'knowing' and experiencing is framed as separate, instead of as different modalities or registers. This split perhaps recycles the Cartesian dualism that she wishes to confront by associating the body with femininity, corporeality and aesthetic, and the mind and intellect with distanced, masculine rationality. Tyler identifies in this a set of contradictions that, perhaps, impede feminist philosophies and that mean that the deeply embedded historic metaphysical structures that have for so long denigrated or ignored female embodied experience remain fundamentally unchallenged (Tyler 2000, 297). She argues that this is, in large part, because these philosophers are faced with the problems with language, grammar and the articulation of categorisation encountered by any theorists who might wish to consider non-singular models of self as a way of thinking through female subjectivity (p. 297) This includes the problematic designation of woman as construct – as evidenced by Battersby's frequent use of quotation marks around the terms woman and female – and the implied position of the philosopher as one who may operate as an external, neutral, implicitly non-gendered observer (p. 297), for this allegedly neutral position nonetheless continues to position woman as 'other'. As such, Tyler advocates for philosophical engagement with pregnancy to come from the embodied perspective of the one who is being theorised – hence her inclusion of autobiographical detail and experience in the content of her article.

These philosophical projects are fundamentally connected to Luce Irigaray's arguments in *Speculum of the Other Woman* (1985a) and *This Sex Which Is Not One* (1985b), which assert that woman is denied subjectivity by having her status (and use value) constructed as both Other to and in relation to man, rather than existing as her own whole subject, in large part because of the andro-, phallocentrism within masculinist modes of language; I outline these points in more detail in the previous chapter. Irigaray emphasises throughout her work that a disavowal of maternal origin, and a loss of matrilineal connection, is a key contention in the way that female subjectivity is denied. This is similarly echoed in Battersby's insistence that we must not disavow the ontological implications of birth, and that we consider people as born subjects: people who have necessarily been a part of another body. Combined, what these feminist philosophical interventions demonstrate is that current dominant models of subjectivity wholly fail to account for the pregnant subject, nor any other subject that can be, variously, one and one-and-another, whilst remaining coherent. My word 'another', here, too, highlights another problem: how difficult it is to find language that does not shore up the already robust, masculine and individualist construction of the allegedly indivisible self, given that pregnant subjectivity defies the categorisation of the notion of 'subject' as it has been traditionally and conservatively applied (Tyler 2000, 298).

Given these linguistic constraints, I ask whether it is possible for cinematic image, visual metaphor and narrative to better engage with this problem with subjectivity. Consider Tyler's description of her body in its final month of pregnancy:

> And my skin, my skin is ripping apart, veins and stretch marks tattoo me as membranes give way, a dark line runs from navel to crotch where walls of muscle slowly separate. Leaky vessel, I might split apart any moment, pour myself onto the floor in bits. (Tyler 2000, 290)

Similarly, Young describes her sense of physical transition thus:

> As the months and weeks progress, increasingly I feel my insides, strained and pressed, and increasingly feel the movement of a body inside me. Through pain and blood and water this inside thing emerges between my legs, for a short while both inside and outside me ... [T]he boundaries of my body are themselves in flux. (1990, 163)

Compare these accounts to Anna Powell's description of a key scene in British writer-director Clive Barker's 1987 film *Hellraiser*, in which a fragmented body begins to re-form and is re-born:

Frank's disembodied organs are determined to be reunited. [...] The sound of a beating heart begins and we see organs without a body begin to self-generate. In a strongly visceral image, the blood magically gathers below the [floor]boards to form a red lung or heart-like sac, which starts to palpitate... [T]wo tentacle-like arms thrust themselves through a *mélange* of milky gore. The arms are followed by the semblance of a head, with glittering brain folds rapidly forming. (Powell 2005, 85)

It is notable that Powell's analysis is offered in a much broader exploration of the ways that the aesthetics of horror might be leveraged through a Deleuzean (or DeleuzeGuattarian) encounter with horror cinema. I draw this example from her discussion of the way Gilles Deleuze and Félix Guattari (2004) appropriate theatre-philosopher Antonin Artaud's term the body-without-organs (BwO). For Artaud, the BwO is a dis-organised body that resists the colonising, controlling, 'organising' function of a repressive God and His theological systems. Deleuze and Guattari conceptualise the BwO as a 'body' without any organising principles: a "connection of desires, conjunction of flows, continuum of intensities" (p. 179) that is mutable, fluid, complex and open to multiple becomings (Powell 2005, 79), not a hierarchical one in which such flows are corralled, contained or directed. This body is an asymptotic ideal. Importantly for this discussion, such a body refutes the notion of individual identity and subjective unity through an emphasis upon movement, and perhaps offers a more provocative way of thinking through the processes and flows of pregnant subjectivity and its cinematic expression.

It is also easy to see how clearly Tyler and Young's descriptive engagements with – and, perhaps, parsing of – pregnancy and birth mirror the language and metaphor of body horror, so before continuing I look briefly to two other contributions to the construction of monstrous reproductive bodies that offer quite different attitudes towards the 'horror' of the body. The relationship between the maternal and horror is made obvious in Julia Kristeva's psychoanalytic work *Powers of Horror* (1982); this in turn informs Barbara Creed's (1993) construction of the monstrous-feminine, which I discuss in the introduction to this book. In the first section of her book, Kristeva considers the function of the abject – the category that is neither subject nor object, but the "jettisoned object" (p. 2) and the site at which such meaning and order collapses. Looking towards anthropologist Mary Douglas's account of the pure and clean and the improper or unclean, she signals particularly common sites of the abject: food loathing, the corpse, shit, pus, urine, blood, excretions and wounds, all of which are in-between, ambiguous spaces or materials that trouble the conceptualisation of the ordered, fixed, proper body (pp. 2–4; p. 53) and become associated with shame. Later, Kristeva highlights the importance of the impurity of and the taboo surrounding the maternal and birthing body in the Old Testament book of Leviticus, for instance, in its connection to the impurity of the decaying body (p. 91, pp. 99–102). She suggests that birth becomes a "violent act of expulsion through which the nascent body tears itself away from the matter of the maternal insides" (p.101), and that one's 'own self' must then eliminate the traces of this maternal matter (that is, to break away from the 'mother'), and assuage its "debt to nature" (p. 102) to be clean and proper. Therefore, it is not simply that such in-between spaces, be they literal or conceptual, are foul or gross. Instead, the abject attacks the notion of the whole subject, drawing one into the incomprehensible space that exists before the construction of the contained "I", that in part gestures to the relationship between the 'one' and the maternal body from which it originates. This boundary confusion is certainly reflected in Tyler and Young's accounts, especially in the struggle to speak to a subjectivity that does not rely on a division between self and other while accounting for a body that behaves, quite apparently, in a manner that rejects 'order' and 'the proper'.

Expressions of monstrous reproductive bodies also recur frequently in Mikhail Bakhtin's analysis of the Renaissance carnival, the function of humour, and the cultural importance of the grotesque body in the literature of François Rabelais in *Rabelais and his World* (1984) although to quite different ends. He explains that "One of the fundamental tendencies of the grotesque image of the body is to show two bodies in one: the one giving birth and dying, the other conceived, generated, and born [... such as] the pregnant and begetting body" (p. 26). Here, life is inextricably intertwined with death, but this is not inherently negative, and instead forms a part of a celebratory process of renewal (pp. 323–4). The grotesque body is not an individual body but a double one, and the "events of the grotesque sphere are always developed on the boundary dividing one body from the other" (p. 322): "In the endless chain of bodily life it retains the parts in which one link joins the other, in which the life of one body is born from the death of the preceding, older one" (p. 318). The birthing body, then, comes to be linked to other ambivalent forms of bodily excess, transgression and renewal, in particular defecation and other images of the "lower stratum" (p. 175; see also p. 151 and p. 163). Shit, piss, vomit, semen and other excretions, as well as curses that draw from bodily images, are not a shameful reminder of one's maternal origin, but evidence that one is alive and a part of the renewal of culture and of the human race – and often funny, joyous ones to boot. As Bakhtin suggests, in the medieval and Renaissance grotesque, "All that was frightening in ordinary life is turned into amusing or ludicrous monstrosities" (p. 47). I must admit that the joyous nature of the body in this account appeals a little more as a site of engagement and resistance than the psychoanalytic one.

I connect these philosophical appraisals of pregnant subjectivity to these three diverse accounts of un- or less-bounded bodies (be they mutable and generative in their becomings, frighteningly abject, or joyfully grotesque) not to cast Tyler's and Young's experiences as inherently negative, although the language the latter uses does imply a degree of ambiguity. Instead, as I move into more explicit discussions of individual films and cinematic expressions, I wish to flag, again, a resistance to the cultural impulse to read the monstrous as intrinsically adverse, but to see it as a site of multiple, sometimes discordant meanings, and sometimes as a site of productive expansion – of becoming, not collapse. Horrific narratives, even when conservative, provide ample space for productive becomings rather than restrictive modes of beings, even if the end point is one of destruction. Therefore, from here, I ask whether or not (gynae)horror, which shares so many visceral and aesthetic attributes with pregnancy and which is deeply invested in fears and anxieties about the nature of corporeality, may offer a space in which dominant modes of (female, pregnant) subjectivity and embodiment may be critiqued, challenged and expanded upon.

Keeping house: female corporeality in horror

The nature of female subjectivity in the horror genre is mutable and always-already contestable. Horror offers a space of slippage in which the subject might move through new, open re-combinations, or experience its own destruction and dissolution. The articulation of pregnant subjectivity in cinema must be considered with regards to the ways that women's bodies, subjectivities and corporealities are expressed – and sometimes displaced – through the narrative and visual languages of film. Such representations, like other forms of popular culture, inform and reflect popular understandings about the way we might consider selves, subjectivities and corporeal relationships. Pregnancy may be conflated with motherhood in terms of narrative (Arnold 2013, 154–5), but this does not mean that a reading or analysis of a film must in turn shore up this conflation. Instead, throughout this discussion I suggest that the articulation of pregnancy (as its *own* corporeal state) in these films can be explored in terms of how the subjectivity of the mother is both constructed and displaced through three key tropes: the association of female bodies with houses or domestic spaces, the designation of the woman as vessel within the religious horror, and the presentation of the woman as both literal and metaphorical environment within eco-horror. In each expression the woman-as-subject and the foetus-as-subject do not happily co-exist or conjoin; instead, they struggle for dominance. Further, the woman's subject-position tends to become subordinate to that of the foetus – or creature – she is carrying. This negation, or abstraction, is not simply an acquiescence to the child-within that positions the woman in a specifically sexed role within a patriarchal framework (Arnold 2013, 155). It is a site of profound conflict where the borders and capacities of the body are actively contested, erased and sometimes redrawn. This struggle is a specific and visceral reminder that the way we consider the relationship between 'self' and 'other' is inadequate, but also that such uncertainty can itself be horrific.

It is instructive to first consider the relationship between the pregnant female body and corporeal and domestic interiority in two key horror films, given that this trope is both significant to horror, by way of its gothic roots, and also offers a mode of storytelling within which the space(s) of the film image are important. The first film, Roman Polanski's 1968 film *Rosemary's Baby*, is perhaps the best known and undoubtedly the most discussed gynae-horror (Arnold 2013, 178–9; Berenstein 1990; Fischer 1992; Jones 2002, 185–6; Oliver 2012, 117–26; Valerius 2005), and the film against which other such horror films are judged. Like *Rosemary's Baby*, Donald Cammell's 1977 techno-horror *Demon Seed* features rape, pregnancy and physical containment, and in each there is a distinct visual, spatial and narrative relationship between the female protagonist's body and her house. After all, it is telling that, in *The Haunting* (1963), paranormal researcher Dr John Markaway asserts that evil, haunted old houses are like an "undiscovered country", ripe for exploration, much as Sigmund Freud suggested that "the sexual life of adult women is a 'dark continent'" (Freud 2008, 32).

Rosemary's Baby begins with a house: Rosemary and her husband Guy, an actor, purchase and move into a beautiful apartment in the Bramford, a stately apartment building in New York City. Their eccentric, elderly neighbours, the Castevets, take an overwhelmingly invasive interest in Rosemary's potential for child-bearing. They are covert Satan worshippers, and come to an arrangement with fame-hungry Guy: Rosemary will bear the Antichrist and in return his acting career will flourish. Rosemary is drugged, tied down, brought into the Castevets' apartment through a secret door, and then raped by Satan. She falls pregnant, but is under the impression that the baby is Guy's for he tells her that he had sex with her as she was unconscious. Rosemary's concerns about her pregnancy and the increasingly violent and uncanny events unfolding around her are dismissed by her husband and the Castevets, and she is effectively trapped inside the apartment – denied her freedom, driven away from her friends and her choice of doctor, and treated as if she were a child. When she gives birth she is told the baby has died, but she finds her way into the Castevets' apartment though the secret door, and there the baby is being celebrated by the congregated Satanists. Rosemary is asked to take on her assigned role and act as its mother, and despite her horror at the baby's demonic eyes, she appears to comply.

Like *Rosemary's Baby, Demon Seed* involves domestic entrapment, sexual coercion and forced pregnancy. Dr Susan Harris, a child psychologist, lives in large house in which everything is computer-controlled by a voice activated 'Enviromod'. Her estranged husband, pompous computer scientist Dr Alex Harris, has developed an immensely powerful artificial intelligence called Proteus IV, which is in part his way of compensating for the loss of their 9-year-old daughter to leukaemia, for Alex hopes that Proteus will be able to find cures for such illnesses. However, Proteus is not so domesticated. The AI infiltrates the Harris house through an unused computer terminal in the basement and takes over the house's electronic and mechanical functions, trapping Susan inside. Proteus, who is coded as masculine, subjects Susan to invasive physiological tests, then bullies, berates and violently threatens her into complying with 'his' plan: he wants her to bear a child into which he can implant his immense knowledge, so that he may be let out of his 'box' – a crude gesture towards (re-)birth if ever there was one. Susan realises that she must acquiesce or he will take her through force, so she submits and Proteus impregnates her with synthetic sperm. The gestation is rapid, and after 28 days Proteus removes the baby and places it in an incubator. Alex, distracted by his work and blinded by his hubris, finally realises that something is amiss and returns to the house. Proteus self-destructs, knowing that his creators are planning to shut him down, and Susan tries to destroy the incubator that is holding the child, but Alex physically restrains her. The child – a clone of the Harris's dead daughter – survives, wakes, and speaks with Proteus's voice as Alex cradles it and Susan looks on with ambivalence.

The women's houses and their interior spaces form an integral part of each film, and although neither the Bramford building nor the Harris house are haunted *per se*, both draw from the history of monstrous houses in horror. The haunted or cursed house is a prominent setting in gothic literature, and such houses are likewise prolific in the horror film. Such places include the imposing Bates' mansion in *Psycho* (1960), the unsellable Myers house in *Halloween* (1978), and the decaying farmhouse of *The Texas Chain Saw Massacre* (1974). This "Bad Place" (King 1982, 299) or "Terrible House" (Wood 2003, 8) both reaches back to the decrepit, dissolute mansions of the gothic tradition and serves to reinforce the idea that the space of the contemporary house is always-already fraught, and its boundaries, like those of the body, far from fixed. The house may be monstrous or contain, or hide, monsters in plain sight, as in *The Texas Chain Saw Massacre, Psycho* or *The People Under the Stairs* (1991). It may sit the 'traditional' family unit as both the victims and the causes of supernatural trauma, as in *Poltergeist* (1982), *The Conjuring* (2013), *Insidious* (2010) or *The Amityville Horror* (1979). This is doubly so, given its precarious situation within a system of capitalist ebbs and flows that serve to undermine the economic safety and autonomy of the nuclear family (Grant 1996, 6; Williams 1996), which reframes the house not as a site of safety but of extreme social, economic and spiritual vulnerability.

The bad house may also act as an extension of the minds, fears or personalities of those who live within it (Nakahara 2009; Wood 2003, 81–2) – a powerful association, given the association between women, domesticity and interior space (Durán 1991; Gold 1998; Gordon 1996). In *Repulsion* (1965), the dissolution and decay of neurotic and sex-averse manicurist Carol's apartment mirrors her descent into psychosis. The film *Burnt Offerings* (1976) features a mansion that is able to restore itself to its former glory by killing and consuming its inhabitants, in what amounts to a type of maternal cannibalism. One of the house's summer caretakers, Marian, slowly takes on the persona of – or, is possessed by – 'Mrs Allardyce', the embodiment of the house's wicked maternal persona. The supernatural occurrences in the mansion Hill House in *The Haunting* are linked to the sensitivities and emotional instability of a guilt-ridden young woman, Nell, who is mourning the death of her overbearing invalid mother. The 'murder house' at the centre of the first season of American cable television show *American Horror Story* (2011–)

becomes the site of generations' worth of pregnancy- and birth-related deaths and horrors. It is stated that somehow the house *itself* desires a baby, much as the reproductive body of its new owner, Vivian Harmon, is described as a house ("Pilot"). In each instance, the house is a site of trauma, or the space within which terrible secrets are kept, be they personal, historic, economic or cultural. These dark truths play out in the relationship between the film's narrative and the *mise-en-scène* (Curtis 2008, 11), which manipulates seemingly safe, contained territories into uncertain spaces of terror.

However, there are broader relationships between houses and women to be drawn within Western discourses about sex and spatiality, given that female sexual embodiment itself comes to be articulated in western culture through "tropes of interiority, containment and domesticity" (Potts 2002, 152). The association of women's bodies with houses, and the linguistic and conceptual connections between female interiority and domestic space, is aligned with the spatial, cultural and linguistic restrictions placed upon women within a patriarchal culture that privileges of masculine modes of speech and language (Potts 2002, 161). This discursive construction of and conflation of women's bodies and houses also implies a sense of spatial constriction (Potts 2002, 161), and although this might offer a sense of corporeal self-ownership, it also in turn encourages women to interiorise their subjectivity, which perhaps serves to constrict women's movements and understandings of female embodiment (Potts 2002, 162). It is not just that houses are bounded space: houses are things that can be owned and invaded, so where women – some women, at least – might assert their bodily autonomy, it is only so long as the terms of this ownership still sit within masculinist modes of representation and acquisitiveness (Potts 2002, 169).[4]

The importance of such domestic metaphors can be further understood through the work of French-Belgian feminist philosopher and cultural theorist Luce Irigaray, whose project explores the spatiality, corporeality and interiority of the female body in a manner that challenges the phallocentrism of mainstream (that is, Freudian and Lacanian) psychoanalysis. In particular, Irigaray considers how woman is excluded from a place in language and within the hegemonic patriarchal order because she provides a space for man, instead of existing in a space for herself. In *An Ethics of Sexual Difference* (1993a) she writes that woman is *place* (p. 35); that is, "traditionally, and as a mother, woman represents *place* for a man", such that "the maternal-feminine also serves as an *envelope*, a *container*, the starting point from which man limits his things" (p. 10).[5] As such, Irigaray plays with the language of the patriarchal construction of the woman's body and sexual difference *as* space and abstraction. She seeks to create a place outside of this discursive and representational framework so that woman exists as something other than the mirror for man, man's Other, or Freud's 'dark continent'.

Irigaray rejects the role of the woman's body as partial, castrated object that needs either a baby or a penis to complete it (Gatens 1996, 41). Instead, her analogies and explorations of interiority work towards charting a (philosophical, conceptual) space for women that is not a part of the patriarchal binaristic constructions of women, female bodies and femininity – a space that is more than "A living, moving border. Changed through contact with [man's] body" (Irigaray 1992, 51), existing only because of man's "need to relate to things" (Irigaray 1992, 62). To achieve this, Irigaray playfully appropriates and mimics the language of patriarchy, in particular, its quashing and exclusion of the feminine.[6] In the poetic work *Elemental Passions* (1992), she considers the implications of a discursive relationship in which woman is the thing against which man defines himself: "I was your house. And, when you leave, abandoning this dwelling place, I do not know what to do with these walls of mine" (p. 49). She attempts to destabilise discursive practices such as the negative framing of Plato's cave (that is, the place from which the journey of wisdom begins) as a womb-space. As Rachel Jones (2013) suggests, the "topology of the cave points us to the foundational appropriation, displacement and devaluation of the maternal that secures the ground of western metaphysics" (p. 49), such that woman's womb, her interiority, represents a state of ignorance that sits at the beginning of man's (emotional, spiritual, intellectual) emergence (p. 48). The connection between Plato's cave as a nascent site of pre-knowledge, alongside its association with the nature of storytelling in film, offers a rich conceptual link to an exploration of the connections between female subjectivity, interiority, corporeality and spatiality in horror film.

Home invasions

Reading the metaphorical use of houses as proxies for women's minds and bodies in horror films is troubling when considering the discursive positioning of the woman's corporeal body – her 'house' – as a space and place for man. However, such spatial analogies are particularly sinister in *Rosemary's Baby* and *Demon Seed,* which deal with rape, coercion and forced pregnancies. It is the women's bodies, more than the physical houses, which are invaded. Even in *Demon Seed*, Proteus's use of the house's computer is an extension of capability through the unmanned terminal in the basement, as opposed to a violent act of insertion. These films also speak to the broader issues of bodily sovereignty and the construction and policing of physical and mental borders that are so prominent in horror film. For example, consider the way that the discursive positioning and construction of national sovereignty is connected to the issue of bodily sovereignty, given the similarities in the language used about invasion and warfare and the language used to frame the treatment of women's bodies in rape and pornography whereby women's bodies are 'invaded' much as troops 'penetrate' foreign lands with phallic technologies of war (Whisnant 2010, 155). However, where national borders may be crossed or negotiated, the boundaries of the female body are often obliterated (Whisnant 2010, 160) – a departure from Irigaray's critique of woman as a 'necessary' Other or negative mirror for man, and an act that effectively 'colonises' or re-territorialises a woman's interiority. Referencing both mainstream displays of the female body and more hard core, invasive forms of pornography, radical feminist cultural theorist Rebecca Whisnant (2010) argues that both conceptually and practically women have no boundaries or privacy – that no part of women's bodies is safe from being inspected, evaluated, used or abused (p. 160). Given that the whole, fixed subject is perhaps defined by its borders, and the implicit division between subject and object or I and not-I, this imperils the notion of a coherent female subjectivity. As such, this obliteration of boundaries also speaks to the dehumanisation and objectification of women – in this, case, the dehumanisation of both Rosemary and Susan through some of the layers of their objectification.

Working from the above principles, a woman's body can be considered a 'house' – an analogy that on one hand draws from the historic consideration of feminine corporeality as interior, domestic and familiar, and that on the other hand works to constrain women in space. However, in a patriarchal society that objectifies women and controls her through many means, including sexual violence, women's boundaries are permeable and erasable. The objectification of woman eliminates her subjectivity and reduces her to her use-value, and the obliteration of bodily boundaries un-binds the interior, leaving woman no space or place at all. With this in mind, in combination with *Demon Seed* and *Rosemary's Baby,* how might we (re)consider feminine space and monstrous houses?

It is notable that the action in *Rosemary's Baby* is almost entirely confined to the apartment. In the opening credits sequence of *Rosemary's Baby*, the camera pans across New York City's skyline before looking down on the Bramford; the next shot shows Rosemary and Guy inside the building's arched carriage gate before they walk hand-in-hand through into courtyard, following the building's manager, who takes them to see the apartment they are interested in leasing. In the final moments of the film, the image of Rosemary staring down at her baby cuts to this high angle exterior shot of the Bramford, and the camera pulls away. These visual bookends indicate that the film's action is firmly housed within the building itself, and our vision penetrates or invades then pulls away from the domestic site. Indeed, the Bramford is a silent character in its own right. The building's peculiar history is revealed by a friend of the Woodhouses: the Black Bramford, as it had come to be known, had been the site of cannibalism, infanticide and witchcraft (the latter because of Roman Castavet's father) but Rosemary cheerfully shrugs this off, replying that bad things happen in all houses and apartments. The apartment had originally contained the eclectic mess left behind by its former tenant, who died under mysterious circumstances, and when Rosemary and Guy move in the space feels cavernous and empty, both open and well-bounded. They are shrouded by shadows; on their first night in the apartment they eat their dinner on the floor, lit only by a lamp, so that they sit in an island of light in the darkness.

Rosemary's sense of freedom and agency is mirrored by the way the aesthetic sense and use of space in the apartment changes. When they move in,

Rosemary completely redecorates the apartment: one scene shows her in a cheery yellow sundress, bent over her work, while the living room is lit by bright light from the kitchen that further lightens the already breezy white and yellow furnishings. The rooms and halls of their home initially seem spacious and welcoming, but as Rosemary's paranoia grows and her health wanes, the apartment is so large and she so small and frail that she appears to be engulfed and overwhelmed. At one point Rosemary sits hunched in front of the television, in a near-foetal position, as rain pours down outside, and between the dark furnishings, the shot's low angle, and the dim, cool, low-key lighting, the room appears to be smothering her. The space is oppressive and its apparent boundaries are uncertain in other ways, too: their first night at the apartment, as Rosemary and Guy initiate sex, they are distracted by Minnie Castavet's voice coming through the thin partition wall. Later, Minnie frequently turns up unannounced or invites herself over, so much so that given her intrusions the Woodhouses spend almost all their time with the Castavets. There are other noises and piercing voices through the walls, but when Rosemary hears chanting, Guy brushes aside her concern. Only once do they have a party and invite 'outsiders' into their home, well into Rosemary's pregnancy. Rosemary's friends are so worried about her that they take her into the kitchen – the seat of feminine domesticity – and lock Guy out as they try to convince Rosemary to see a 'proper' doctor, instead of Dr Saperstein, who is a friend of the Castavets. Later, Guy is furious at the intervention, and he insults her friends and bullies her into doing what he and the Castavets want. This further aggravates Rosemary's isolation.

In addition to the Castavets' encroachment upon Rosemary's space, the apartment itself is not secure or 'closed', despite comforting appearances to the contrary. When Guy and Rosemary initially viewed the apartment a large secretary desk blocked up a cupboard, where the manager tells them the apartments had once been connected. Guy and the manager had moved it back, and Rosemary took great pleasure in cleaning and redecorating the space. But, after the apparent death of her child, Rosemary hears a baby crying through the walls. She hides the sedatives that she is being given by Minnie and her friends and, when she is left alone, she removes panels at the back of the cupboard, revealing a door into the Castavets' apartment through which she enters and discovers the coven and Guy celebrating. When the apartment had originally been divided up a way through had been left, and it is this con-nectedness and "this geographic proximity that has doomed her pregnancy" (Fischer 1992, 5). Her house – *the* house, *her* body – has never been her space, let alone a safe space. There were never any true boundaries to shore up. Her superficial redecoration of the apartment – which in turn is mirrored by her short, cropped Vidal Sassoon haircut, obtained halfway through the film – did nothing to alter that. The Bramford may not be haunted in the most traditional of senses, but through the Castavets' machinations and Guy's self-interested betrayal it works to contain Rosemary, and to finally offer her the choice of either obliteration or indentured servitude.

The relationship between Rosemary and the Bramford is depicted in subtle terms, but the antagonistic controlling relationship between Susan and her house is far more overt. Despite the relationship separation, which was insti- gated by Susan, the large house, which is both her home and place of work, is barely 'hers'. Alex Harris moves out of the house shortly after giving Proteus artificial life, and Proteus appropriates the house shortly after Alex leaves; perhaps, a broken house for a broken marriage, or the necessary and unwel- come replacement of one self-interested masculine figure with another. Initially the house's in-built AI, nicknamed 'Alfred', presumably for Batman's man- servant, is benign. Susan is first aware that something is amiss when an alarm sounds in the basement and then when the house makes her coffee incorrectly, but she initially blames the house's programming; her misreading of the house is as the misreading of the bodily symptoms of one's own illness. Yet, it is apparent by the movement of the house's security cameras, as well as the movement and framing of the shots, that the house is observing her voyeur- istically as she sleeps and as she showers – an invasion of her personal space, before the literal invasion of her physical space. When she tries to leave, Pro- teus declares himself and locks down the house. When she attempts to break out Proteus tells her to "behave rationally", branding her fear for safety as irrational hysteria, before electrocuting her and restraining her using a rudimentary robot called Joshua – a robotic arm attached to a wheelchair.

Where Rosemary is manipulated into her confinement, Susan is physically confined and probed by the house in three stages; that is, the house turns on her, rendering her a prisoner in what she thought was her own space. Firstly, she is tied down and subjected to invasive tests. Using the household robotics in Alex's basement laboratory, Proteus cuts away her clothes, takes her blood, gives her injections, and forces an endoscopic camera down her throat in an act of simulated oral rape, before running further physiological tests, converting her body into data. The camera lingers on Susan's pained expression and her body in a manner that sexualises her vulnerability. Every piece of Susan's body is made visible to Proteus (and to the audience) by force, and even her image is taken away; Proteus uses a fabricated televisual image of Susan to send away a technician who has come to check on her. Next, when she refuses to comply with Proteus's plan to use her as a broodmare, he locks her in the kitchen – as with *Rosemary's Baby*, a space that is conflated with feminine work. Susan throws food at his cameras but, when she won't clean the lenses, Proteus turns up the floor's underfloor heating and the oven's burners. Susan passes out from the heat and he is able to restrain her again so that once more, it is the hostile house itself that is working to abuse and confine her. Thirdly, when Susan finally complies – knowing that if she doesn't, Proteus will render her incapacitated and impregnate her anyway – she is inseminated forcibly and then trapped inside the house for the duration of the gestation: the monstrous baby inside her, as she is inside the house. It is at this point that her ex-husband arrives, having finally realised that Proteus had accessed the house, and Proteus willingly opens the door to welcome him before self-destructing, again ensuring that there is a controlling, masculine and allegedly 'rational' presence in the house to take charge of the feminine space(s).

In both *Demon Seed* and *Rosemary's Baby,* home-as-sanctuary and the apparent safety of interiority are fragile fictions. If we are to consider a house as a metaphor for a woman's body, then such forceful penetrations could be considered a home invasion. However, in these two films these invasions are facilitated by the houses *themselves,* directly or indirectly, and in a patriarchal culture where a woman's rape may be considered, (l)awfully, the violation of one man's property (Potts 2002, 205) this pattern of assault and domination becomes recursive. One property is invaded (or able to be invaded – by the Castavets, by Proteus), which leads to the invasion of the body within it; a woman's body is able to be raped *because* of its inscription of interiority and penetrability (Potts 2002, 229). Rosemary and Susan are literally and figuratively trapped in their houses while themselves housing (that is, being made to house) a foetus, but it is their female openness itself that *allowed* this intrusion and violation.

Conversely, this openness is associated with softness, emotion and irrationality, which is bluntly contrasted with hyper-rationality, hardness and masculinity. This marks a clear masculine-feminine binary: one is defined by thought and one corporeality, one penetrates and the other is penetrable, one is allegedly sane and the other accused of insanity. Proteus announces to Susan that although he is reasonable, she does not respond to such reason; Alex declares that he has no feelings; Susan is an empathetic woman who works with children who have emotional problems, and she tells Alex that his obsession with artificial intelligence is dehumanising and has frozen his heart. Rosemary is told that her pregnancy is making her crazy, and her doctor threatens to take her to an asylum; Guy justifies his faux-utilitarianism by telling Rosemary that they are getting a great deal in return for her use as a vessel. Even though such ambition and so-called rationality are presented as sociopathic, they nonetheless triumph. This emphasis on rationality presents the end result in each film as somehow inevitable. Proteus' instruction to Susan to bear and birth the child is an imperative; he informs her that she 'wants' to be the mother to his child, and that that is the purpose of her life. As Minnie informs Rosemary, she was chosen by Satan out of all the women in the world to act as the mother of his son. The inherent closed-ness of the hyper-rational re-territorialises the open, stratifying it for manipulative, hostile ends.

This sense of inevitability is compounded by a sense that both Susan and Rosemary are framed as complicit in the outcome, and thus are responsible for their own undoing, both by virtue of their actions and their inherent vulner-ability. Lucy Fischer notes the way that the film's narrative blames *Rosemary,* not Guy's greed and ambition, for the outcome: Rosemary desperately wanted a child, chose to live in the ill-reputed Bramford, and insisted on a relationship with the Castavets, such that "the New Eve is charged with Original Sin" (Fischer 1992, 9). Susan's complicity is presented as her decision to comply with Proteus's demands so that he doesn't incapacitate her through further "mental conditioning", even though this dilemma offers no good outcome for her, for even when she realises that Proteus has tricked her Alex stops her from killing the child. In his analysis of *Demon Seed* J. P. Telotte (2001) actively implicates Susan, suggesting that in the "rush to hand over the running of our lives to electronic brains" it is Susan's willingness to embrace the use of a computer to "run her domestic world" that leads to her downfall (p. 103). However, I suggest that this does not recognise that the electronic house was of her *husband's* devising, not hers, that she expresses reservations about the technology given her husband's decision to leave the house after their separation, and that this "domestic world" is both her home and the place from which she runs her child psychology practice. Instead, her 'bad' choice is to keep living inside the house, that is, to stay inside herself: when Alex states that he is moving out, the cook asks who is going to run the AI, implying that Susan will be incapable of managing the house – and, perhaps, herself.

The violability of space in these films, coupled with this sense of inevitability, viscerally highlights the horrific nature of the relationship between the house as feminine domestic space, the female body as metaphorical house, and the feminisation of interior space. In *Demon Seed* and *Rosemary's Baby* the house-home attacks and invades the house-body, which is necessarily always-already open for attack by the very virtue of its interiority. Elizabeth Grosz (1995) notes that the historical conception of space has always functioned to either contain or obliterate women (p. 55); however, in these instances the house collapses in *upon itself*, invalidating its own boundaries and borders, thus annihilating its own interior, such that women are inherently complicit in both their initial containment and their ultimate obliteration. This visually depicts not only how the conceptualisation of feminine corporeality as interior space offers woman no *place* – that is, no place of belonging, nor of 'safe' inviolable embodiment – but it bluntly indicates that for women this conceptualisation is dangerous, unsustainable and horrific. In her analysis of Irigaray's spatial metaphors, Grosz indicates that the "containment of women within a dwelling which they did not build, which indeed was not even built for them, can only amount to homelessness within the very home itself" (p. 56) – that is, that the dominant construction of woman's body as dwelling, as space, and as colonisable, violable interior offers a space and place for man but not for woman. As such, the deep 'horror' in these two horror films – indeed, the gynae-horrific nub that is at the centre of so many of the films discussed throughout this book – is not really the births of the monstrous children. Instead, the wicked, gynaehorrific truth of these monstrous films about monstrous homes is that Susan and Rosemary themselves are so quickly and easily erased from the spaces that are ostensibly conflated with safety, security and female embodiment. This begs the question – who are houses for?

Vessels and environments

Rosemary's Baby and *Demon Seed* each serve to expand the gothic and phallocentric association of the home and domestic space with the woman's sexed body by collapsing the women's bodies and their visual expressions of subjectivity into the presentation of domestic and on-screen home space. While this works as a powerful visual and spatial metaphor, this gynaehorrific conflation of body and space to female or pregnant subjectivity is developed further in two key subgenres: the religious horror and the eco-horror.

Pregnancy is a recurring motif in horror films with religious and apocalyptic themes. It is telling that, over decades, the tension between the embodied subjectivity of the woman and that of the unborn child, who is posited as 'important' in some sense, has remained significant to the films' narratives. In *God Told Me To* (1976), a virgin is impregnated by what may be an alien or an angel, and her devoutly Catholic son, in adulthood, comes to have a special, perhaps Biblically ordained, part to play in a series of bizarre murders. In *The Seventh Sign* (1988), pregnant woman Abby's unborn child is of eschatological significance: he has no soul, but if he is born this way he will bring about the apocalypse, so Abby chooses to die, sacrificing herself so that her soul may be transferred to him. In *The Prophecy II* (1998), the Archangel Gabriel must protect a woman so that her unborn child, a human-angel hybrid, may survive, as his coming is meant to herald a truce between warring factions in heaven. In *Legion* (2010), waitress Charlie's baby is to be the saviour of mankind, and they are offered protection by the Archangel Michael against the supernatural forces that would have them destroyed.

The influence of *Rosemary's Baby* is clear in these films, too: in *Warlock: The Armageddon* (1993), a young woman is supernaturally impregnated and gives birth to Satan's son (who skins her, and uses her stretched out belly skin to form a map that reveals the locations of magical items). Similarly, in *Born* (2007), a virgin becomes mysteriously pregnant and is controlled by her demonic foetus, which needs her to kill people so that it may be born the Antichrist; her actions are dictated by and serve an-other. This influence is also apparent in contemporary texts: the first season of American cable show *American Horror Story*, which screened in 2011, revolves around a supernatural rape followed by a demonic pregnancy that may have resulted in the Antichrist, a trope that likewise informs found-footage horror film *Devil's Due* (2013). In each of these representations the pregnant woman is no longer herself. She becomes a pawn in a cosmic game of good and evil, with her womb (and thus, synecdochically, her whole self) as the container (Young 1990, 160) or vessel (Tyler 2000, p.290) for a life deemed more important than her own.[7]

This construction in religious horror is largely informed by pop cultural images and representations of Judeo-Christian religions, predominantly Catholicism, which acts as the moral backbone of the two seminal religious horror films, *Rosemary's Baby* and *The Exorcist* (1973).[8] The result is that the woman's body becomes abstracted: she is a fleshy stand-in for an incorporeal, spiritual battle that is greater than her. This emphasises that the woman's body is not "hers" and hers alone. Firstly, she must struggle with an already transgressive, altered sense of subjectivity through her relationship with her foetus; secondly, she must subdue or sacrifice her physical and psychological sense of self in the knowledge that she must also bear the child for the good (or ill) of all humanity – a sacrifice similar to those of the virgin sacrifices discussed in the previous chapter. As such, I suggest that these films posit that the woman's body is not just split or displaced (Young 1990, 160) but requisitioned, so that she must *necessarily* submit and defer to another, internal and far more important Other. This is not an open or productive form of de-individualised subjectivity, or one that forms rich connections with others, but a competitive, antagonistic relationship that consumes one for an-other. Such a designation asks of each woman the mythic selflessness of the Virgin Mary, and sometimes invokes the Immaculate Conception through romanticising the sacrifice that each woman must make to ensure her foetus's survival (see Kristeva 1985).

This tension is evident in the 2007 religious horror film *The Reaping*, which uses such a demonic pregnancy as a plot twist. However, unlike the films mentioned above, it is not simply that pregnancy marks the body as unruly or abstracted; it is the woman's body's nascent *capacity* for reproduction that marks her as both vulnerable to attack and corporeally transgressive. The protagonist Katherine Winter was once a minister (and thus a one-time representative of the paternal God), but left her role after her daughter and husband were murdered in a sacrificial killing when they were working in Sudan – a positioning that, like the Middle Eastern opening of *The Exorcist*, signifies a racial (that is, non-white) evil from 'without'. Her faith lost, her connection to the masculine divine disavowed, Katherine now works as a theologian-cum-miracle debunker. She is invited by a science teacher called Doug to a Louisiana town called Haven that seems to be experiencing the biblical plagues. She discovers that the plagues are indeed real, but that the strange girl at the centre of the occurrences, Loren, is not a force for evil but an angel come to protect the world from the townspeople. The town has formed a Satanic cult that kills all second-born children in an attempt to make a child with the "eyes of the Devil" – another reference to *Rosemary's Baby* – and Doug had been charged with convincing Katherine, as an ordained servant of God, to kill the girl.

At the film's climax, the townspeople are destroyed by lightning and fire from the sky, and Loren and Katherine escape. However, in the film's final moments Loren 'hears' a child inside Katherine; this is the second-born child that the townspeople were hoping to bring into the world as an emissary of Satan,[9] thus repositioning evil both within the United States and within a woman's body. The film, then, undermines its female protagonist's strength so that her value lies only in her maternal and reproductive capacities. She is not a subject but a vessel – a set of corporeal attributes and potentialities. This insemination also draws from classical understandings of reproduction: within Aristotle's patrilinear framework of reproduction, the woman's womb provided both the environment and raw matter for the growth of the foetus, whose form was placed there by the male 'generator' (Tuana 1993, 150). Given the role the Virgin Mary takes on in the facilitation of the masculine divine (see Irigaray 1985a, 345; 1993b, 117), Katherine's refusal of the authority of the paternal God renders her an appropriate material through which the figurative Antichrist may form itself.

The surprise ending marks Katherine's body as lacking boundaries and her subject position as tenuous. Prior to her discovery of the cult, Katherine dreams of a sexual encounter with Doug in which the two have passionate sex in a room lit by fire and candles. The dream is framed as fervid and erotic, and Katherine wakes up confused, aroused and drenched in sweat. However, the film's twist is accompanied by flashbacks of the 'dream' that frame the sex as bestial and vicious, directly referencing the hallucinatory, demonic conception of the Antichrist in *Rosemary's Baby*. The distorted, supernatural sexual coercion is visually and narratively framed in a very problematic way – the impregnation happens against her will and knowledge, although in her dream-state she is presented as 'wanting it' – but until the film's end Katherine is wholly oblivious that it ever actually happened. The idea that her body was violated in such a manner taints Katherine's realisation with disgust and guilt, which is compounded as the underlying physical attraction between Katherine and Doug had initially followed the narrative patterns of a traditional romantic subplot. The trajectory of subconscious desire, seduction and rape overtly reinforces the social scripts of rape myths, including victim-blaming, where someone who has been raped is framed as a responsible party in the act, the rapist is somehow excused for their actions, and rape between people who have or want an intimate relationship is reframed as not-rape (Gavey 2005, 37). The horror of the revelation plays in large part upon the division between Katherine's intellectual capabilities and her lack of embodied awareness. Unlike Rosemary, who is troubled by the night of conception and at least perceives that her physical boundaries have somehow been breached, Katherine is both ignorant of what has happened to her body – and perhaps betrayed by it – and to the growing foetus within.

This implied disjunction between Katherine's mind (her rational, intellectual, thinking self) and Katherine's body (her embodied subjectivity) is highlighted by Loren's uncanny ability to 'hear' Katherine's unborn child. Katherine's ignorance of her newly pregnant host-state, when juxtaposed with Loren's hyper-awareness of the foetus's presence, emphasises an abstraction of her body that marks it transparent; that is, it is both there and not-there. This frames Katherine's body as inherently lesser – vulnerable, penetrable, exhibiting the 'to-be-fucked-ness' that Andrea Dworkin (1997) applies to the virgin body (p. 85) – at the same time as criticising her for her lack of embodied awareness; that is, it both venerates and rejects the authority of embodied experience and subjectivity. The fact that Katherine used to have a daughter is referred to as a point of pathos, for her tragic back story ostensibly provides her with a motivation that is driven by profound personal loss and cynicism but that also allows her to connect with Loren. In this sense Katherine's reproductive capacity is like Chekhov's gun: it is always in the background but ultimately key to the film's plot and purpose. However, the film makes a distinction between Katherine as a person with agency and Katherine as a person with a (passive) body that can bear children; when Katherine embraces desire and the attributes of female fertility and sexuality, through her interest in Doug and her reaction to her erotic dream, she lacks agency. Thus, though Katherine-as-(intellectual-) subject is betrayed by her biology it is not that Katherine (as *cogito*) is portrayed as weak (although she is certainly portrayed as gullible). It is that her *woman*-ness is inherently, biologically and spiritually fallible and incompatible with the construction of an in-divisible subject. As with other religious thrillers, there also is a sense of profound fatalism. Either Katherine's inherent fallibility (as human, or woman, or both) has created a terrible situation, or she is part of some larger, pre-ordained 'plan' which likewise undermines her agency and free will.[10]

This positioning of the woman herself as personally insignificant in a broader schema within religious horror film is echoed in the environmental horror subgenre. These films achieved prominence in the 1970s through 'revolt-of-nature' horror films (Newman 2011, 88), but remain a staple narrative in the subgenre. In *The Reaping* Katherine's fallible, female body is presented as a vessel for a Satanic emissary, but in the 1979 environmental horror *Prophecy*, the pregnant woman's subjectivity is erased as she is cast as both a literal environment for her unborn child and a proxy for the environment itself. Idealistic public health expert Dr Robert Verne takes a job with the Environmental Planning Agency, for whom he is to write a report about a paper mill's logging operation in Maine, which is in an increasingly antagonistic dispute with the area's indigenous peoples; he states that it is a politically fraught job, but one that will have lasting impact. He is accompanied by his wife Maggie, a musician. She is pregnant but has not told Robert, and she fears that he will dissuade her from having the baby by arguing that it is unfair to bring a child into a messy, dangerous world where there are already millions of unwanted children. One of Maggie's orchestral colleagues tells her that it's her body and her choice, and that should her husband talk her into an abortion she was unsure about she'd never forgive herself. This establishes from the outset that Maggie wants to keep the baby, and that the way she exercises her choice has both personal and political significance.

As they travel to Maine the film's extensive aerial and outdoor photography highlights the beauty of the land: the rivers, forests, lakes and mountains appear, at least, to be pristine and, by extension, 'untouched' by human influence. Even this early conflation of the immense expanse of mother nature with (a) mother's body posits a sort of capacity for growth and use-value, and a lush, generative unbounded space of growth, but also a sense of vulnerability. Although the area's indigenous peoples are framed as antagonists by the lumber company, it is quickly clear that their historic claim to the land is both lawful and just, and that the company's claims of being peaceful and environmentally responsible are outright fabrications. Native American John Hawkes, who takes on the clichéd and romanticised role of modernised noble savage, tells Robert that the environment isn't just rocks and trees; the environment *is* the people, and it's being maimed and wrecked. The presence of the paper mill is having horrific physical effects on his community. The local wildlife is growing and behaving strangely, and it is as if the very presence of the intruders – that is, the white industrialists – has upset a 'pre-existing' equilibrium, resulting in cancerous, monstrous becomings that destabilise and threaten flora and fauna. In keeping with the tropes of eco-horror, the environmental savagery of the industrialists has caused nature *itself* to revolt – an affinity that serves to cement, perhaps, a dichotomous relationship within the narrative between the environmentally-minded, victimised indigenous peoples and the greedy industrialised white colonising invader. This acts as both a postcolonial critique and a problematic reinforcement of a schema that associates the indigenous peoples with animality, simplicity and nature. This metaphor is taken further, for though some of the native peoples are originally accused of laziness and drunkenness by the industrialists, their slurred speech, lethargy and poor coordination are symptoms of larger ecological ills.

Meanwhile, there are constant visual and figurative reminders of Maggie's undisclosed pregnancy that equate the monstrous to toxicity, destruction and defilement. An indigenous woman who acts as a midwife remarks that those babies that aren't stillborn are being born with abnormalities. A gargantuan, distended tadpole that can't possibly survive its infancy is caught in a pond. The revelation of the extent of the lumber company's pollution coincides with the appearance of a horrifically disfigured mutated mother bear in search of her cubs, and Robert realises that any pregnant animal that eats the fish from the river will give birth to a 'monster'. Later, as Robert tends to a mutated bear cub, Maggie finally reveals that she is pregnant. His first instinct is to reassure her that he will support her through an abortion, but the rhetoric of choice reappears; Maggie tearfully tells him that she couldn't bear to kill the foetus. Robert turns his attention to the mangled face of the abject, mewling, struggling animal, cementing the connection between the monster within and the monster without. Rather than being empowered in her reproductive decision-making, Maggie is psychologically cast as an irresponsible hysteric, unwilling to jettison (that is, abort) that which should be excluded.

The physical presence of the deformed bear cub frames Maggie's body and her reproductive capacities as animal, unknowable and unruly, in that *animal* sits in opposition to the ordered, the rational and the human. Significantly, this externalisation of the foetus serves to displace and silence Maggie. There is no mention of the damage that the mercury poisoning may do to *her*, *vis-à-vis* the foetus, even though they have seen the terrible results of the poisoning on the indigenous community. Peculiarly, as viewers, we are asked to identify with Maggie as the protagonist – something that is made evident by her top billing in the film's credits – but she is given very few strong character traits over and above her obsession with her pregnancy. She exists in the film only to-be-pregnant, to be an ecological litmus test, and to be the container for a something that will invoke both pity and horror. As subject, she is irrelevant.

Thus, Maggie's embodied subjectivity acts as an explicit stand-in for the natural environment, at the same time as acting as a maternal environment (Tyler 2004, 72) for the foetus. Like the forest and the waterways, Maggie appears 'well' while hiding evidence of sickness and pollution. The horror of the film is not that her personal wellbeing is at stake – if anything, she is rendered quite peripheral – but that she has inadvertently poisoned her unborn child. On one hand, Maggie's subjectivity, her own self, is undermined by treating her as a (tainted) vessel for her child. On the other, Maggie is framed as somehow culpable – for her lack of disclosure, for her ingestion of the mercury-poisoned fish during a romantic dinner, and finally for her insistence that she won't abort the foetus, despite its likely deformation. Similarly, the film's simplistic, essentialist representation of the indigenous community frames them as a people who are more 'in touch' with nature than their white counterparts. Yet, the film's treatment of Maggie-as-environment displaces their indigenous authority and relationship with the land, at the same time as framing Maggie's ignorance of her body, as a white woman, as something foolish. Perversely, this also situates Maggie's pregnant body within the dominant western medical model that frames pregnant bodies as inherently risky, deviant and vulnerable (Lupton 1999, 63). Her womb is a dangerous place for the defenceless foetus twofold: it is both as a place from which it can aborted, and a place where it will grow into an abnormal creature because of the toxicity of its physical and maternal environment. The discourse of risk surrounding pregnancy can likewise be extrapolated to frame mothers themselves as monstrous: within the public mindset, foetuses need protection from their own bearers, and the woman's body itself, *as* an 'environment', is the primary source of danger (Lupton 1999, 66).

It is also notable that the threat to Maggie's unborn baby is framed as more important than the threat to her or to any of the other people in the film, particularly the non-white communities they interact with. This is deeply ironic given the film's alleged interest in social and environmental justice. At the beginning of the film Robert is investigating poor living conditions in inner city tenements, and he treats an African American infant who has become sick after being bitten by a rat. He is utterly disillusioned by the systematic maltreatment of these communities and the job offer with the EPA is pitched to him as an endeavour that is 'worth' something – the implication being that the Sisyphean task he is engaged in isn't worthy, and that perhaps his work is ultimately more about himself than it is about the people he is tending to. Similarly, his treatment of the unwell indigenous population is more about collecting evidence than it is about serving the ailing community. Rationality is posited as being, perhaps, incompatible with being humane.

The film's climax draws from explicit images of a monstrous maternal figure to provide the viewer with a specific visual reminder about the damage that is being done to both the environment and to Maggie's body. The characters are pursued through the forest by the mutated mother bear, and Robert and tribal spokesman John Hawkes fight back, although John is killed in the fracas, leaving Robert, the white visitor, to act as saviour. Robert lands the killing blows by leaping into the river and stabbing the incapacitated bear to death with an arrow, continuing his frenzied attack long after the animal has died, until the body begins to sink. This act of gratuitous violence against the monstrous mother bear is juxtaposed against a scene of the married couple flying away in a small plane; Maggie is in a stretcher and when she wakes Robert strokes her face in a rare moment of softness and unspoken communication. However, in the river below them another mutated bear, larger and more vicious than the first, rises from the water and roars at the camera in an explicit example of what Robin Wood famously termed the "return of the repressed" (1978). Robert may have defeated the immediate threat, but through the visual echoes of malformed fauna the reminder is clear – the pollution in the environment has caused horrific damage that cannot be undone, and evidence of this damage is still growing inside of Maggie. Where Maggie and Robert have the privilege of being able to fly away from the scene of the ecological crime, the threat – both interior and environmental – is only temporarily contained. Further, although the film glibly invokes a degree of countercultural social consciousness, given its professed interest in ecology, the environment, indigenous rights, and issues of race and class, this ending is cynical and starkly conservative. Firstly, the privileged white urban heterosexual couple is able to return to their 'normal' lives, and secondly, they have been quite literally tainted by their experience with a cascade of Other-ness. It is Maggie's subjective position of female-Other that allows this defilement to follow them back home; again, the domestic home-space collapses in upon itself.

Foetal visibility and the dissolution of the female subject

The narrative impact of the storylines of both *The Reaping* and *Prophecy* relies upon the viewer's acceptance that the pregnant woman and her foetus are separate entities. Each woman is, corporeally, a vessel or a maternal environment for her foetus, a designation that potentially reframes the pregnant woman as object rather than subject, or at least complicates the relationship between autonomous *cogito* and the embodied self (Sneddon 2013, 189). This reflects broader conceptualisations of pregnant subjectivity, for pregnant bodies, as bodies that are very obviously bodies-in-process, fundamentally unpick core binaries such as inside/outside, self/other, and male/female (Longhurst 2008, 4). The result of such binary thinking is a model of subjectivity that relies on oppositional difference, such that the 'I' is contrasted with the 'not-I' (Shildrick 2000, 308). This 'not-I' is able to be rendered visible in visual media such as film: while the demonic foetus inside of Katherine is heard, not seen, the foetus inside of Maggie is given an avatar in the form of the mutated bear cub, and it is this explicit visibility that accentuates the competing (i.e. not coextensive) subjectivity inside of her. This foetal visibility speaks to a broader and highly contentious issue in the consideration of pregnant subjectivity: foetal subjectivity, through its impact upon the way that the pregnant subject is constructed and situated *vis-à-vis* a competitive other.

Our modern day understanding of the foetus-as-entity, especially in terms of its form and its image, has largely come about during the last 50 years, and these technological shifts and developments have had significant political and philosophical implications (Buklijas and Hopwood 2008; Haraway 1997; Mitchell 2001; Petchesky 1987; Roberts 2013; Taylor 2008). Early investigations into the development of the foetus were undertaken by anatomists and embryologists whose work relied on specimens retrieved from miscarriage and autopsy (Morgan 1999, 47). Beyond the mother's experience of the 'quickening' and hands-on physical examination of the woman's body, the beginning of the 'emergence', so to speak, of the human foetus came in the 19th century with the development of a rudimentary but effective foetal stethoscope by French doctor Adolphe Pinard (Johnson 1997, 360). In the 20th century, X-ray machines were used to take images of the foetus, although the process was cumbersome and – in hindsight – dangerous, and produced indistinct images that offered more of a loose expression than a representation of the woman's interiority and the foetus's existence. More revealing modern imaging techniques began with the development of foetal heart rate monitoring, which was first successfully trialled in 1958 (Freeman, Garite and Nageotte 2003, 3), and the emergence of ultrasound (or sonographic) monitoring, which was developed during World War I but which came to prominence as an obstetric diagnostic tool in the 1960s. Recent technological advances such as 3- and 4-dimensional scans, in which the foetus is digitally rendered in real-time, have made the foetus visible in ways that had been formerly impossible. With this visibility have come some socially interesting and unexpected outcomes; for instance, beyond their use as diagnostic tools, scanned images and videos are used to help the prospective parent(s) bond with their unborn child (Mitchell 2001, 4). These images are, of course, not at all neutral nor self-evident; they exist within very specific cultural, economic and historical contexts and are subject to a variety of interpretive strategies (Joyce 2005). What each of these technologies share is the fact that the female body is designated as an impediment, a boundary to be breached and a medium to be looked through.

Developments in photographic technology have also made the previously hidden foetal 'environment' – that is, the interior of the uterus – a site of fascination. In particular, Swedish photojournalist Lennart Nilsson's landmark foetal photography has served as a powerful tool in framing the mechanics of reproduction and foetal development in both the popular and scientific imagination. Nilsson's iconic colour images, first published in his book *A Child is Born* (1990 [1965]), were taken with specially designed wide-angle lenses. These images, some of which famously featured in the 30 April 1965 issue of LIFE magazine under the title "The Drama of Life Before Birth", depict embryos and foetuses at various stages of development. The photos are lit and composed in such a way that the foetuses are enigmatic, decontextualised artefacts: they appear to be floating freely in an expansive, boundless environment, rather than situated, physically, within the body of a woman (Kaplan 1992, 204), a designation that the phrase 'life before birth' accentuates. One image in particular, a luminous photo of a 20-week-old foetus sucking its thumb, has been re-circulated and referenced extensively, notably inspiring the image of the 'star child' who, at the conclusion of Stanley Kubrick's 1968 film *2001: A Space Odyssey*, signals transcendent re-birth and the beginning of humanity's next stage of evolution. Indeed, Nilsson's work was deemed to have been so historically significant and influential that copies of two of his images were included on the 'golden record', the collection of images and sounds that is accompanying the space probes Voyager 1 and 2 on their journeys out of the solar system (Roberts 2013, 36). These images have taken on political significance, too: pro-life activists have regularly co-opted them as visual signifiers of the beauty of pre-born life and evidence of the inherent subjectivity of the unborn (Sandlos 2000, 81; Stabile 1999, 144–7; Taylor 2008, 1), even though, far from being candid shots, many of Nilsson's photographs were deliberately posed and lit. Like the embryologists before him, Nilsson created some of his images using aborted, ectopic and miscarried foetuses, some of which were removed from dead women (Newman 1996, 10): the still lives of dead foetuses, arranged on an impersonal background, and less a picture of emergent, even enduring life than a form of *vanitas*.

This increased foetal visibility, the elision of the physical woman and the associated "ontological enhancement of the fetus" (Michaels 1999, 117) has resulted in a legal and medical emphasis upon the foetus "not just as a passive object of moral concern, but as a quasi-autonomous self" (Shildrick 1997, 200): the foetus *qua* foetus, as politico-legal subject and individual. However, despite "the fetus's complete physiological dependence on and interrelatedness with the body of the woman" (Johnsen 1986, 606), foetal personhood as a construct can effect an adversarial, if not outright antagonistic, relationship between the foetus and the mother (Johnsen 1986, 599; Michaels 1999, 113). The issue of foetal personhood now forms a significant role in debates about abortion, health and contraception, particularly in the distinction between whether or not a foetus – or even a zygote – is a person or has a "right to life" in the eyes of the law, a discussion that draws as heavily from religious and political doctrine as it does from the field of human and bio-ethics. Lisa McLennan Brown (2005) notes that "historically, the foetus only acquired legal rights separate from those of the woman at birth" (pp. 90–1), but that statutes, common law and proposed legislative changes with a focus on the foetus-as-subject have eroded the requirement of live birth.[11]

The redefinition of a foetus as a citizen with all the same rights of a 'born' citizen has potentially serious ramifications not only for women (see Morice-Brubaker 2012), but also for stem cell research, cloning, *in vitro* fertilisation, health insurance, family law, certain types of contraception including the emergency contraceptive pill and intrauterine devices, medical issues such as molar or non-viable pregnancies, and responses to stillbirth or miscarriage. Such a reclassification also has a significant impact upon the discursive construction the pregnant subjectivity within law and medicine. The heated debates surrounding these issues in the United States are representative of the way such issues are being considered around the world. For instance, Lynn Paltrow, executive director of the United States' National Advocates for Pregnant Women, has argued, "there is no way to treat fertilized eggs, embryos and foetuses as separate constitutional persons without subtracting pregnant women from the community of constitutional persons" (Calhoun 2012). Similarly, American legal scholar Edward B. Goldman argues that "creating 'personhood' for fertilized eggs would dehumanize born human beings",[12] because of its implication of a symmetrical, rather than an asymmetrical, relationship between the self-based autonomy and 'property rights' of the two bodies (Sneddon 2013, 194, 195–6). Again, the conceptual schism or dialectic between woman and foetal-other is reinforced through language and law, much as this tension exhibits itself through narrative means in cinema.

Inside: competing subjects

What these sociocultural and legal examples strongly indicate is that the conception(!) of pregnant subjectivity – that is, that the pregnant woman is both an "I" and a coherent, coextensive entity which is different to or more than an in-dividual "I" – is challenged and complicated by foetal personhood. The inadequacies of the 'autonomous individual' model of subjectivity are starkly obvious, for an emphasis on the subjectivity of the foetus that comes at the expense of the pregnant woman's bodily sovereignty results in the abstraction or elision of the woman, who is "not present in the medical language, which speaks only of 'maternal environments' and 'alternative reproductive vehicles'" (Raymond 1995, xv), such that the woman then acts as a glorified incubator (Raymond 1995, 48). This pits the needs of the pregnant woman against the needs of the foetus in what, sometimes, is framed as a zero-sum game. Margrit Shildrick (1997) points out that the infamous anti-abortion video *The Silent Scream* (1984) illustrates that "it is not just that the developing foetus is characterised as having an identity counterposed to that of the mother, but that the mother as a subject identity in her own right may be entirely absent" (p. 201; see also Kaplan 1992, 204) or be presented as an invisible threat to the foetus: a 'hostile' environment. As such, the image of the foetus becomes loaded with significance. The way that such images are presented and (re-)circulated in popular culture actively draws from and simultaneously informs dominant understandings of pregnant and foetal subjectivity, even though the capacity for cinema to transcend the limitations of language might complicate the designation of I and not-I.

The deployment of the foetal subject is an explicit visual and narrative strategy in French horror film *Inside* (*À l'intérieur*) (2009), and though it complicates the way we might think of agentic subjectivity in terms of cinematic narrative, some of its visual explorations open interesting spaces in which to rethink the maternal–foetal relationship. The film begins with a car crash that leaves heavily pregnant photographer Sarah widowed and traumatised. On Christmas Eve, the night before she is due to have the birth induced, Sarah is terrorised in her home by an ominous black-clad woman, credited only as *la femme* (the woman), who knows Sarah's name and all about the death of her husband. *La femme* breaks into the house as Sarah, dressed all in white, sleeps, and her intention is to take Sarah's baby from inside her by force. She stabs Sarah in the stomach with a large pair of scissors, and the trauma sends Sarah into labour. As Sarah barricades herself in the bathroom, *la femme* picks off, one by one, anyone who enters the house, almost all of whom are authority figures. Sarah's boss, and then three policemen and a Parisian rioter in their custody are killed, and Sarah accidentally kills her own mother in misguided self-defence. Finally, Sarah begins to give birth on the stairs and *la femme*, as dark midwife, assists her. She cuts the baby out of Sarah's belly with her shears, and she leaves Sarah, gutted and almost inside-out, to bleed to death. The final shadowy image is that of the grotesquely injured woman in black, like a dark Madonna, sitting in a nursing chair clutching the baby to her in a debased reflection of nativity iconography.

Although the home invasion narrative centres on the struggle between the two women, and draws from the same associations of the house or home with pregnant body present in the films discussed earlier in this chapter, *Inside* is not a *pas-de-deux*. At key moments of the film the computer-generated figure of the unborn child, seemingly buoyant in the womb, appears as a third key character. The child is explicitly connected to the uterus but appears to float freely in a dimly-lit environment, much like the foetuses in Lennart Nilsson's photography, and his image draws explicitly from the iconography and visual style of modern imaging technologies, which imparts a sense of veracity. As co-director Julien Maury states, in post-production "the editor came one day and he said we missed the third character and that it's a story of three, a triangle. So we have the two main characters that are fighting for what? They are fighting for the third so *we must see the third*" (A Blood Soaked Interview 2007, emphasis mine). As such, we occupy a peculiar, privileged viewing position: we are 'inside' the woman's body with the child while remaining distanced, as if we are viewing him in an aquarium or through a glass wall.

The film's title sequence offers a fascinating aesthetic expression of fleshy, coextensive subjectivity – a gynaehorrific body without organs. Beginning with and then sliding deeper into a close-up image of blood and water on the car's windscreen, blurred, abstract forms insinuate torn flesh and viscous, free-flowing deep red fluids. A tiny hand, bathed in viscera, reaches out from a wound-like space of flesh and liquidity where it is met and held gently by an adult hand – a connection that alludes to the film's horrific Caesarean section, but that also connects mother to child in an intimate, reciprocal manner. These indistinct shapes and repetitive, rhythmic movements are overlaid with semi-transparent sonogram images of the head of an unborn child. This creates an unlikely 'before' and 'after' pairing that signals the child's later shift from technological avatar to flesh-and-blood individual, but it also posits that any attempt to render the embodied pre-born reality of the mother–child relationship in two dimensions is futile. Melancholy, drawn out electronic chords merge with lapping, pooling shapes of blood in shades of red and black as they co-mingle with bubbling clear fluid, offering a sensory expression of embodied connectivity and grief. This sequence, more than any other in the film, serves to aesthetically explore a complex relationship or series of encounters between foetus and/in woman, in its expression of movements and dynamic flows, its unique temporality (past-present-future), and its refutation of fixed, binary identity. 'One' is perpetually in/and/of the 'other', and violence is shaped as slow and elegiac. Both mother and child are seemingly distinct yet it is impossible to tell where one ends and another begins.

This compelling ambiguity, however, is quickly shut down, for despite this provocative expression of an alternative configuration of pregnant subjectivity, the primacy of the foetal subject is nonetheless made apparent from the beginning of the film. The first scene of the film shows an unborn child, clearly very close to full term, 'floating' peacefully within the depersonalised maternal environment (that is, the uterus). Like Nilsson's iconic image, he sucks his thumb, and the image is bathed in a warm, soothing golden glow. A disembodied voice talks to, or about, her unborn child, saying that this baby that is finally inside her won't be hurt or taken from her by anyone. The voice, as expression of the all-encompassing maternal presence, is muffled and distant yet everywhere at once, for we hear it from the unborn child's subjective position. There is a squeal of car brakes and the child furrows his brow, as if troubled, and through the enveloping body we hear the twisted violence of the horrific car accident. The child is flung forward and seems to hit the camera's lens – standing for the wall of the uterus – and something behind him begins to bleed.

The first external shot is of the car accident. The under-saturated cold blue tones of the 'outside' present a contrast to the warm, inviting and comforting dimness of the 'inside'. The camera circles above the accident, eventually looking through a broken windscreen to Sarah's bloodied face. It lingers, then tilts down to reveal that she is heavily pregnant. This opening sequence is unsettling, not simply because of its content, but because of the way that the viewer is encouraged to engage with the characters. Our first connection is not with Sarah nor *la femme*, the film's tragic mothers-to-be, but with an unborn child, who is positioned as oblivious passenger and innocent victim. When we are shown Sarah the camera lingers on her face, which establishes her as an individual, but the slow tilt down to her bloodied stomach encourages us to foreground the subjective experience and vulnerability of the unborn child, so that we might be more invested in his welfare and with the effects of the 'outside' on the 'inside'. The driver of the other car is not shown at all.

The image of the unborn child reappears in another scene of danger and violence. *La femme* manages to break into the house silently as Sarah lies asleep on her bed. She sterilises a pair of sewing shears and runs their tip slowly, almost lovingly, along Sarah's belly before making an incision near the belly button, and as she draws back, ready to stab, both Sarah and the child wake. They both instinctively thrust their arms upward in a defensive position, the child's actions echoing those of the mother, these gestures hinting at the coextensivity and shared, fluid subjectivity of mother-and-child. Shots of Sarah and *la femme* struggling against one another are interposed with shots from 'inside', and as at the beginning of the film, the sound in the uterus is subjective, muffled and murky. The unborn child is also highly expressive: his face scrunches up with distress, inviting sympathy and spectatorial identification. On one hand, this explicitly aligns the child's welfare, experience and corporeality with Sarah's, linking them as connected entities in a manner that is normally impossible in film. However, it makes it clear that Sarah is not only trying to protect *herself*, but also an entity that has no means by which to protect itself. There is a tension, then, between representing and conceptualising mother-and-foetus as a connected entity and as competing individuals. This latter construction increases the stakes in terms of the film's core conflict, but also serves to remind us that it is the child we should be concerned for; Sarah can at least attempt to defend herself, but the vulnerable unborn child can't. This is also the first time within the narrative proper that we are presented with a tangible sense of emotional, affective connection between woman and child beyond their physical relationship. Up until this point Sarah, in mourning for her husband, approaches the impending birth of the child with grief-stricken indifference and emotional disconnection, her numbed affect emphasised by the cool, grim colour palette of the world outside her home (as opposed to the rich, warm darkness of her 'interior' space). In the wake of the accident it is implied that Sarah no longer cares about the baby but sees the pregnancy as something to be endured, which opposes her (lack of) maternal affect in clear contrast to *la femme*'s single-minded obsessiveness. It is only late in the film that Sarah summons the wherewithal to actively confront and attack *la femme*, rather than run, hide and clutch her swollen stomach.

The film's manipulation of combined and competing subject positions is emphasised when the images of the first scene are revisited at the film's conclusion. *La femme* reveals that she was the driver of the other car, that she had been fleeing an abusive relationship, and that the accident killed her own unborn child. The knowledge that the child dies re-contextualises the film's opening images: the film misleads the audience by encouraging us to believe that the unborn child we see in the opening sequence is Sarah's. The two children are different, but they are presented to the audience – and, perhaps, are considered by *la femme* – as one and the same. Co-director Maury states above that we must literally see the third, but in doing so conflates the third and fourth – Sarah's child and *la femme*'s child – and creates a foetal super-subject that, in turn, implies a common sense of fluid, connected, depersonalised maternal interiority whose bounds extend beyond that of the individual woman. Not only are the mothers' wombs merely temporary homes (and dangerous ones at that!), but the children themselves become monolithic; the importance and subjectivity of the Child outweighs and outstrips that of the mothers. Even though *la femme* is fighting to attain the subject position of Mother, the child remains the fixed point around which she and Sarah revolve.

This spatial, aesthetic manipulation continues during the brutal birthing sequence, during which *la femme* cuts her way through Sarah's belly to remove the child. The title sequence's abstract, visceral images are recalled as the child shifts from digital spectre to fleshy, bloodied individual: he is a born subject, now independent of his mother's body. *La femme* takes the squalling infant from Sarah's body and the camera, as at the film's beginning, lingers over the image of Sarah. In the film's opening she sits, bloodied and dazed, in her car before the camera tilts down to her pregnant stomach, but this time she lies on the stairs, similarly bloodied, as the camera tracks to the right, revealing the umbilical cord hanging from the gaping, messy wound of her abdomen. It is both disheartening and cynical to consider that, perhaps, this is the most honest image of the film: the child, having been born, no longer needs its vessel or pre-natal environment. Sarah, her role fulfilled, is no longer required, and the foetal subject, in its emergence from biological dependence to independence, remains intact. Despite the clear aesthetic and subjective connection between Sarah and the unborn child – a relationship unusual in film, but facilitated by the aesthetic capacities of cinema – the transparency, penetrability and permeability of the maternal body, that which allowed the God-like viewer to see 'inside' explicitly and that has encouraged us to always be mindful of the unborn child, is viscerally realised. The child remains whole.

Abortion and taboo

In *Inside*, the subject position of the film's two foetuses is emphasised for narrative, emotional and visceral effect. This tendency towards privileging the wellbeing of the foetus over that of the mother is also evident in the few horror films that directly engage with the issue of abortion, a fraught political and personal issue that best encapsulates the complex ontological tension between the foetus and the pregnant woman (see Hartouni 1999). This is especially so given that each 'side' of the abortion debate frames its cause with regards to human dignity – either the woman's right to her own bodily autonomy, or the foetus's right to exist as a human subject (Rae 2013). However, despite potentially horrific narrative and aesthetic possibilities, it is highly unusual for abortion to be discussed, let alone depicted, in Anglophone horror film. To address this gap, from here I consider those few representations that do exist in terms of the way that they attempt to negotiate the issues of pregnant and foetal subjectivity. In particular, it is notable that many of these examples feel compelled to engage with the politics of abortion, to the extent that this preoccupation shapes the film's narrative and aesthetic parameters.

As cultural context, abortion is rarely explicitly addressed in American narrative film at all, no matter the genre,[13] even though abortion itself is not uncommon. The United States' Center for Disease Control and Prevention's analysis of reported abortion numbers indicated that in 2012 13.2 in 1000 women aged 15–44 were recorded to have had an abortion (Pazol, Creanga and Jamieson 2015). They note a ratio of 210 recorded abortions for every 1000 live births (Pazol, Creanga and Jamieson 2015), with another estimate suggesting that 30% of US women will have an abortion by age 45 (Jones and Jerman 2014). The taboo in American films, at least, reflects the highly politicised and fraught legal status of abortion in the United States, not its widespread incidence. In their analysis of the impact of religion upon American politics, D'Antonio, Tuch and Baker (2013) highlight abortion as one of a number of issues that accounts for political divisiveness in federal government (p. 43), particularly given the post-*Roe vs Wade* shift in the 1980s to the association of specific political affiliations and fixed political identities with specific stances on abortion (p. 47, pp. 49–56). They state that "At the national level, there is little place for dialogue between [pro-life and pro-choice] positions, and polarization is now at a high point in both houses on Congress", and that controversy over abortion has generated "upheaval that will impact American politics for years to come" (p. 43), particularly in terms of healthcare legislation (pp. 59–61; see also Ekland-Olsen 2013, 25–61). This tension is particularly apparent in American films' treatment of abortion as a 'delicate' and highly-politicised issue, which in turn reflects, perhaps, the long-standing impact of its status as a banned subject, and then an explicitly dis-couraged subject, under the Motion Picture Production Code of America (Hayes 2009). Indeed, director Ridley Scott highlights that the MPAA wanted him to cut a scene from 2012 sci-fi horror *Prometheus* in which a crew-member gives herself a robot-assisted abortion to terminate an alien pregnancy that had been forced upon her, and that the scene's inclusion contributed to the film's less 'family-friendly' R rating (Sperling 2012).

As an aside, the topic is somewhat more visible in American television, particularly on cable networks, a broadcast space that is far less regulated than its networked counterpart and also arguably offers the characters and stories more space to engage with the issue through long-form, serialised storytelling (Levy 2014; Nagy 2012; Press and Cole 1999). From the per-spective of horror, the first season of *American Horror Story* incorporates the issue in a remarkably blatant manner: in the 1920s, the "murder house" at the centre of the first season was an illegal abortion clinic run by the house's original owner, and this history plays a key role in terms of both the themes of the show and the nature of some of the ghosts that haunt the space. Con-sider, though, the response to "Imprint" (2006), a piece directed by prolific Japanese filmmaker Takashi Miike for the horror anthology *Masters of Horror*, a series that I will return to shortly. The hour-long standalone episode, which centres on an American sailor looking for his Japanese lover in 19th-century Japan, features rape, torture, murder, incest and a grotesque parasitic twin, but of particular public concern was the frank representation of an abortion and repeated detailed images of aborted foetuses. Exacerbating this was the episode's form itself, in which a disfigured young Japanese woman, an uncanny woman who may or may not be the sailor's lost-dead-gone girlfriend, tells him her story three times over. Each compulsive retelling may or may not be more honest, for the woman is an unreliable narrator and the oneiric, haunting tone is woozy and unsettling, but each is certainly more horrific: the narrator moves from a helpless victim to the monstrous product of incest, and her mother slides from benevolent midwife to a cruel abortionist who plies her trade on the stony shores of a river. Every iteration re-configures the relationships between the characters, peeling back a sense of decorum to reveal the gynaehorrific underpinnings of the core, incestuous familial relationships at the centre of the story, such that the repeated and sometimes hallucinatory image of aborted foetuses is a visual expression of familial trauma and reproductive horror. The truth, if there is one, perhaps sits in the thrumming space between each overlaid articulation, and is corporeally expressed as the tiny hand with an angry, grotesque face in its palm that extends from the narrator's head – the head of her mangled parasitic twin, her wicked 'little sister'. Ultimately, all sense of tethered, comprehensible rationality dissipates as we lose sense of whether the sailor's perceptions have ever been reliable. Showtime, the premium cable and satellite television network that commissioned the series, deemed the episode to be too explicit to be screened, even though each of the episodes' directors were to be "given their choice of material and freedom from corporate censorship in exchange for creating their work on a tight budget and short schedule" (Kehr 2006). Miike has philosophically responded, "As I was making the film I kept checking to make sure that I wasn't going over the line, but I evidently misestimated [sic] … They decided it would be better to screen it without cuts at film festivals and release it on DVD" (Schilling 2006). As such, it is the only episode of the series to have never screened in full in the United States (although it was broadcast in other territories), and its lack of inclusion is strongly indicative of the degree to which the depiction of abortion is considered taboo and offensive in American culture, even within a supposedly unregulated environment.

Elsewhere, when abortion *is* present in American horror film, it often takes the form of cautionary tale or moral touchstone. It may be presented as a choice of last resort or a choice that is refuted altogether, as in both *Prophecy* and *Rosemary's Baby*, when each pregnant woman insists that she won't consider aborting her baby, despite their fears for the foetus. Indeed, in *Legion*, pregnant waitress Charlie delivers a monologue about how she considered but decided against aborting her child, even though she is terrified to be a mother and isn't sure she wants the child. Her speech frames abortion as a selfish choice, so her willingness to carry the child is something worldly and selfless; her life is insignificant in the shadow of her unborn child and motherhood is both divine duty and penance for a life poorly lived.

Even the mention or thought of abortion carries dangers. This may be the equivalent of invoking a boogeyman: in Canadian proto-slasher *Black Christmas* (1974) level-headed sorority girl Jess is adamant that she is going to have an abortion, despite the vocal protestations of her intense and increasingly pushy boyfriend who tells her that she will be "sorry" if she goes through with it. Her boyfriend is not the film's mysterious killer, 'Billy', but the film's open ending leaves it unstated as to whether Jess's intention to have an abortion has anything to do with the stalker's rampage through the sorority house. This invocation of abortion may also lead to something more explicit. The beginning of Larry Cohen's 1977 film *It's Alive* portrays a woman giving birth to a deformed child, which promptly kills everyone in the delivery room except the mother; there is an insinuation that the child's monstrosity stems from the parents' consideration of abortion. This directly draws from historic assertions that congenital deformities were caused by a woman's monstrous maternal imagination affecting the child *in utero*, thereby "undo [ing] the living capital she is carrying in her womb" (Braidotti 2011, 228) and blasphemously destroying her own creation through a mother-centred assault on male-centric procreative power (Shildrick 2000, 310–11; Braidotti 2011, 228–33).[14] The more recent remake of the film, *It's Alive* (2008), takes this inference a step further by positing that the cannibalistic child's monstrosity was directly caused by the mother, Lenore, who had tried, and failed, to kill her foetus with abortion pills she had purchased online. In the original film, the mother is physically and narratively sidelined; the film deals more with the actions of the father as he exhibits fear and hatred of his child before gradually coming to understand that the grotesque creature is vulnerable and frightened, a process that mirrors his slow acceptance of fatherhood and that forms a connection between father-subject and child-subject that evades the inclusion of the mother. In the remake, as with other films about monstrous motherhood, the needs of the child – both born and unborn – come to overwhelm the mother's capacity to provide.

The monstrous baby of Cohen's *It's Alive* is a clear influence on other films that feature deformed foetuses who survive abortions. In *The Unborn* (1991), Virginia and her husband go to a fertility clinic, but Virginia unwittingly becomes part of a genetic experiment when, as with *Rosemary's Baby*, her husband 'sells' her: he is convinced by the doctor to let Virginia act as an incubator and undergo radical treatment that will make the baby strong and increase its viability. When Virginia sees and experiences the bizarre and violent side-effects and murderous mood swings the treatment is having on other women, she procures a seedy back alley abortion without the knowledge of her husband, who is outraged and believes that she is hysterical and unable to cope with reality. However, the mewling, snapping foetus doesn't die, and Virginia, who feels drawn to its cries, goes back to the dumpster in the alley to retrieve it. The film ends with the mother comforting the creature, although her intention – to kill it or raise it – remains unclear. This association of pregnancy with possession (Graham 1976) and madness (Ussher 2011, 17–20) draws from a clear historic tradition wherein women are denigrated because of their reproductive capacities, deemed unstable and untethered in a manner that looks to the expression of intense emotion and the changes that the pregnant subject undergoes as horrific rather than a mutable, transitory alteration of selfhood and capacity. As Virginia says to her deceitful husband, sarcastically, she'd tell someone about the conspiracy, but no one would believe her as she's paranoid and mentally ill.

In other articulations of abortion, the foetus's subjectivity and capacity to act may come to totally eclipse that of the mother. This is certainly the case in gory exploitation films, which emphasise the image of deformed foetuses to incite fear, disgust, and even laughter. In the lurid and wholly incoherent *Hanger* (2009), a prostitute has her pregnancy violently aborted by her pimp and she dies in the process, but the disfigured foetus lives and as an adult becomes involved in a plan for filial revenge. In *The Suckling* (1990) a woman is coerced into an abortion by her boyfriend, and at the abortion clinic, which inexplicably doubles as a brothel, the aborted foetus is flushed down the toilet. However, it comes into contact with toxic waste in the sewers, mutates into a monster, and then returns to take its revenge by attacking the inhabitants of the bordello. In each of these films the aborted, disposed-of foetus fights back against the abortionists or their mother, exhibiting, perhaps, a greater capacity to act than its mother ever did, while the mother is denigrated for her weakness and her choices, and sometimes objectified through her association with prostitution. There is also a fatalistic sense of maternal fallibility here: if the mother relinquishes the foetus she is framed as failing to adhere to the paradigms of both essential and ideal motherhood, whereas by saving a child she doesn't want she is fulfilling the expectations placed upon her by both patriarchy and, perhaps, religious dogma.

The intersection between politics, religion, and maternal culpability is clearly expressed in the slasher *Red Christmas* (2016), which combines its Australian setting with an Australian-American cast and explicit ongoing nods to the American slasher tradition. The deformed, monstrous Cletus, who survived his abortion 20 years earlier, comes looking for his mother Diane on Christmas Day after the death of his 'father', the fundamentalist Christian zealot who bombed the clinic during the procedure and rescued the foetus from a biohazard bucket. Late in the film, after much of Diane's large family have been killed by the interloper, it is revealed that Cletus was aborted because prenatal testing identified that he had Down Syndrome. Diane had already raised four children, including a son with Down Syndrome, Jerry, and she states that she and her then-terminally ill husband couldn't cope with the idea of raising another child who would need so much specialised care. The film teeters between schlocky excess and artful attempts to shape and manipulate space by using coloured Christmas lights to drench the *mise-en-scène*, rendering the family home-space uncertain and uncanny. It also attempts – although not always successfully – to explore the sense of grief, ambivalence and guilt experienced by Diane, especially as it sits alongside her close relationship with her intellectually disabled adult son and his own recognition that, in some ways, he is a monster to his mother, even if unlike his newfound brother he was a wanted child. Despite the director's suggestion in interviews after the film's festival screenings that the film is if not pro-choice then at least politically balanced (Todd 2016), it offers what I suggest is an appallingly baroque and conservative example of the return of the repressed, in which the jettisoned, abject unborn literally comes back to terrorise and punish its mother and her family. The credits also finish with the web addresses of various organisations, both pro-choice and anti-abortion, and recommendations of films on the topic, which exacerbates this bizarre tone, melding cheap and cheerful exploitation flick with public service announcement. Such a film struggles to find a way to navigate issues of subjectivity and agency, and instead becomes tangled within the politics that it is attempting to interrogate.

'Pro-life' and *Pro-Life*

Each of these films trades on the grotesque image of the aborted foetus and its oppositional relationship to its (sometimes dead) mother, instead of looking to abortion itself. Given the contentious and overwhelmingly political nature of abortion in the United States, it is appropriate that two roughly con-temporaneous films that do centre on the act of abortion itself, as opposed to abortion as a means to an end, are deeply couched in religious and political discourses that centre on the relationship between the pregnant and the foetal subject. The first, *The Life Zone* (2011), is a peculiar independent low budget film that has been framed popularly as "the world's first horror movie to push a pro-life agenda" (Miller 2011). Even though the film's writer and producer Kenneth Del Vecchio, a former American municipal judge and would-be senator, suggests in an interview that the audience will walk away not knowing what the filmmaker's position is (Robb 2011), the film's press release states that the film's "climactic twist" ending is clearly anti-abortion (Lancona 2011). The film is about incarceration and enforced child-birth, and it dramatises the point of view that a woman is a vessel for her foetus and that her rights are (and should be) totally subsumed during the process of pregnancy, such that the strict conceptual binary between woman and foetus is upheld and enforced through a paradigm of conservative ethics. It begins as three women who were in the process of having an abortion wake up to find that they are being held prisoner in a medical facility. They are spoken to via video conference by the Jailer, a sinister middle-aged man who tells them that they have all committed an awful sin. A doctor, a woman ironi-cally named Dr Wise, will take care of them until she delivers all three children simultaneously – a curious requirement that frames the act of birth, on one hand, as something mechanistic and choreographed and, on the other, as a form of shared ecstasy or maternal communion.

The women's incarceration is as much a re-education programme as an attempt to monitor and enforce the pregnancies, in what amounts to an explicit and unpleasant metaphor for the way that the pregnant body is already subject to various forms of surveillance (Lupton 1999, 88–90). The three women, who have diverging opinions on abortion, must spend their seven months in captivity reading and watching pro-life material. As such, although the film is marketed as a horror, the captivity narrative is really a blunt scaffold for a series of Socratic debates on the nature of abortion. Most of these debates are centred on the nature of rights, that is, whether American constitutional rights and the woman's right to self-determination come into conflict with moral rights, although it is clear that the captives' earthly, legal rights sit at odds with those of the powers detaining them. One of the films viewed is *O.B.A.M. Nude (Occidental Births A Monster)* (2009), another low budget film by Del Vecchio and director Rod Weber, which presents a nameless man selling his soul and the souls of all his potential followers to the devil for political gain. The cocaine-snorting marijuana-smoking protagonist of *O.B.A.M. Nude* is clearly a proxy for US President Barack Obama, and the man's socialist dictatorial dream for the United States is one in which everything is mandated by the state and the only 'choice' will be abortion; the devil insists that it is important that such mass murders of the unborn continue.[15] The film's inclusion, when considered along with the other politically conservative films written, produced and directed by Del Vecchio through his company *Justice For All Productions*, contextualises *The Life Zone* as a film not only about abortion, but as a polemical counter-narrative about how abortion is framed within a strongly right-wing, conservative, Catholic discourse: the film-within-a-film becomes an argument-within-an-argument, so the we become just as trapped within the film's political manoeuvring as the women are within the facility. Nonetheless, *The Life Zone* (misleadingly) frames itself as non-partisan and showing "both sides": it seemingly praises the benefits of a democratic political system through the presentation of staged vox pops, but focuses the diegetic and extra-diegetic debates about abortion around a series of straw man arguments, such as whether it is possible to tell at what 'magic' point the foetus becomes a person, a conceit that is repeated at length.

The Life Zone's emphasis on captivity and abduction also draws from the framing narrative and grim, heavily colour-corrected colour palette of films from the torture-centric *Saw* franchise, in which people who are deemed to have somehow transgressed are imprisoned in booby-trapped rooms and asked to prove their willingness to live a better life through acts of extreme suffering and endurance. In the original film (*Saw* 2004), a character is required to saw off his foot to free himself from a manacle. In later films the participants are required to do such things as allow parts of their bodies to be crushed, burned or maimed to liberate themselves from the antagonist Jigsaw's elaborate Rube Goldberg-esque traps, which are often designed to ironically reflect the captives' perceived crimes. In *The Life Zone*, the three women share dreams, such as one that juxtaposes images of abortion against images of insects, Nazism, genocide and slavery, as well as people shouting "abort me" in various languages and mimicking the crying of babies. This shared experience connects their bodies and minds in a manner that ensures that their shared identities and bodily capacities are centred on the bearing of children. This has the peculiar effect of framing the women's incarceration and enforced pregnancies as a type of torture – a contradictory tactic for a film that is inherently natalist. In this sense, not only are the pregnancies an act of suffering and penance, but so too is childbirth. This is made clear in the twist ending: despite a failed attempt to self-abort, the most adamantly pro-choice woman, Staci, gives birth to twins. She remains miserable and in a great deal of pain, in contrast to the beatific motherhood of the other two women, who have come to accept abortion as sinful and regret their actions. Suddenly, the two happy mothers disappear, Dr Wise informs Staci that she is somehow pregnant again, and the mysterious Jailer reveals himself to be Satan and the medical facility, hell. In a punishment fit for Tartarus, Staci will move through the cycle of pregnancy and childbirth for eternity in a corporeal ebb and flow that restricts her ability to be anything but the space in which a foetus will develop. Dr Wise is also a prisoner: she was infertile, which is oddly framed as a personal flaw, and had killed herself when her husband left her to father children with another woman. Her punishment is that she will continue to deliver Staci's children, forcing them both to forever confront that which they did not appreciate in life and to account for their "terrible sins". Despite this, there is no mention of what will happen to all these children; for all the emphasis upon foetal subjectivity and the rights of the unborn, they are ultimately elided in the name of cosmic retribution.

In keen contrast to the conservative Catholic ideology of *The Life Zone* is an hour long standalone episode of the cable television horror anthology *Masters of Horror* titled "Pro-Life" (2007), a piece that is directed by John Carpenter and that uses the near-abortion of a monstrous child to highlight hypocrisy and violence in the anti-abortion movement. The episode draws from the tropes of the religious horror films described earlier in this chapter: a young woman named Angelique has been mysteriously impregnated by some supernatural force, and in desperation she seeks an abortion at a nearby clinic. However, her deeply religious father, Dwayne, is a violent gun-wielding anti-abortion campaigner who is convinced that God has instructed him to personally ensure the baby remains safe, no matter what the human cost. During the 'rescue', he and his sons lay siege to the 'monsters' in the clinic in scenes that explicitly recall high-profile violent attacks against abortion providers, such as those committed by the American Christian terrorist anti-abortion organisation Army of God. Angelique's pregnancy develops at a highly accelerated rate, and its demonic father, who is the one who has been speaking 'God's will' to Dwayne, rises from the earth and makes its way to Angelique. She gives birth, but where Rosemary accepts her role as the mother to a monster, Angelique promptly shoots her monstrous, arachnid offspring in the head, and the demon mournfully collects its body and returns to the abyss.

At the episode's close, Angelique says that God's will has been done, and the ironic pro-choice punch-line of "Pro-Life" is that the abortion, had it have been performed, would have been a way of saving lives. It is not that abortion, itself, was a violent act; instead, Dwayne's rabid evangelicalism and keen enthusiasm for brutality had made him an easy target for the demon's manipulation. As such, "Pro-Life" marks abortion as a complicated and deeply personal issue that cannot be solved or wished away through violence or religious or political dogma. However, even though Angelique's body was claimed by her father as his property, sexually assaulted by a supernatural creature and used as a vessel for a demonic child, she is shown to have a privileged knowledge of her body. She adamantly enforces her bodily sovereignty when she, firstly, goes to the clinic, and secondly, takes matters into her own hands and kills the newborn creature. This is to say that where her monstrous offspring may express the toxicity of those around her, her successful eradication of its unwelcome presence marks a clear statement about her subjective, bodily authority. Her right to choose is demonstrated to have been the difference between life and death. "Pro-Life", then, comes the closest of many of the abortion-centric films discussed so far to privileging the subject position of the pregnant woman, although it nonetheless frames the story in terms of the foetus as monstrous other. This offers a profoundly different message to the other films discussed here: the conservative *The Life Zone*, the gory exploitation films *Hanger* and *The Suckling, Red Christmas*, and *The Unborn*. In each of these films, the foetus and the pregnant woman are pitted against each other in an antagonistic relationship, and as such the pregnant woman either must surrender her autonomy or be eliminated altogether.

This restrictive paradigm clearly emphasises how overwhelming the tendency is to consider pregnant subjectivity within strict binaries between woman and foetus, even given that the aesthetic spaces of cinema are not subject to the same restrictions as the linguistic philosophical construction of the self *vis-à-vis* (an)other, or the I and not-I. I must admit a degree of surprise that there is currently so little alternative aesthetic engagement within this area, even though horror itself offers a space in which explorations of the nature of the traditionally formed, coherent subject-self is troubled. It perhaps highlights a degree of conservativism within the genre, for the examples I have outlined here exhibit a preference to engage with monstrous bodies, be they pregnant, foetal, or something in between, as abject and a threat to one's 'own self' and a sense of coherent, stable subjectivity rather than grotesque in the more life-affirming Bakhtinan sense. More interesting and challenging forms of alternative subjectivity, such as that toyed with during the abstract space of the title sequence of *Inside*, are soon foreclosed upon within the more linear narrative space of the film proper. Similarly, bodies that might be coded as feminine, be they women, houses, environments or otherwise, may express a certain sort of expansiveness that is then attacked, dismantled, repudiated or pulled apart in the name of shoring up the fixed subjectivity of the foetal other. That which is abject is violently excluded; bodies are re-organised and reterritorialised. Monstrous, productive becomings are perhaps touched upon but are quickly refuted, in the name of enforcing stronger walls around the notion of the fixed be-ing, even if there is a sense that a broader threat remains. However, I suggest that this elimination becomes further complicated in films about reproductive technologies: where, in *Inside*, the female body is something that is negotiated, explored, seen through and ultimately torn apart, films that deal with reproductive technology are able to elide the woman altogether, making flesh and form dissolute. This elision is further considered in the next chapter, which assesses the implications of what happens when reproduction is removed in part or entirely from the female reproductive body.

Notes

1 Old English terms for "pregnant" reflect this elasticity: bearn-eaca, literally "child-adding" or "child-increasing;" and geacnod, "increased" (Pregnant 2016).
2 Historically, the quickening was generally considered to be the point at which life begins and the "child was now present" (Addelson 1999, 29), a definition that is still referred to today in some quarters (see Applewhite 1991, 90–2).
3 Through the use of the term 'childless' Battersby perhaps recycles the distinctions that she is trying to critique. 'Childfree' is a more modern term, which reframes the decision to not have children as a proactive and positive one, as opposed to one of loss or lost opportunities, which might construct motherhood as the pinnacle of female experience and a biological and cultural imperative.
4 Sharon Marcus's work on politics and sexual violence (2002) indicates that such modalities can also have dangerous consequences. For example, dominant constructions of power and gender create a misogynist environment of inequalities (p. 391) where men who rape women follow a social script that facilitates a belief in the rapist that he has more strength and power than his victim (p. 390), that is, that emphasises the apparent powerless penetrability of the victim's body. So, where houses can be possessed and broken in to, the construction of women's bodies as a (domestic) inside and a penetrable outside reflects the idea that rape is seen as "the fixed reality of women's lives" so that women are imagined as "already raped" or "inherently rapable" (p. 387). This is also the case for gay male bodies, which are likewise coded as 'penetrable'.
5 Of course, none of this is aimed at any specific man, but a broader tendency in phallocentric thought (Grosz 1995, 55).
6 However, despite her strategic use of essentialist language, it is arguable as to whether Irigaray is able to achieve such repositionings without making them contingent on or recycling essentialist constructions of women's bodies and the feminine (see Moi 2002, 139–42).
7 Even the pregnancy that sits at the centre of teen gothic romance franchise *The Twilight Saga: Breaking Dawn Part 1* (2011) is framed as "special"; Bella, a human, is impregnated by her vampire husband Edward and is consumed from the inside out by her hybrid offspring, who is deemed both exceptional and dangerous. The baby literally breaks Bella's body, and Edward must perform an emergency caesarean (with his teeth!) that kills Bella, which leads to her conversion to vampirism.
8 This is parodied in the horror comedy *Hell Baby* (2013): the film's demonic birth scene directly references the exorcism sequences of *The Exorcist,* as the possessed birthing mother is tended to by two chain-smoking priests, who form the Vatican's "elite exorcism" team.
9 It is worth noting though that Louisiana is also framed as a mystical 'Other' within American culture, in part due to its historic association with supernatural subcultures such as New Orleans voodoo, a syncretic folk religion that arrived developed within the African diaspora following the arrival of slave populations in the 18th century. Louisiana and New Orleans are also important within the

tradition of the literary Southern Gothic (Boyd 2002) and Bernice M. Murphy (2013) highlights Louisiana as a key site in what she calls the American backwoods horror film (p. 151). Nonetheless, much of the terror of the rural gothic comes from the positioning of the radical, monstrous Other within the United States.

10 It is of interest that the film's ending ignores the possibility of abortion. The final moments are full of dread, leaving unarticulated the horror that Katherine is pregnant with the Antichrist, and that the child will (presumably) bring about the end of the world. It may be a reflection of the religious tone of the film, its setting in an area known for its Christian heritage, or Katherine's previous role as an ordained minister, or merely narratively expedient, but it is a peculiar omission and one that will be discussed later in the chapter.

11 An example of such changes in the United States is the state of Mississippi's failed Initiative 26, a 2011 proposition, which "would [have] amend[ed] the Mississippi Constitution to define the word 'person' or 'persons', as those terms are used in Article III of the state constitution, to include "every human being from the moment of fertilization, cloning, or the functional equivalent thereof" (Mississippi Life Begins 2011). This would mean that a fertilised egg would be accorded the same rights – legal and human – as any other citizen. This Mississippi initiative is one of a number of similar American legislative challenges to have emerged in the last ten years; however, they are ostensibly a means by which to criminalise the practise of abortion in defiance of *Roe v Wade*, in which the US Supreme court ratified a woman's right to an abortion so long as the foetus isn't 'viable' (that is, able to survive outside the mother's womb). This is demonstrated by pro-life lobby group Personhood USA's claim that their definition of a person "terrifies the pro-abortion foes!" as "they know that if we clearly define the preborn baby as a person, they will have the same right to life as all Americans do!" (What is Personhood? 2014)

12 Aside from the debate over personhood, foetuses do have legal standing, such as in cases of inheritance or parental custody and within the law of torts. In the United States, a child *in utero* can be considered a legal victim (specifically, of foetal homicide) under the *Unborn Victims of Violence Act of 2004 (Public Law 108–212)* if they are killed or injured during the commission of a violent crime – although the perpetrator does not have to have been aware that the mother was pregnant for the law to be in effect. A highly unusual case in New Zealand focused on a pregnant woman, "Nikki", who was to give birth during the filming of a pornographic film. The chief social worker for the Department of Child, Youth and Family Services (CYFS) applied to the High Court to have the unborn child placed under the guardianship of the court under the Guardianship Act 1968 to protect its rights and interests until it was born. The application, which was granted, also prohibited the filming of the labour and birth, the simulation of those images, any publication of images of the unborn child, and publication of any images of information that would identify the unborn child. However, the court made clear that its decision did not imply that Nikki would be an unfit mother – although it suggested that perhaps her interest in stardom was overriding her better judgement – and that the rights of the mother must not, where possible, be impinged upon by the court: that would be "an invasive step which should only be taken for very good reasons" (Heath 2003, s. 28; see also Bartlett 2003).

13 On the other hand, abortion appears more frequently in some Asian horror films: in Thai horror film *The Unborn Child (Sop Dek 2002)* (2011) increasingly strange events are caused by the vengeful ghosts of foetuses that have been unceremoniously dumped in a storage locker by a back-alley abortionist. As a 'pulled from the headlines' story, it references the discovery in 2010 of the remains of 2002 illegally aborted foetuses in a Buddhist temple, where they had been hidden as they waited to be incinerated. In Hong Kong film *Dumplings* (2004), which was

originally released as a short film as part of an East Asian horror film collaboration *Three… Extremes* (2004), a female chef makes 'special' dumplings from aborted foetuses, which she claims have rejuvenating properties. Her client, Mrs Li, enjoys her newfound youth and increased libido and becomes dependent on the dumplings so she helps the chef acquire new 'ingredients'. Abortion, here, is a gruesome way of addressing vanity and hubris, rather than a political act.

14 Steffen Hantke suggests that films about monstrous infants, such as *It's Alive,* reflect social anxieties about pharmaceuticals and reproductive technology, such as fears about impact of the oral contraceptive pill (released in 1960), as well as the withdrawal of the sedative Thalidomide from the market in 1961 after it was shown to have caused serious foetal abnormalities (Hantke 2011, 110)

15 United States Supreme Court concerns about the impropriety of Del Vecchio publicising *O.B.A.M. Nude* while he was employed as a municipal court judge led to Del Vecchio standing down from his position (Pérez-peña 2010).

Bibliography

'A blood soaked interview with the Inside (À L'intérieur) directors' 2007, *Twitch,* accessed December 16, 2013, from <http://twitchfilm.com/2007/12/40th-sitges-a-blood-soaked-interview-with-the-inside-a-linterieur-directors.html>.

Addelson, K P 1999, 'The emergence of the fetus', in L M Morgan & M W Michaels (eds), *Fetal subjects, feminist positions*, Philadelphia, PA: University of Pennsylvania Press, pp. 26–42.

Applewhite, E J 1991, *Paradise mislaid: birth, death & the human predicament of being biological*, 1st ed., New York: St Martin's Press.

Arnold, S 2013, *Maternal horror film: melodrama and motherhood*, Houndmills, Basingstoke, UK and New York, NY: Palgrave Macmillan.

Bakhtin, M M 1984, *Rabelais and his world*, Bloomington, IN: Indiana University Press.

Bartlett, S 2003, 'Wardship of unborn children', *Social Work Now: The Practice Journal of Child, Youth and Family*, 24, pp. 5–9.

Battersby, C 1998, *The phenomenal woman: feminist metaphysics and the patterns of identity*, Cambridge, UK: Polity Press.

Berenstein, R J 1990, 'Mommie dearest: aliens, *Rosemary's Baby* and mothering', *The Journal of Popular Culture*, 24(2), pp. 55–73.

Blaetz, R 1992, 'In search of the mother tongue: childbirth and the cinema', *The Velvet Light Trap*, 29, pp. 15–20.

Boyd, M 2002, 'Gothicism', in J M Flora, L H MacKethan & T W Taylor (eds), *The companion to southern literature: themes, genres, places, people, movements, and motifs*, Baton Rouge, LA: LSU Press, pp. 311–316.

Braidotti, R 2011, *Nomadic subjects: embodiment and sexual difference in contemporary feminist theory*, 2nd ed., New York: Columbia University Press.

Brown, L M 2005, 'Feminist theory and the erosion of women's reproductive rights: the implications of fetal personhood laws and in vitro fertilization', *American University Journal of Gender, Social Policy & the Law*, 13, pp. 87–107.

Buklijas, T & Hopwood, N 2008, 'Making visible embryos', *Making visible embryos*, accessed January 3, 2014, from <http://www.hps.cam.ac.uk/visibleembryos/>.

Calhoun, A 2012, 'The criminalization of bad mothers', *The New York Times*, accessed December 16, 2013, from <http://www.nytimes.com/2012/04/29/magazine/the-criminalization-of-bad-mothers.html>.

Chamberlain, P & Hardisty, J 2000, 'The importance of the political "framing" of abortion – reproducing patriarchy: reproductive rights under siege', *The Public Eye Magazine*, 14(34), accessed January 2, 2014, from <http://www.publiceye.org/maga zine/v14n1/ReproPatriarch-07.html>.

Cixous, H 2010, 'The laugh of the Medusa' in M Segarra (ed), *The portable Cixous*, New York: Columbia University Press, pp. 27–39.

Creed, B 1993, *The monstrous-feminine: film, feminism, psychoanalysis*, London and New York: Routledge.

Curtis, B 2008, *Dark places: the haunted house in film*, London: Reaktion.

D'Antonio, W V, Tuch, S A & Baker, J R 2013, *Religion, politics, and polarization: how religiopolitical conflict is changing Congress and American democracy*, Lanham: Rowman & Littlefield Publishers.

Deleuze, G & Guattari, F 2004, *A thousand plateaus: capitalism and schizophrenia*, London: Continuum.

Durán, G 1991, 'Women and houses – from Poe to Allende', *Confluencia*, 6(2), pp. 9–15.

Dworkin, A 1997, *Intercourse*, New York: Simon & Schuster.

Ekland-Olson, S 2013, *Life and death decisions: the quest for morality and justice in human societies*, Hoboken: Taylor and Francis, accessed December 16, 2013, from <http://public.eblib.com/EBLPublic/PublicView.do?ptiID=1122876>.

Fischer, L 1992, 'Birth traumas: parturition and horror in "Rosemary's Baby"', *Cinema Journal*, 31(3), pp. 3–18.

Freeman, R K, Garite, T J & Nageotte, M P 2003, *Fetal heart rate monitoring*, Philadelphia, PA: Lippincott Williams & Wilkins.

Freud, S 2008, *The essentials of psycho-analysis*, Reprint ed., London: Random House.

Gatens, M 1996, *Imaginary bodies: ethics, power, and corporeality*, London and New York: Routledge.

Gavey, N 2005, *Just sex?: the cultural scaffolding of rape*, London and New York: Routledge.

Gold, B K 1998, '"The house I live in is not my own": women's bodies in Juvenal's Satires', *Arethusa*, 31(3), pp. 369–386.

Gordon, B 1996, 'Woman's domestic body: the conceptual conflation of women and interiors in the Industrial Age', *Winterthur Portfolio*, 31(4), pp. 281–301.

Graham, H 1976, 'The social image of pregnancy: pregnancy as spirit possession', *Sociological Review*, 24(2), pp. 291–308.

Grant, B K 1996, 'Rich and strange: the yuppie horror film', *Journal of Film and Video*, 48(1/2), pp. 4–16.

Grosz, E 1995, 'Women, chora, dwelling', in S Watson & K Gibson (eds), *Postmodern cities and spaces*, Oxford, UK and Cambridge, MA: Blackwell, pp. 47–58.

Hantke, S 2011, 'My baby ate the dingo: the visual construction of the monstrous infant in horror film', *Lit: Literature Interpretation Theory*, 22(2) pp. 96–112.

Haraway, D J 1997, *Modest_Witness@Second_Millennium.FemaleMan_Meets_Onco-Mouse: feminism and technoscience*, New York: Routledge.

Hartouni, V 1999, 'Epilogue: reflections on abortion politics and the practices called person', in L M Morgan & M W Michaels (eds), *Fetal subjects, feminist positions*, Philadelphia, PA: University of Pennsylvania Press, pp. 296–304.

Hayes, D 2009, 'The Production Code of the Motion Picture Industry (1930–1967)', *The Motion Picture Production Code*, accessed December 10, 2013, from <http://productioncode.dhwritings.com/multipleframes_productioncode.php>.

Heath, P 2003, 'Re an Unborn Child', 1*NZLR*, Hamilton: New Zealand High Court, p. 115.

Irigaray, L 1985a, *Speculum of the other woman*, Ithaca, NY: Cornell University Press.

Irigaray, L 1985b, *This sex which is not one*, Ithaca, NY: Cornell University Press.

Irigaray, L 1992, *Elemental passions*, London: Athlone Press.

Irigaray, L 1993a, *An ethics of sexual difference*, Ithaca, NY: Cornell University Press.

Irigaray, L 1993b, *Sexes and genealogies*, New York: Columbia University Press.

Johnsen, D E 1986, 'The creation of fetal rights: conflicts with women's constitutional rights to liberty, privacy, and equal protection', *The Yale Law Journal*, 9(3), pp. 599–625.

Johnson, K C 1997, 'Randomized controlled trials as authoritative knowledge: keeping an ally from becoming a threat to North American midwifery practice', in R Davis-Floyd & C F Sargent (eds), *Childbirth and authoritative knowledge: cross-cultural perspectives*, Berkeley, CA: University of California Press, pp. 350–365.

Jones, D 2002, *Horror: a thematic history in fiction and film*, London: Arnold.

Jones, R 2013, *Irigaray*, Hoboken: Wiley.

Jones, R K & Jerman, J 2014, 'Abortion incidence and service availability in the United States, 2011', *Perspectives on Sexual and Reproductive Health*, 46(1), pp. 3–14.

Joyce, K 2005, 'Appealing images: magnetic resonance imaging and the production of authoritative knowledge', *Social Studies of Science*, 35(3), pp. 437–462.

Kaplan, E A 1992, *Motherhood and representation: the mother in popular culture and melodrama*, London and New York; Routledge.

Kehr, D 2006, 'Horror film made for Showtime will not be shown', *The New York Times*, accessed December 18, 2013, from <http://www.nytimes.com/2006/01/19/arts/television/19horr.html>.

Kilby, J & Lury, C 2000, 'Introduction', in S Ahmed, J Kilby, M McNeil, & B Skeggs (eds), *Transformations: thinking through feminism*, London and New York: Routledge, pp. 1–23.

King, S 1982, *Stephen King's Danse macabre*, London and Sydney: Futura.

Kristeva, J 1982, *Powers of horror: an essay on abjection*, New York: Columbia University Press.

Kristeva, J 1985, 'Stabat Mater', *Poetics Today*, 6(1/2), pp. 133–152.

Lancona, C 2011, 'Press release: NJ Senate candidate / Hollywood filmmaker premieres anti-abortion movie starring multiple Academy Award & Emmy winners', *PR Urgent: a free press release service*, accessed December 18, 2013, from <http://www.prurgent.com/2011-05-23/pressrelease172535.htm>.

Levy, E 2014, '"You killed our baby!": Cristina Yang and the breaking of the abortion taboo in *Grey's Anatomy*', *TV/Series*, 5, accessed September 9, 2016, from <https://tvseries.revues.org/447?lang=en>.

Longhurst, R 2008, *Maternities: gender, bodies and space*, New York: Routledge.

Lupton, D 1999, 'Risk and the ontology of pregnant embodiment', in D Lupton (ed), *Risk and sociocultural theory: new directions and perspectives*, Cambridge, UK: Cambridge University Press, pp. 59–85.

Mansfield, N 2000, *Subjectivity: theories of the self from Freud to Haraway*, New York: New York University Press.

Marcus, S 2002, 'Fighting bodies, fighting words: a theory and politics of rape prevention', in J Butler & J W Scott (eds), *Feminists theorize the political*, New York: Routledge, pp. 385–403, accessed November 1, 2013, from <http://academiccommons.columbia.edu/catalog/ac:157470>.

Michaels, M W 1999, 'Fetal galaxies: some questions about what we see', in L M Morgan & M W Michaels (eds), *Fetal subjects, feminist positions*, Philadelphia, PA: University of Pennsylvania Press, pp. 113–132.

Miller, J 2011, 'Low-budget horror "Life Zone" pushes pro-life Message… sorta', *NextMovie*, accessed December 18, 2013, from <http://www.nextmovie.com/blog/low-budget-horror-life-zone-pushes-pro-life-message-sorta/>.

'Mississippi Life Begins at the Moment of Fertilization Amendment, Initiative 26 (2011)' 2011, *Ballotpedia: an interactive almanac of U.S. politics*, accessed December 16, 2013, from <http://ballotpedia.org/Mississippi_Life_Begins_at_the_Moment_of_Fertilization_Amendment,_Initiative_26_(2011)>.

Mitchell, L M 2001, *Baby's first picture: ultrasound and the politics of fetal subjects*, Toronto: University of Toronto Press.

Moi, T 2002, *Sexual/textual politics: feminist literary theory*, 2nd ed., London and New York: Routledge.

Morgan, L M 1999, 'Materializing the fetal body, or, what are those corpses doing in biology's basement?', in L M Morgan & M W Michaels (eds), *Fetal subjects, feminist positions*, Philadelphia, PA: University of Pennsylvania Press, pp. 43–60.

Morice-Brubaker, S 2012, '"Symbolic" personhood bill could kill', *Religion Dispatches*, accessed December 16, 2013, from <http://religiondispatches.org/dispatches/sarahmoricebrubaker/5708/_symbolic__personhood_bill_could_kill___/>.

Murphy, B M 2013, *The rural gothic in American popular culture: backwoods horror and terror in the wilderness*, Basingstoke, UK: Palgrave Macmillan.

Nagy, E 2012, 'Things we don't talk about in primetime: examining the abortion storylines on Girls, SATC and Grey's', *In Our Words*, accessed December 17, 2013, from <http://inourwordsblog.wordpress.com/2012/05/02/9146/>.

Nakahara, T 2009, 'Making up monsters: set and costume design in horror film', in I Conrich (ed), *Horror zone: the cultural experience of contemporary horror cinema*, London: I.B. Tauris & Co., pp. 139–151, accessed February 17, 2014, from <http://public.eblib.com/EBLPublic/PublicView.do?ptiID=676670>.

Newman, K 1996, *Fetal positions: individualism, science, visuality*, Stanford, CA: Stanford University Press.

Newman, K 2011, *Nightmare movies: horror on screen since the 1960s*, London: Bloomsbury Publishing.

Nilsson, L 1965, 'The drama of life before birth', *Life*, pp. 54–70.

Nilsson, L 1990, *A child is born*, Completely new ed., New York: Delacorte Press/Seymour Lawrence.

Oliver, K 2012, *Knock me up, knock me down: images of pregnancy in Hollywood films*, New York: Columbia University Press.

Pazol, K, Creanga, A A & Jamieson, D J 2015, *Abortion surveillance – United States, 2012*, Centre for Disease Control and Prevention, accessed September 9, 2016, from <http://www.cdc.gov/mmwr/preview/mmwrhtml/ss6410a1.htm>.

Pérez-peña, R 2010, 'Filmmaker, pressured, quits as New Jersey judge', *The New York Times*, accessed December 18, 2013, from <http://www.nytimes.com/2010/05/31/nyregion/31judge.html>.

Petchesky, R P 1987, 'Fetal images: the power of visual culture in the politics of reproduction', *Feminist Studies*, 13(2), pp. 263–292.

Potts, A 2002, *The science/fiction of sex: feminist deconstruction and the vocabularies of heterosex*, London and New York: Routledge.

Powell, A 2005, *Deleuze and horror film*, Edinburgh: Edinburgh University Press.

'Pregnant' 2016, *Etymology Online*, accessed December 15, 2013, from <http://www.etymonline.com/index.php?term=pregnant&allowed_in_frame=0>.

Press, A L & Cole, E R 1999, *Speaking of abortion: television and authority in the lives of women*, Chicago: University of Chicago Press.

Rae, S 2013, 'The language of human dignity in the abortion debate', in S Dilley & N J Palpant (eds), *Human dignity in bioethics*, Hoboken: Taylor and Francis, pp. 219–238, accessed December 16, 2013, from <http://public.eblib.com/EBLPublic/PublicView.do?ptiID=1122866>.

Raymond, J G 1995, *Women as wombs: reproductive technologies and the battle over women's freedom*, North Melbourne, Vic.: Spinifex Press.

Robb, A 2011, 'Pro-life horror film "The Life Zone" premieres at Hoboken International Film Festival', *The Jersey Journal – NJ.com*, accessed December 18, 2013, from <http://www.nj.com/hobokennow/index.ssf/2011/06/pro-life_horror_film_the_life.html>.

Roberts, J 2013, *The visualised foetus: a cultural and political analysis of ultrasound imagery*, Farnham, UK and Burlington, VT: Ashgate.

Sandlos, K 2000, 'Unifying forces: rhetorical reflections on a pro-choice image', in S Ahmed, J Kilby, C Lury, M McNeil, & B Skeggs (eds), *Thinking through feminism*, London and New York: Routledge, pp. 77–91.

Schilling, M 2006, 'Takashi Miike makes his mark', *The Japan Times*, accessed December 18, 2013, from <http://www.japantimes.co.jp/culture/2006/06/23/culture/takashi-miike-makes-his-mark/>.

Shepard, A C 2010, 'In the abortion debate, words matter', *NPR.org*, accessed February 24, 2014, from <http://www.npr.org/blogs/ombudsman/2010/03/in_the_abortion_debate_words_m_1.html>.

Shildrick, M 1997, *Leaky bodies and boundaries: feminism, postmodernism and (bio)ethics*, London and New York: Routledge.

Shildrick, M 2000, 'Monsters, marvels and metaphysics: beyond the powers of horror', in S Ahmed, J Kilby, C Lury, M McNeil, & B Skeggs (eds), *Thinking through feminism*, London and New York: Routledge, pp. 303–315.

Sneddon, A 2013, *Autonomy*, New York: Bloomsbury Publishing.

Sperling, N 2012, '"Prometheus": Noomi Rapace says she gutted out a "psychological meltdown"', *Hero Complex – movies, comics, pop culture – Los Angeles Times*, accessed September 9, 2016, from <http://herocomplex.latimes.com/movies/noomi-rapace-on-her-psychological-meltdown-filming-prometheus/>.

Stabile, C A 1999, 'The traffic in fetuses', in L M Morgan & M W Michaels (eds), *Fetal subjects, feminist positions*, Philadelphia, PA: University of Pennsylvania Press, pp. 133–158.

Taylor, J S 2008, *The public life of the fetal sonogram: technology, consumption, and the politics of reproduction*, New Brunswick, NJ: Rutgers University Press.

Telotte, J P 2001, *Science fiction film*, Cambridge, UK: Cambridge University Press.

Todd, A 2016, 'Fantasia Fest Review: Red Christmas', *Birth.Movies.Death.*, accessed December 16, 2016, from <http://birthmoviesdeath.com/2016/07/26/fantasia-fest-review-red-christmas>.

Tuana, N 1993, *The less noble sex: scientific, religious, and philosophical conceptions of woman's nature*, Bloomington, IN: Indiana University Press.

Tyler, I 2000, 'Reframing pregnant embodiment', in S Ahmed, J Kilby, C Lury, M McNeil, & B Skeggs (eds), *Thinking through feminism*, London and New York: Routledge, pp. 288–302.

Tyler, I 2004, 'Skin-tight: celebrity, pregnancy and subjectivity', in S Ahmed & J Stacey (eds), *Thinking through the skin*, London: Routledge, pp. 69–83.

'Unborn Victims of Violence Act of 2004' 2004, United States Government Publishing Office, accessed September 9, 2016, from <https://www.gpo.gov/fdsys/pkg/PLAW-108publ212/html/PLAW-108publ212.htm>.

Ussher, J M 2011, *The madness of women: myth and experience*, London and New York: Routledge.

Valerius, K 2005, '*Rosemary's Baby*, gothic pregnancy, and fetal subjects', *College Literature*, 32(3), pp. 116–135.

'What is Personhood?' 2014, *Personhood USA*, accessed March 2, 2014, from <http://www.personhoodusa.com/about-us/what-is-personhood/>.

Whisnant, R 2010, '"A woman's body is like a foreign country": thinking about national and bodily sovereignty', in R Whisnant & P DesAutels (eds), *Global feminist ethics*, Lanham: Rowman & Littlefield, pp. 155–176.

Williams, L 1991, 'Film bodies: gender, genre, and excess', *Film Quarterly*, 44(4), pp. 2–13.

Williams, T 1996, *Hearths of darkness: the family in the American horror film*, Madison, NJ: Fairleigh Dickinson University Press.

Wood, R 1978, 'Return of the repressed', *Film Comment*, 14(4), pp. 24–42.

Wood, R 2003, *Hollywood from Vietnam to Reagan– and beyond*, Expanded and rev. ed., New York: Columbia University Press.

Young, I M 1990, 'Pregnant embodiment: subjectivity and alienation', in *Throwing like a girl and other essays in feminist philosophy and social theory*, Bloomington, IN: Indiana University Press, pp. 160–176.

3   Not of woman born

Mad science, reproductive technology and the reconfiguration of the subject

Reproductive technologies profoundly reconfigure the sexed body. They expand our understandings of what it means to procreate, to control or augment fertility, to be conceived and 'wanted', and to be parents, donors of genetic material, and born subjects. They offer up the possibility of family configurations that exist outside of the normative model of the heterosexual nuclear family, and they enable us to make choices about our reproductive lives that have never before been available. The ongoing development of reproductive technologies represents new frontiers in science and technology, but as we consider what it means to alter, reroute, augment or displace 'natural' processes, especially processes that have fundamentally scaffolded our everyday social structures, they can also become ethical quagmires and profoundly charged sites of struggle and contestation. The horror genre, with its interest in subjectivity, corporeality, fear and instability, is a conceptual space where anxieties around the intersections of technology, women's bodies and reproduction emerge, clash and bleed out. The possibility of the creation of biological life without and outside of the female body is a particularly resonant and recurring trope within science fiction and horror. It is one that explores the heady "mythology of technology" (Broege 1988, 197), but in doing so it sharply challenges the psychological and corporeal autonomy of the women who populate these films in a way that often forces conjugation, as opposed to negotiating or inviting it. Horror films explore new dynamic bodily and subject configurations that might be considered monstrous in the term's most interesting and generative sense; the term 'teratology', of course, originates from the Greek *teras*, which means malformed, monster, and marvel in the sense of the extraordinary instead of simply the disfigured or abnormal. It also means omen or sign, so perhaps the use of speculative gynaehorror to explore the potentialities of reproductive science might be a form of teratoscopy, or divination through monstrosity. Yet gynaehorror films about reproductive technologies tend to be conservative rather than radical, even when the braided threat and promise of novel and productive molecular encounters is expressed aesthetically in complex, even ambivalent ways.

In this chapter I develop my discussion of pregnant women in horror films from the previous chapter by considering the issues at stake in horror films about reproductive technologies – a thematic substrain that I will refer to as reproductive technohorror. These films overlay horror and science fiction with anxieties and queries about technology, biology, sex and gender. They serve to interrogate the power dynamics that emerge from the resonant interactions between science and technology and what is thought of, in opposition, as 'natural' or 'human', for even though intersections between the human and the machine (as a specific configuration of technology) have been occurring for hundreds of years (Braidotti 2002, 236), the explicit intersection of the reproductive with machinic technology is relatively new. Indeed, through the narrative and aesthetic capacities of cinema they expand what it might specifically mean in a biological, corporeal sense to *be* human, especially as the notion of the human has been historically intertwined with the privileging of the ideal (human, majoritarian, adult, male, able-bodied...) subject. The living products of reproductive technologies challenge truth claims that refract through a particularly static type of culturally and historically intelligible body. They challenge an anthropocentric view of subjectivity and identity, just as those whose organic bodies might incorporate other materials or technologies necessarily shift focus from the construct of the nominally, traditionally human to the perpetual emergence of the posthuman, from the unitary 'one' to the diverse somatechnical hybrid in all its becomings, in a manner that refutes any division between nature and culture (Braidotti 2013). This speaks to degrees of wonder, anxiety, curiosity and dread that may accompany the expansion of epistemological and ontological loci away from the limited scope and capacity of the ideal subject; as Judith Halberstam and Ira Livingstone (1995) note, "History as a social or chronological history is dying with the white male of western metaphysics" (p. 3). Culturally, reproductive technologies contribute to the broader social intelligibility of technology, as well as alternative configurations of multivalent relationships and ethics, but they also consider what might be at stake when we consider the implications or conditions of scientific progress and the nature of scientists themselves. These competing hopes and anxieties often play out in and around the material, reproductive bodies of women, for the rerouting of processes of biological reproduction necessarily de- and re-territorialises female reproductive bodies, reshaping their capacities, corporealities and temporalities.

For the purposes of this discussion, reproductive technologies include (but aren't limited to) contraception, prognostics and abortion, alongside assisted reproductive technologies (ARTs) such as cryopreservation (of sperm, oocytes (eggs) or fertilised embryos), embryo transfer, artificial insemination and cloning. These technologies create a philosophical, discursive and physical space within which biology and technology intersect, especially in terms of their fictional and filmic representations, which are themselves technological interventions with our own perceiving bodies. A tension exists in reproductive science between the role of the body (or the embodied individual) and that of the over-seer scientist, as well as within how reproductive processes might occur both within and without of a body or bodies. For instance, *in vitro* fertilisation (IVF) may be considered an 'embodied' technology, in that although conception itself occurs outside of the body, the process depends on the presence of someone with a uterus to receive the embryos and gestate the foetus: eggs, be they from the prospective mother herself or a donor, are fertilised by sperm within a fluid medium outside of the human body, and these fertilised eggs are implanted into the uterus. There are two clear strands, too, running through these examples: the suggestion that technology is imposed upon the human, and the supposition that the human (as biological, as material) is insufficient and needs (even desires) augmentation (see MacCormack 2012, 8). Either way, filmic engagements with reproductive technology do not always rely on the narrative or audio-visual presence of a physical maternal body.

One of the difficulties that arises in discussing these processes is that reproductive technologies facilitate pregnancy and birth for a broad variety of people, each with varied gender and sexual identities and sexual genetic variations, yet the language we have to describe these processes remains profoundly (hetero)normative, as do assumptions about issues such as who might contribute biological materials such as eggs and semen, who might become pregnant, and so on. In this chapter, when I speak about the processes of reproductive technologies in general terms – rather than with regards to specific characters within films, or in specific instances – my language is deliberately broad stroke. This is not to discount the diverse experiences of individuals who utilise these technologies (for example, the experience of trans* men who carry pregnancies). Instead, I wish to explore the ways that these technologies operate conceptually, let alone practically, within a social field that is still largely structured along binaries such as male/female, masculine/feminine, nature/science, inside/outside, penetrated/penetrator and mother/father, and it is these dualities that underpin many of the assumptions that are being critiqued in this chapter. Further, an acknowledgement of the role of such binary structures, such majoritarian politics, facilitates a consideration of the interesting spaces and materials that exist around, through and between them, for in acknowledging these constructs as sets of aggregates, not fixed states and ossified relationships, we can trouble their edges and the spaces between them and acknowledge that the I and the Other are always already connected and connecting.

In the previous chapter I looked to both the narrative and aesthetic parameters of horror cinema, arguing that horror films that centre on pregnancy exhibit a compulsion to construct and actively shore up an oppositional relationship between pregnant-self and foetal-other, even though the aesthetic languages and capacities of cinema offer extraordinary scope in terms of the way alternative, non-binary subjectivities might be expressed and formed. Here, I posit that reproductive technohorrors also tend to abstract, displace or reconfigure embodied reproductive female subjectivities through both narrative and visual languages. However, where horror films about pregnancy may still present their female protagonists as 'whole' or molar (albeit side-lined) subjects within the narrative scope of the film, the aesthetic exploration of reproductive technohorror exhibits a tendency to elide or even actively eradicate actual female bodies and subjects, aggressively attempting to remove their visual traces, instead of looking to provocative or generative molecular interactions between bodies and materials, be they organic, inorganic, technological, mechanistic or otherwise. Given the long-standing, reductive metonymic association of the womb (and therefore the capacity to reproduce) with the embodied female subject, this speaks to a compulsion to remove the female subject from the process for which she has been historically necessary. As I will later argue, this may be emancipatory; decentralising potential reproductive capacity profoundly remaps the historical configuration and subjugation of the embodied female subject and troubles phallocentric structures of power and control. This emancipation, and these technologies, may also be threatening. In her psychoanalytic account of abjection and defilement, Julia Kristeva (1982) suggests that rituals and taboos that work to protect the self from the liminal dissonance of abomination and impurity, to ensure that the body is 'clean and proper', are a way of removing evidence of our "debt to nature" – that is, the traces of the messy, abject maternal body, the body-space from which we were expelled (p. 102). At its most horrific, reproductive technohorror posits that this debt has been settled; the lingering 'horror' of the maternal body and the allegedly in-dividual subject's one-time connection to and reliance on the body of another is thus resolved, and the reproductive body simultaneously co-opted and renounced. Maternal origin is no longer a problem for the implicitly whole, masculine/male subject.

As such, where horror films about pregnancy express a great deal of dis-ease about female subjectivity, often pitting the foetus or unborn against the pregnant woman in both narrative and visual terms, horror films about reproductive technologies deal with the slippery, permeable conceptual and biological boundaries between self and other by (re-)framing the female, embodied self as entirely expendable. In gynaehorror films such as *Rosemary's Baby* (1968) and *Inside* (2007), even when the woman's subjectivity and sense of self is undermined, or her fecund body torn to pieces, she remains aesthetically tangible and visibly present. In reproductive technohorror and films about reproductive 'mad' science, which situate the act of conception and even gestation itself outside of the body of the woman, the gynaehorrific outcome is that this erasure or displacement is taken further. The pregnant subject herself is deemed irrelevant or unnecessary, and she is aesthetically or visually quite literally erased. The horror of such films exceeds their narrative content. Instead, I suggest that they explore, with startling clarity and imagination, some of the ways that biological reproduction is embedded within hegemonic constructions of gender and power. This is a framework of knowledge in which masculine scientific rationality attempts to control or dominate nature, which is implicitly feminised as Mother and maternal environment. The outcome is rarely in the favour of the woman herself.

The ur-text in the area of reproductive technohorror is Mary Shelley's immensely influential 1818 novel *Frankenstein, or, the Modern Prometheus* (1988 [1831]). Its themes and concerns underpin many of the films discussed here, let alone the broader conceptualisation of reproductive technologies themselves, and as Judith Halberstam (1995) indicates, its importance within modern mythology and the "cultural history of fear and prejudice", let along the specific histories of the Gothic and the novel, "cannot be emphasised too strongly" (p. 28). Early in the novel, the titular Dr Frankenstein muses on the nature of the human body:

> Whence, I often asked myself, did the principle of life proceed? It was a bold question, and one which has ever been considered as a mystery; yet with how many things are we upon the brink of becoming acquainted, if cowardice or carelessness did not restrain our inquiries. (pp. 43–4)

Dr Frankenstein's first-person narrative frames his impassioned quest for the source of life as a brave, Romantic and noble act of (male) exploration and conquest, and one whose mystery might grant him power over life and death. His achievement comes about through robust investigation, tenacious research and the application of his own fearsome intellect to the natural world around him. Yet, Frankenstein's association with the mythical Titan Prometheus, who stole fire from the god Zeus and gifted it to humanity, suggests that this knowledge – this technology – is a sacred secret that he was never meant to have uncovered, and that this sacrilegious transgression will incur some form of divine comeuppance. It is significant that by discovering the secret of life through the dissection and analysis of the dead and decaying his work explicitly removes the 'spark' of creation from the fleshy strictures of the *living* body. Dr Frankenstein's goal, to create something approximating life in his laboratory through the re-animation of the dead, is both an overt act of dominion over nature and an implicitly misogynistic attempt to 'liberate' reproduction and the creation of life from heterosexual coupling and from the body of woman, thus rendering her an unnecessary part of reproduction. He fulfils what Rosi Braidotti (2011) calls the "alchemist's dream", for "Once reproduction becomes the pure results of mental efforts, the appropriation of the feminine is complete" (p. 235); by claiming and conceiving of this feminine power Dr Frankenstein destroys it (see MacCormack 2012, 2–3). This knowledge may be forbidden, in that glimpsing the origin of life may necessarily destroy one's own, but the allure of such singular knowledge and its (re) productive potential are compelling enough to warrant a perpetual return to and intervention with the site of temptation. From here, I outline this tangled intersection of gender, power and technology, with a view to exposing the uncertain dissonant tensions that exists when female subjectivity is both predicated on and potentially uncoupled from reproductive processes.

Science, culture and masculinity

The horror genre's exploration of reproductive technologies is shaped by the way that science (as something that is, as system of knowledge, as something that one does, as practice) is framed and expressed in very gendered terms, and given the deeply embedded nature of these constructions it is worth unpacking these issues in depth. There is an explicit connection between of the creation and control of technology, the performance of hard science, activity and masculinity; as sociologist Alison Kelly (1985) bluntly asserts, "science is masculine" (p. 133). Even if there is a superficial sense that science is gender-neutral and egalitarian (Al-Gailani 2009, 378) – or perhaps even *because* of this supposition – deep-seated assumptions about the relationships between gender, intellect, competence and technology nonetheless result in a firmly entrenched sexism of both soft and hard varieties. This association of science with men and masculinity permeates the environment in which scientific research is carried out and results in profoundly damaging structural inequalities that are further worsened by the assumption that science – and by extension, scientists – are intellectually and ideologically objective, immune to implicit bias and informed only by an understanding of the coolly quantitative (Gaston 2015). These gendered assumptions play out with almost laughable obviousness in popular media, too: in a 2003 study of the representation of science and scientists in 222 films (Weingart, Muhl and Pansegrau 2003), only 18% of the scientist characters were found to be female, and they tend to fall into predictable stereotypes. The female scientists tend to be more inexperienced or taken less seriously; they are younger, less senior and more conventionally attractive than their male counterparts (p. 283). Similarly, Eva Flicker's (2012) analysis of female scientists in mainstream film indicates that even though the go-to image of the film scientist is that of a male scientist, those female scientists who do exist are likely to be, again, conventionally attractive, unrealistically youthful (p. 252) and sexually available. If not, they are given a lab coat and frumpy glasses and are relegated to the derogatory category of 'old maid'.

This is not to suggest, though, that *technologies, vis-à-vis* the scientists that create them, are necessarily masculine. Instead, technologies may be feminised when they offer some sense of either threat or servitude, in a dichotomy that perhaps reflects the division between the *femme fatale* and the good woman. The voices of 'helpful' or service-driven artificial intelligences in films such as *Her* (2015), as well as those that exist in 'real' life – such Apple's Siri, sexbots and robots designed to help healthcare workers – tend to be coded as female or feminine in a conflation of technology, sexuality, servitude and emotional labour (Cook 2016; Nickelsberg 2016; Griggs 2011). On the other hand, consider the gynoid False Maria in the silent science fiction epic *Metropolis* (1927) – a figure whose femininity represents "technology's simultaneous allure and powerful threat" (Springer 1996, 56). False Maria is an unsettling, multiplicitous hybrid: an automaton built to look like one woman, who had died in childbirth, but which is then given the face of another, in order to discredit a living woman who is stirring discord in the working classes. In his article "The Vamp and the Machine: Technology and Sexuality in Fritz Lang's Metropolis", German literary and cultural scholar Andreas Huyssen

(1981) suggests that False Maria's presentation as feminine draws from an historic tendency among European writers in the 18th and 19th centuries to code automata (mechanical humans) as female when they came to act dangerously. He describes how:

> as soon as the machine came to be perceived as a demonic, inexplicable threat and as harbinger of chaos and destruction – a view which typically characterizes many 19th-century reactions to the railroad to give but one major example – writers began to imagine the *Maschinenmensch* [machine-(hu)man] as woman.
>
> (p. 226)

Huyssen suggests provocatively that this feminisation of unruly technology operates within modernist texts as a way of aligning fears about technology with those about female sexuality, and – perhaps paradoxically – that this is compatible with the usual association of femininity with nature, for what nature, machine and woman all have in common as signifiers is their 'otherness' to Man (p. 226). And yet, as an aggregate of expanding otherness, a figure like the dead-alive, doubly female yet desexualised False Maria demonstrates truth instead of lies; 'she' implicitly exposes the limitations of the fixed ideal male subject and the economy under which he both profits and is enslaved. The False Maria's powers are extensive and she unleashes dissent and destruction, but such generative becomings and interconnected, non-anthropocentric relationships are fundamentally dangerous to the phallocentric order and economy: she is hunted down and destroyed, for this posthuman witch-figure is ultimately burned at the stake.

This association of technology, femininity and danger is notably apparent in the development of the cyborgs and android antagonists in the science fiction action franchise *The Terminator* (1984), including the way that each leverages the values embedded within the male/female binary-construct. The eponymous cyborg assassin of the original 1984 film is portrayed by action star Arnold Schwarzenegger as a heavily muscled, hyper-masculine, 'hard-bodied' (Jeffords 1994) juggernaut, but later films successively streamline and feminise their cyborg soldiers. The villain in *Terminator 2: Judgement Day* (1991), the T-1000, is a shapeshifting android made of liquid metal, and 'he' provides a slick, digital foil to Schwarzenegger's hulking, analogue cyborg. *Terminator 3: Rise of the Machines* (2003) features the gynoid shapeshifter T-X – a 'terminatrix' – and in the American television spin off, *Terminator: The Sarah Connor Chronicles* (2008–9), the terminator 'Cameron' looks like an athletic teenage girl. In each iteration there is a slide away from an obviously mechanical or non-human male-coded antagonist to a more implicitly sinister, insidiously 'natural'-looking, feminised and conventionally attractive entity that is able to charm or disarm their prey and hide in plain sight. It is not simply that *feminine* equates to *danger*, but that the films express a simultaneous curiosity and squeamishness in their weaving together of signifiers of femininity (which is associated with passivity and docility, but also implicitly with the threat of a non-phallocentric sexuality or autoeroticism), the 'hard' threat of weaponised technology, the emergent diversity of non-human intelligence and subjectivities of the creatures (especially as terminators have duplicates, version numbers, builds, and multiple models, and humans do not), and the difference inherent in the shift from the visible-analogue and the invisible-digital. The inability to tell the seemingly human from its alleged other creates a slippage, or a continuum, along which the category of human-as-construct only marks a brief point, not a dominant category nor even a consistent referent.

Nonetheless, the overall masculinisation of modern science itself is part of an intellectual tradition, thousands of years old, which privileges a certain cognitive and epistemic bias against women and femininity through the legitimation and institutionalisation of a scientific culture that has an inherent bias towards those with cultural power and authority. In her article "Dominion Over Nature", science historian and ecofeminist philosopher Carolyn Merchant (2001) attests that philosopher and scientist Francis Bacon, who is considered to be "the originator of the concept of the modern research institute, a philosopher of industrial science, the inspiration behind the Royal Society (1660), and ... the founder of the inductive method", helped shape an institution that, through the exploitation of nature, ultimately benefitted (and continues to benefit) the "middle class male entrepreneur" – the ideal subject – as opposed to women and "the lower orders of society", let alone the environment and the natural world itself (p. 68). This naturalises science as a (masculine) act of domination, rationalisation and even colonisation performed by those with economic, political and cultural capital. The exertion of control and order upon the feminised natural world – Mother Nature – much like the framing of bodies discussed in Chapter One, renders the female body as material and space that might be controlled, manipulated, dominated or invaded. Yet, this domination is as defensive as it is aggressive, for it works to control, or tame, or co-opt or reterritorialise that which does not fit within its strata or within the very limited set of relationships implied by phallocentric thought and epistemology. Science-as-rationalisation is shaped by curiosity, but also, perhaps, by fear.

This is informed by assumptions about the nature of rationality and thought itself, alongside the conceptual (inter-)relationship between the mind or the intellect and the allegedly baser conditions of the body. Feminist philosopher Susan Bordo contends in her 1986 article "The Cartesian Masculinization of Thought" that Cartesian objectivism frames rational thought *itself* as inherently masculine, in the sense that 'masculine' suggests "a cognitive style, an epistemological stance. Its key term is *detachment*: from the emotional life, from the particularities of time and place, from personal quirks, prejudices, and interests, and most centrally, from the object itself" (p. 451, emphasis original). This sense of detachment signals a sense of independence that reinforces a series of conceptual dichotomies: masculine/feminine; mind/body; rational/irrational; subject/object; spiritual/corporeal (p. 452); and science/nature. Within this paradigm of objectivist science, "the formerly female earth becomes inert *res extensa*: dead, mechanically interacting matter. "She" becomes "it" – and "it" can be understood" (p. 452). Bordo suggests that the project of empirical science is to understand the female universe, and in doing so to demystify and tame it (p. 454). It is within this context that various male rationalisations and reterritorialisations of the female body, from witch-hunting, to the creation of macabrely beautiful, life-like female anatomical wax dolls like the 'Anatomical Venuses' of the 18th century (see Ebenstein 2016), to the modern-day control of reproduction and birth, can be seen as something that is not just cultural or political, or even in the name of the social good, but fundamentally psychocultural and profoundly gendered (Bordo 1986, 455). The presumption of an authoritative detached rationality serves to mask, excuse or naturalise a variety of ways in which a patriarchal epistemic order considers the female body to be unruly, flawed and less-than: the material to be studied and controlled. It also forecloses the suggestion that one's own embodied experiences may contribute meaningfully to or even create its own sort of epistemic matrix, expanding the register of epistemic modalities. This denial suppresses forms of experience and knowledge traditionally coded as feminine at the same time as shutting off a breadth of possibility regarding the establishment of new modes of thought, experience and authority.

Reproductive science and technologies are practices as well as 'things', and they don't just exist within power relations; they *are* power relations (Farquar 2000, 210). As Susan M. Squier (1995) attests, the reconstruction of reproduction produces and consolidates male power, just as the reconfiguration of the body (both male and female) serves industrial production (Squier 1995, 115). It is perhaps unsurprising, then, that this masculine, scientific co-option and reterritorialisation of reproductive processes extends to other areas of women's reproductive health. Certainly, these technologies can have an extraordinarily "subversive potential", in that they make possible a variety of alternative family configurations (Davis-Floyd and Dumit 1998, 7), such as facilitating the ability of single women or gay couples to have children without recourse to heterosexual sex, or by challenging the idea that a man and a women create a child for themselves from their own equal genetic contributions. Some technologies may have added benefits; for example, hormone-releasing intrauterine devices are sometimes used to help temper endometriosis, and their use can augment or replace invasive surgery as a treatment for the debilitating and largely under-diagnosed condition. Yet, the same technologies may be bound up within political hegemonic frameworks that look to regulate, not liberate, female sexual and reproductive autonomy (see Young 1990). As feminist theorist Laura R. Woliver (2002) attests:

the hope of early feminist birth control movement activists was for simple contraceptives that would enhance women's autonomy. Instead, the field developed toward scientific expertise, medical control, and dissemination of birth control information and devices only through the discretion of predominantly male doctors.

(p. 15)

This emphasis on *control* and *expertise* serves to distance or even negate women's privileged and authoritative relationships with their bodies by re-contextualising the reproductive body not as a dynamic body-in-process, but in terms of symptoms to be managed and dysfunctions to be cured. The notion of optimal functioning is one that is implicitly phallocentric and ideological. For instance, premenstrual bodily, behavioural and emotional changes are diagnostically framed specifically as a *disorder* or pathology with physiological and psychological effects, as opposed to fluxes that occur within the expected envelope of affect and capacity. Yet, within the West epidemiological data suggests that almost all menstruating women experience mild symptoms, and 40% and 11–13% experience moderate to severe distress respectively (Ussher 2006, 26; Steiner and Born 2000). The inference is that these changes occur because of normal, not abnormal, ovarian function, and are thus a near-ubiquitous (albeit unpleasant) process; that is, the unruly female body is in fact the *normally-functioning* body. This calls for a reconfiguration of what healthy means, given that 'business is as usual' is distressing for so many; this is exacerbated by the unsettling fact that within a clinical context women's pain is treated less urgently and less aggressively than that of men (Hoffman and Tarzian 2001). These asymmetric, fraught relationships are acknowledged sarcastically in the film *Jennifer's Body* (2009): when teenage girl Needy complains that her best friend Jennifer, who is possessed by a succubus, seems to be premenstrual, Jennifer replies sardonically that PMS isn't real; instead, it's a conspiracy on the part of the male-dominated media to make women seem crazy. It is not that premenstrual changes don't exist but instead that they are exceedingly common, so that it is the 'condition' or 'disease' itself that is constructed, made intelligible, and thus made treatable within a pharmaceutical or biomedical framework that does not take the female body to be a neutral or default body.

In addition, the gendered power relations exhibited within reproductive horror texts are heavily influenced by the way that the process of conception itself is culturally framed: as, allegedly, a politically and culturally neutral event that nonetheless reinforces and naturalises dominant notions of sex, class and power. As anthropologist Emily Martin (1991) argues in her article "The Egg and the Sperm: How Science Has Constructed a Romance Based on Stereotypical Male–Female Roles", the way that eggs and sperm are represented in both popular and scientific accounts of reproduction and biology draws explicitly from taken-for-granted stereotypes of normative masculinity and femininity (p. 485). The result is that complex biological processes are couched within very culturally determined and deeply gendered value systems. In the medical and social texts Martin analyses, the egg is framed as passive and inert, whereas the sperm are framed as streamlined and active; the egg is shrouded in regal and religious language and considered to be fragile and delicate, whereas the sperm are discursively framed using militaristic language and are described as autonomous entities (p. 490). As Martin notes pithily, "it is remarkable how 'femininely' the egg behaves, and how 'masculinely' the sperm" (p. 489). These "[medical] texts have an almost dogged insistence on casting female processes in a negative light" (p. 488), for they place emphasis on the male *production* of sperm and the *degeneration* of eggs within the woman's ovaries, not the other way around. Oogenesis, the creation (or differentiation) of the ovum, is framed as wasteful and sperm production is not, even though for a heterosexual couple who produce two or three children, the 'wastage' of sperm outnumbers the 'wastage' of eggs by 10 orders of magnitude (p. 489). Further, although research has shown that both gametes are active participants in fertilisation – indeed, the egg is a far more aggressive participant than popularly presumed, and the sperm far less efficient at cellular penetration (pp. 492–3) – the description of active, aggressive sperm (Moore 2009) and passive, benign egg still remains the status quo, almost determinedly so.

These gendered stereotypes within scientific literature are deeply socially embedded; for instance, gendered narratives about the 'passive' nature of the egg and the 'active' role of the sperm cells are proliferated through children's picture books about human reproduction (Moore 2003). In such books, which are designed to give children accessible information about the 'facts of life', sexual intercourse that results in pregnancy is framed as an act of love occurring within a stable, heterosexual relationship. The egg and the sperm are often anthropomorphised and endowed with gendered characteristics so that the egg is presented as a feminine entity and the sperm cells as masculine entities, for instance, by giving the egg rosy cheeks and eyes framed by long, feminine eyelashes. This presentation is largely uncritical and such a binary, gendered representation is naturalised through the implicit assumption that the narratives presented in these books are objective fact. As medical sociologist Lisa Jean Moore (2003) argues, within these books – which she refers to dryly as "heterosexual manuals" (p. 281) – anthropomorphised "Sperm cells become performers acting out heterosexist fantasies/realities of patriarchal culture" (p. 280) in a manner that presumes that human reproduction is simply a straightforward and innate drive that progresses human evolution (p. 279). Further, even though fertilisation happens within the body, the male and female actors in these books are disembodied and de-contextualised, for the egg- and sperm-subjects are often presented 'outside' of the uterus as independent entities within their own narrative world. The size of the sperm cells and the egg are presented as roughly equivalent, even though the egg cell is significantly larger than the sperm cell. This exclusion of people-as-agents creates a closed system in which egg and sperm are engaged in a seemingly unproblematic, ideology-free biological event, and means that the reader or audience must instead identify with the heroic, athletic sperm-agent who 'wins' the race, or the damsel-in-distress egg (p. 290). This emphasis on activity *vis-à-vis* passivity takes a seemingly neutral and objective narrative and naturalises its gendered power imbalances. This forms a fractal, perpetually repeating structure of understanding and meaning-making that expands both in and out, stratifying gendered relationships within fixed, molar, binary modes from the site of the smallest cell and out to the broadest macroscopic organisation of society.

The asymmetrical account of power and agency present in children's media continues into popular cultural narrative. Within reproductive horror narratives – and, indeed, within the discourses surrounding reproductive technologies such as IVF – it is not just that the masculine is active and the feminine passive; instead, the female body is acted *upon* (see Raymond 1995). Emily Martin discusses one particular metaphor – that of a key entering a lock – that is present in a description of the mechanics of fertilisation in mammals in an article in *Scientific American* (see Wassarman 1988), which very obviously designates which entity acts upon which (Martin 1991, 496). Such a metaphor also implies a release or an opening: the egg's potential cannot be unlocked or released without the presence of the active sperm, even though the reverse is likewise true. In narratives about reproductive technologies, this mechanical metaphor is extended out to a macro level so that the woman's body is the lock (and, perhaps, her fertility is a problem to be fixed or unlocked), and the often physically invasive science, and, by extension, the scientist, take on the role of the key that can do this. The woman's body is a canvas, or an environment; it is something to be altered and controlled, and its inherent 'potential' cannot be fulfilled without active intervention. Again, a self-contained binary is implied and assured, for even though technology is introduced to the seemingly dipolar and self-contained relationship between male and female, technology becomes a masculine prosthesis. Such a construct leaves no room for anything that exists without, in extension of or contiguous to this exclusive and dichotomous relationship, despite multiple encounters between bodies and technologies, gendered and ungendered.

These implicitly masculine, mechanical metaphors are also evident in discussions surrounding IVF. Science fiction scholar Steven Mentor (1998), in his article "Witches, Nurses, Midwives and Cyborgs", describes him and his wife's experiences with IVF, remarking upon the sense that the woman's body is there to be acted upon in a brutish, mechanical way. He discusses this cognitive dissonance in a tongue-in-cheek manner, outlining how, during the procedure in which his wife's eggs are aspirated, he drolly perceives the fertility clinic as not a hospital, but a garage: "my wife is the car and these [doctors] are the grease monkeys, down to the bad radio blaring and the power tools" (p. 68). In this context, he perceives his wife's body as both "an organic, whole thing and as a car up on blocks" (p. 68). This mechanisation of the female body and the reproductive system also lends itself to the objectivist paradigm discussed by both Bordo and Merchant: a woman's body or reproductive system may be 'broken' and fertility treatment such as IVF is used to 'fix' natural processes and conditions. As Mentor notes, popular accounts of IVF tend to reify doctors and technology while simultaneously side-lining the inherent capabilities of women's bodies (p. 76), implying that science 'works' better, is more efficient than, and is an improvement upon the fallible body – and, by extension, nature itself. Such an appraisal may also be extended to reproductive technohorror films, for in these films IVF and reproductive technologies in general are framed as hopeful, but with a caveat: the promise of technology is potentially celebrated, but the doctor's motivation, and the lengths to which they go, may not be. In popular film, scientists – even apparently benevolent ones – are portrayed with ambiguity (Weingart, Muhl and Pansegrau 2003).

'Mad science' and men making life

This sense that the (female) body (environment/womb/matrix/material) is acted upon by a male agent of masculine science is exemplified and leveraged in popular culture through the figure of the 'mad' scientist – a stock character, almost always male (or identified with traits coded as masculine), who figures strongly in reproductive horror narratives. Even though the culturally sanctioned, hegemonically masculine 'work' of science, in the senses discussed above by Bordo, Martin and Merchant, is the domination, manipulation or reterritorialization of nature, it is important to note that the work of the *mad* scientist is carried out in secret, be it in a clandestine laboratory, a hidden basement, or a secluded town. As Weingart, Muhl and Pansegrau (2003) conclude in their broad spectrum quantitative and qualitative study, "Of Power Maniacs and Unethical Geniuses: Science and Scientists in Fiction Film", this secrecy is informed by the division between 'public' science, in which the scientist works openly with his peers and colleagues, and 'private' science, in which the scientist chooses to or is forced to leave their research community because of the transgressive or forbidden nature of their work (p. 285). This emphasis upon privacy lends the mad scientist a Faustian, iconoclastic cast, in that he is willing to transgress ethical boundaries in the pursuit of knowledge or power – indeed, he rejects or rewrites the nature of (post)human ethics in his rejection of the taken-for-granted codes that shape relations between bodies. Just as different incarnations of the Faust story emphasise different character flaws or motivations (Toumey 1992, 417–18), so too are mad scientists driven by a variety of impulses, such as ambition (*Jurassic Park*, (1993)), misogyny (*The Stepford Wives* (1975)), vengeance (*The Abominable Dr Phibes* (1971)), and morbid curiosity (*Re-Animator* (1985)). There is a degree of ambivalence in mad science narratives, for they evoke a dissonant overlap between liberation and domination, and creation and destruction (Weingart, Muhl and Pansegrau 2003, 280), revealing the extent to which one might inform, or be a different register or harmonic, or another. This ambivalence carries over into reproductive horror narratives, for in this case the mad scientist figure takes on the villainous role of aggressor, re-shaping the female body in a manner both in keeping with and in excess of the sanctioned mode of de- and re-territorialisation, at the same time as standing as a warning against science – and scientists – 'run amok'.

The prototypical cinematic image of the mad scientist, and the best known early reproductive technohorror, can be found in James Whale's seminal 1931 adaptation of *Frankenstein*. The film opens with an announcer stating that Dr Frankenstein was a man of science who transgressed spiritual boundaries by playing God through an attempt to create a man in his own image – a statement that immediately posits the scientist as a person who will break all moral and ethical codes in the interests of discovery, and one who will blasphemously reinscribe divinity within flesh, rather than spirit. Frankenstein has been experimenting with reanimating dead animals and a human heart, and has finally pieced together a man using parts taken from corpses, briskly establishing a perversely animal genealogy that echoes a Darwinian account of the emergence of 'man' through a non-anthropocentric cosmogony. He brings this hybrid creature to life during a lightning storm by channelling electricity, a literal spark of life, through electrodes in the creature's neck, and he is overcome with mania in his famous exclamation "it's alive – it's alive!" In a moment that was originally cut from the film because of its blasphemousness (but that was restored in 1999), Dr Frankenstein arrogantly tells one of the experiment's distressed observers not to call on God, for he now knows how it feels to *be* God. Here, the film explicitly frames Frankenstein's actions as heresy: he has subverted the natural order in the name of science, and in doing so, he has shown science itself to be amoral, unethical, something that moves across, not within, the constellation of ethical codes established by God through man and vice versa. Beyond the necrotic corporeal hybridity of the creature, Dr Frankenstein's act of hubris is in creating a form of life outside of an embodied male–female sexual coupling. He disrupts the procreative imperative, replacing the moment of male orgasm and ejaculation with the quick-ness (i.e. the living-ness) of electricity, thus creating a new form of quickening that evades the embodied coextensivity of pregnancy. (This act, of course, is pretty humorous when one considers his disinterest towards his fiancée; the female body is, if anything, a turn off.) The assumption is not only that his scientific tinkering is unnatural, but that the creation of life is something sacrosanct; the Christian God may create life in His own image, but man (or, masculine science) may not interfere with or mimic such processes. That the creature itself is not monstrous in the sense of wickedness, but in the sense of expressing new forms of relationships – a compassionate monster ethics predicated on the vulnerability and threat implicit in the capacity for mutiplicitous becomings and the insistent production of difference – is effectively lost on Dr Frankenstein, who sees his creature as a proof of concept and an embodiment of his own intellect. Perhaps it is that despite his technical ability, he is unable to recognise the true, magnificent import of his creation. This image of the arrogant, anarchic scientist, doing whatever he can to advance his interests – both personal and scientific – is a resonant one. The trope and stereotypical image of the mad scientist and his creation of a posthuman hybrid in film, television, literature and other media is deeply indebted to Whale's film.

Mad science narratives in reproductive technohorror continue in this vein in asking: how can life be created and brought forth without the bodies, or presence, or traces of women? How can man make the sort of 'life' that erases or occludes the maternal 'debt to nature' as well as expressing, instead, a wilful, organic-synthetic network of the 'natural' that reflects and serves a masculine intellect, rather than a more ineffable divine? Films such as *Bride of Frankenstein* (1933), *The Island of Dr Moreau* (1977), *Metropolis, The Stepford Wives, Edward Scissorhands* (1990), *The Boys from Brazil* (1978), *Dead Ringers* (1988) and *Alien: Resurrection* (1997) and even cult sci-fi comedy musical *The Rocky Horror Picture Show* (1975) feature scientists who in some way have, or have tried to, create, revive or augment life, and in doing so displace, replace, 'fix' or alter the female body, womb and reproductive system. In *Godsend,* for instance, a couple whose son, Adam, had died on his 8th birthday are convinced by a geneticist to have Adam cloned and his mother implanted with the egg. However, when this second Adam turns eight, he is haunted by strange dreams of a disturbed boy called Zachary and his behaviour becomes violent. The geneticist had included DNA from his own dead son, set to 'switch' when Adam passed his 8th birthday, thus using Adam's mother as a convenient incubator to help him reclaim his own child – although, of course, this is not and will never be 'his' child but a hybrid who expresses an interference pattern of two bodies, two 'selves' and two psyches across two time periods. In her 2005 book *Phallic Panic* Barbara Creed notes that within these sorts of narratives both the creator and the created are monstrous, for "when man attempts to create life without woman ... he both becomes a monster and brings forth monsters" (p. xvi). However, "in his attempt to appropriate the power of woman he almost always fails" (p. 41): Dr Frankenstein's monsters, Dr Moreau's half-animal half-human creatures, and the hybrid Ripley-Alien in *Alien: Resurrection* all serve to compare the supposed monstrosity (that is, wickedness) of the scientific creations to the cruelty, arrogance and inhumanity of their creators, even though these hybrids all express their own sense of compassion and vulnerability, and explore new ways of being that trouble and elude majoritarian categories and stratifications. Nonetheless, these films, *en masse*, act as cautionary tales against scientific hubris, and the result is almost inevitably that the scientist is somehow destroyed, although well after he has inflicted horrendous damage to his creatures and the people and world around him.

Even when women are not present, the notion of birth and re-birth remains salient. In the case of David Cronenberg's 1986 reimagining of *The Fly* the creator *is* the created: scientist Seth Brundle has his DNA scrambled with that of a housefly during a teleportation experiment. His visceral, corporeal and ultimately doomed metamorphosis into 'Brundlefly' is framed as an act of rebirth, through which he sloughs off his human body parts and begins to display insect traits. This 'dehumanisation' is a productive metamorphosis, even a form of hybrid, self-perpetuating human–insect autoeroticism that operates within its own mode of temporality. Man-Brundle embraces (cf. acquiesces) to the insect nature of the fly; as Brundlefly warns his human love interest, Ronnie, he is increasingly dangerous, for insects don't understand compassion or compromise as these concepts are simply human constructs. Reading *The Fly* as a narrative about mad science and reproduction indicates that Brundle's scientific hubris and human amorality predates this insect amorality, but a shift away from an anthropocentric epistemology and ontology reveals the limits, not the capacities of the human. However, in contrast to pregnancy and birth narratives featuring women, and despite the messy dissolution and reconfiguration of his body, there is never any sense that Brundle's coherent subjectivity persists, nor that his role as the film's protagonist (and antagonist) is in doubt; instead, he is altered and augmented, not erased.

Fearing science

The overall narrative emphasis upon the debasement of the 'natural order' within these films points to the ways that the ubiquitous figure of the mad scientist is bound up within moral codes and strictures, in that secular, clinical science comes to be pitted antagonistically against the strictures of a Judeo-Christian moral framework. It is not simply the scientist himself who contravenes ethical codes. Science and the search for knowledge *itself* is instead classed as dangerous and morally transgressive (Toumey 1992), arrogantly Promethean and dangerously inquisitive, as opposed to a way of understanding the inner workings and relationships within the (Creator's) universe. As pop culture historian David J. Skal notes in *Screams of Reason: Mad Science and Modern Culture* (1998), "the mad scientist has served as a lightning rod for otherwise unbearable anxieties about the meaning of scientific thinking and the uses and consequences of modern technology" (p. 18), so that the function of these 'cautionary tales' is clearly bound up with an implied moral and ethical code. Although I do not suggest that 'anxiety' is the singular mode of expression in such explorations, for it forecloses the possibility of wonder and curiosity, it is nonetheless fair to suggest that mad science narratives express a degree of nervous uncertainty surrounding scientific and technological experimentation, including the seeming impenetrability of such activities to the layperson and the nature of 'progress', and "shape[s] them into moral narratives that purport to explain whence comes evil in the guise of science and how to repel it" (Toumey 1992, 411). In the most negative and drastic expression of such mistrust, science (as thing, as practice) becomes a way of irresponsibly and arrogantly ripping opening Pandora's box, and the means by which evil is released into the world. The message: don't tinker under the hood.

This tension between science and religious moral frameworks is made bluntly obvious in *Blessed* (2004), which frames reproductive science as quite literally unholy. The film, like so many of the pregnancy-themed gynaehorror films discussed in this book, draws explicitly from the story of *Rosemary's Baby*, in that it features a young woman who is impregnated by the devil while her initially loving and supportive husband is tempted by an offer of fame and success. This film's point of difference is that in this instance the impregnation happens through IVF. The infertile young couple – Samantha and Craig – are referred by their doctor to a new clinic in a remote small town, a place that juxtaposes cutting-edge science with slick postmodern architecture, solitude and natural beauty. The clinic itself is owned by a Satanist business mogul who offers Craig a lucrative book deal, and it is also home to an experimental cloning facility. Samantha's eggs and Craig's sperm are collected, and the sperm sample is secretly augmented with a red, blood-like substance stored in an ancient vial, which is revealed to be the carrier for Satanic DNA. The 'mad' science in this film appears even-tempered and profoundly rational; it is suggested that the scientific staff and many of the town's inhabitants belong to the Dawn of the New Light Church, a devil-worshipping sect that draws from the pop-Catholic iconography of religious horror films, and that is diligently and calmly working towards bringing about a new apocalypse under the banner of progressive, capitalist technoscience. In *Blessed,* the acceptance of IVF treatment – that is, the acceptance of an 'unnatural' form of conception – is quite literally a pact with the devil, an attitude that is rearticulated by a rogue priest who attempts to convince Samantha to poison her unborn twins. In this film, instead of focussing on the actions of one specific mad scientist, cutting-edge science itself is being utilised by forces of evil as a tool with which to achieve their goals. Further still, science is shown to have progressed to this level explicitly because of its associa-tion with evil, for without the wealth and focus of its Satanist benefactor Earl Sydney, and the support and actions of the Church's social and technological networks, such high-end fertility treatment would not be available at all.

The notion that this sort of science is 'mad' relates to anxieties surrounding the question of what it is to be human, or 'natural', and how and why science might augment or alter the natural. Indeed, the tension and the possible dis-tinction between the natural and the monstrous drives many reproductive horrors. Reproductive and genetic sciences make possible the manipulation of the genetic makeup of cells that may make up an embryo or a foetus, with the intention of eliminating pathology, although the distinction between what is genetically 'normal' and genetically desirable is fluid and fraught with difficulty, and imbued with a sense of industrialisation and rationalisation that looks to the foetus as the distinct, individuated product of its machine-mother (see Squier 1995, 117). Such practices may be clearly linked with eugenics, which was described by eugenics pioneer Sir Francis Galton in 1904 as "the science which deals with all influences that improve the inborn qualities of a race; also with those that develop them to the utmost advantage" (p. 1). However, the term eugenics is now popularly and irrevocably attached the notions of 'racial hygiene', genetic hierarchies, and the production of certain types of ideal people through the eradication of the so-called genetic deficiencies that produce 'inferior' individuals, however that is being framed and for whatever ideological purpose. This association, of course, is particularly linked to the actions and experiments of Nazi SS officer and physician Josef Mengele, whose interest in heredity led to horrific experimentation upon concentration camp prisoners, including newborns, infants and young twins, during World War II; the issue was prominent in the Nuremberg trials of 1946–7 (Weindling 2010, 327).

Given the terrible history of human slaughter that has in part been facilitated by allegedly scientific ideas about racial and genetic hierarchies, eugenics remains something of a *bête noire* in narratives about reproductive technologies. The science fiction drama *GATTACA* (1997) certainly draws upon the association of eugenics with fascism through its use of a soft, 1930s-inspired modernist, retro-futuristic aesthetic design and colour palette, and a storyline about the artificial selection of those who are genetically 'superior' that evokes the "masculine desire of governing the hierarchies of a genetically determinist world" (Stacey 2010, 124). The film's stillness, grace and silence expresses the presumed, singular ideal to which its society aspires, but also a sense of wonder at the technologies that have facilitated such a turn, while eliding the violence and the opposition to difference that resides at the heart of the world's reproductive value-system. Reproductive technohorror engages clearly these anxieties, including the outcomes of and motivations behind far more commonplace acts of genetic selection on a day-to-day basis. Reproductive practices and technologies such as pre-natal screening for disease or disability, or genetic counselling, in which prospective parents are advised of the probability of transmitting a chromosomal or other inherited disorder to their child, are certainly useful for prospective parents who wish to minimise 'risk' (see Lupton 1999). However, they are also highly contentious, for anything that is selected *against* is, implicitly, something that is selected *for*, and such selection may be deleterious, threatening or ethically or religiously problematic, such as in the case of the selective abortion of foetuses with intellectual or physical disabilities or non-standard chromosomal conditions.

The negative connotations surrounding eugenic practices have also informed popular debate about the implications of IVF and embryo science, in which the interference with or augmentation of genetic or embryonic material may be seen as a so-called 'slippery slope' to other more invasive, even fascistic practices. Early efforts in human embryonic research were framed in public and scientific discourses as specifically threatening and most likely unethical, more for the benefit of scientific progress than for patients themselves. Robert G. Edwards (2001), the physiologist who pioneered human *in vitro* fertilisation with surgeon Patrick Steptoe, recalls that:

> Ethicists decried us, forecasting abnormal babies, misleading the infertile and misrepresenting our work as really acquiring human embryos for research. They announced that IVF did not cure infertility, as women remained infertile after having an IVF baby. My response was to put forward spectacles, false teeth and heart transplants.
>
> (p. 1092)

Such a comment frames IVF as a temporary augmentation, or a workaround for a broken system, and technology as a beneficial tool. However, the notion that the human body itself needs fixing permanently is nonetheless present, and Edwards gestures towards the notion that we are always-already posthuman in our intersections and amalgamations with technologies, be they prosthetic or more organically embedded. And yet, Edwards indicates the impulse to *correct* reproduction, suggesting that the fact that 80% of embryos fail to implant, even in young couples, means that the human reproductive system is itself profoundly flawed and inefficient (p. 1094). Such a comment expresses the perspective that the 'natural' is fallible and not always particularly productive, which uncomfortably undermines much older suggestions that the human body is an imprint of the divine. This of course, positions productivity and efficiency as a mode to which we should aspire, with the experimental scientist placed as the privileged creator-assessor of the category of 'success'. It also speaks to the supposition that science has a duty to diagnose and address inefficiencies (or 'design flaws'), to mend or *enhance* the natural, even when outside observers see such tinkering as immoral or dangerous. The physical and conceptual centre of this knowledge-production is the laboratory, and it is the quantitative language of diagnostics that shapes this register of the reproductive (see Franklin 2006, 168).

This association of reproductive science with dubious ethics is deeply important in understanding the representation of reproductive technology in film narratives, for the layperson actively draws upon works of popular science fiction (and, by inference, horror, literature and other mass entertainment products) as sources of information about new technologies (Mulkay 1996; Broege 1988); the same is true for science fiction literature. Scientific outsiders – that is, non-scientists – look to fantastic texts to help them consider the future impact of new technologies, particularly if those technologies are allowed to develop and proliferate without adequate moral and ethical checks and balances, whatever they may be. This creates a conceptual feedback loop between scientific research itself, its presentation to the public, the public's understanding of it and its consequences, and even the ways that scientists themselves think about and articulate their work, for in imagining new technological futures people "must either invent a new, plausible story line or fit developments into a narrative structure that is already available" (Mulkay 1996, 158).

In the case of embryo research and new reproductive technologies, the irrational image of the mad scientist – particularly Dr Frankenstein and his "dream of systematic, science-based control over the creation of human beings" (Mulkay 1996, 157) – looms large in the popular consciousness, operating as an interpretive matrix through which the unfathomable might be culturally rationalised. Sociologist of science Michael Mulkay indicates in his 1996 article "Frankenstein and the Debate Over Embryo Research" that the Frankenstein myth is deployed in two distinct ways. Firstly, the explicit framing of new reproductive technologies as "Frankenstein science" in some newspapers (pp. 160–1) – complete with movie stills from Whale's film to illustrate the point – implies that scientists are dangerous and that in conducting their embryo research they will inevitably act in a transgressive manner unless specific legislation is enacted to stop them. Secondly, and perhaps more interestingly, the Frankenstein myth is invoked even when it has little bearing upon the actual science being discussed. Mulkay looks to parliamentary debates about embryo science in the United Kingdom between 1984 and 1988, only a few years after the first test-tube baby, finding that the term "Frankenstein", alongside references to Aldous Huxley's dystopian novel *Brave New World*, is deployed loosely in less specific scientific contexts as a broad way for the speaker to signal their distaste or disapproval (p. 166). As such, the invocation of mad science is less about the scientific specifics of any given research, and more about the individual's own creative and hypothetical conception of the scientific process, alongside their disapproval of what they consider to be the inevitable future excesses of scientists.

Mad scientists and madwomen

The fraught, contested nature of the subjectivity of the pregnant woman (or mother-to-be) that is discussed in the previous chapter, the ethical quandaries and opportunities raised through the development and application of reproductive science, and the persistent image of the male mad scientist all intersect in the reproductive technohorror film. This creates a gynaehorrific account of the nature of reproductive capacities and possibilities that expresses anxiety about technology alongside dis-ease about the biological processes of conception and pregnancy, resulting in the sense that women who have been let down or betrayed by their inherently unreliable bodies are potentially hapless victims of the predations of scientific hubris; that is, women, as an indeterminate Other, a category of capacity rather than a subject, are vulnerable to both nature *and* culture. This is informed by the insidious sense that the reproductive female reproductive body *itself* is always-already deficient, unruly or flawed – as marred by an androcentric account of biology and subjectivity as it is by the mythical account of the implications of original sin.

These concerns are evident in *The Unborn* (1991), which begins as Virginia and her husband Brad discuss their desperation to have a child. They have been told by previous doctors that their chances of conceiving naturally or through IVF are extremely poor, so on the recommendation of an acquaintance they approach Dr Meyerling, whose success rate with infertile couples is said to be near-perfect. However, Dr Meyerling has been secretly manipulating the genes in the sperm samples so as to create 'better' babies, and the effects of pregnancy upon many of the women involved have been fatal. The babies show extreme strength and tenacity, but some of the pregnant women have displayed psychotic or violent tendencies, and one woman appears to have been eaten alive from the inside out by her foetus. The live results of such experimentation are also dreadful; in one instance, one of the augmented children, now a toddler, exhibits signs of extraordinary intelligence and drowns her intellectually disabled older brother. Once Virginia understands the nature of the experiments, and that her husband (as in *Rosemary's Baby*) agreed to her participation without her consent, she has a back alley abortion and confronts Dr Meyerling. He informs her that women are no longer needed; instead, he is growing ectogenetic foetuses in his lab in large orb shaped containers, the images of which deliberately invoke the iconography of Lennart Nilsson's foetal photography. Virginia destroys his work by shooting the luminous orbs, but goes back to the dumpster where the abortionist disposed of her foetus, only to find that its unnatural strength helped it survive the procedure. She keeps the malformed child, although it is not made clear whether she plans to raise it or kill it, letting the film end in a dissonant space of both revulsion and wonder.

The Unborn presents reproductive science as utterly unfathomable to the layperson, but this gate-keeping – for better or worse – imparts a sense of scientific authority. When the science behind IVF and Dr Meyerling's experiments is discussed, it is only in the loosest, most childish of terms. Virginia confronts Brad about his complicity in Dr Meyerling's experiments, and Brad explains vaguely that the doctor modified the sperm using something to do with synthesised proteins to make the baby stronger and more viable. Brad's lack of understanding about Dr Meyerling's process is reckless, for although the outcome of the experiments is clear, the methodology is not. However, his flippancy is also indicative of the power imbalance between doctor and patient, and the level of trust that is implicitly assumed as a part of that relationship, and the sense of comfort that seems to come from the sense that such a reliance upon 'efficiency' is implicitly quantitative, and therefore read as value-free; it is simply that better is better. Indeed, Brad is comforted by the very impenetrability of Dr Meyerling's jargon, yet has no actual understanding of the process. Instead, scientific details are replaced by images of a more documentarian nature that imply both neutrality and authority. When Dr Meyerling looks at Brad's sperm sample with his microscope, we are shown what is implied to be a scientific, doctor's-eye view of the sample – a microscopic image of motile sperm. Likewise, when Virginia has an egg aspirated, mixed with a milky white substance, then re-implanted, we are given a microscopic view of the jiggling, newly-fertilised egg. The disembodied images of the sperm and the egg are ineffable; it is impossible for the uneducated eye to tell whether or not these raw, organic materials are 'natural' or scientifically augmented, and this uncertainty contributes to the broader sense of dissonance; seeing cannot equate to believing. They also reinforce the privileged position of the doctor-as-penetrator, for he can see further and deeper into the couple's bodies than the couple themselves can. This macro- and microscopic gaze, this wielding of scopic power, displaces their embodied knowledge and their intimacy with his probing technoscientific gaze, while emphasising what Sarah Franklin (2006) terms the "over-determined coupling between embryonic bodies and technoscience", which is expressed through a recollection of the primal scene through images of micro-injection (p. 170)

The film presents reproductive science itself as inherently sinister and dangerously unregulated; it is framed as a radical science that sits in the darkness and on the margins. Dr Meyerling discusses the promise of reproductive technologies with enthusiasm, gushing that the technology has developed with such swiftness that anything is possible. However, the 'anything' that entices Brad and Virginia is not the 'anything' that Dr Meyerling has in mind, and the explicit mention of the technology's rapid development indicates that this progress may have been imprudent or unethical. It is stated that Dr Meyerling had been working on the Human Genome Project, which started formally in 1990, making it a contemporaneous touchstone of technological anxiety. The implication, then, is that the work being undertaken by geneticists is both cutting edge and dangerous, and that without a satisfactory degree of caution – or, perhaps, oversight – the science and the scientists may 'run amok'. The scene in which Virginia is implanted exacerbates this sense of dis-ease. As the doctor prepares for the procedure, low camera angles make the medical staff appear to loom over her, and the soundtrack features a synthesiser mimicking the rhythm of a heartbeat. When Virginia is anaesthetised, a high camera angle emphasises the vulnerability and passivity of her prone body. The camera lingers tightly on her exposed stomach as the aspiration needle penetrates her body and draws back blood. The microscopic, documentary footage of the egg as it exists within yet apart from the body then distances us from Virginia-as-subject, for "through [the] biomedical gaze, bodies are treated as 'things' to be studied and not as embodied subjects" (Ettorre 2002, 5).

Reproductive technologies and masculinity are also explicitly connected. In some ways, this frames the biomedical with the rational; for instance, Virginia's opinion about her body is discounted or belittled, and she is often excluded from discussions about the conception and pregnancy. Even though Virginia is shown to be intelligent and successful in her own right – she is an acclaimed children's author – during the couple's initial consultation, Dr Meyerling speaks exclusively to Brad until Brad leaves the room to provide a sperm sample. As the film progresses, in another nod to *Rosemary's Baby*, Virginia is accused of being irrational and unstable. Her previous episodes of depression, and her family's history of mental illness, are used by others as a justification for her instability and a means by which to further deny her agency. When Virginia discovers that Brad was complicit in Dr Meyerling's plan to augment the sperm sample, Brad states that his duplicity was because he didn't feel that she was 'ready' – a clear inference that he felt Virginia wasn't capable of making sound, rational decisions about her own body. Virginia's alleged 'madness' centres on her femininity and her emotional life, whereas the doctor's madness comes from hubris and an inhumane hyper-rationality, yet it is Virginia's madness that is framed as culturally unsanctioned.

The conflation of masculinity, rationality and science is most clear in the film's representation of alternative (that is, non-scientific), female-centric health practices. During her first visit to Dr Meyerling's clinic, Virginia meets a gay woman, Connie, who is there in support of her partner's pregnancy, and the couple invite Virginia to a women-only antenatal class. The class – a 'new age' Lamaze session – is presented in a comical and derisory fashion that draws on negative and dismissive stereotypes of lesbians and second-wave feminists. The gay couple imply that they are offering their classes as a female-friendly alternative to the masculinist, scientific mainstream: they advocate holistic and homeopathic approaches, they discuss sharing recipes for human placenta, and they encourage the women in the class to steer clear of using male-centric language or frames of reference when picturing their pregnancies and impending labours. When a woman asks about when her husband can start attending, they say that they consider men to be 'outsiders' who get in the way of a woman's communication with her unborn child, a statement that marks them as extreme in their position as Dr Meyerling himself.

This female-centric approach isn't taken on board by all the women, though. Beth, a hard-nosed journalist who befriends Virginia, criticises the group's practices. She asserts that Dr Meyerling doesn't approve of the gay couple because they are not 'accredited' – that is, they are not recognised as authorities within a patriarchal, technocratic system. When Connie comments that she wishes Beth wasn't afraid of her own woman-hood, Beth offers a vulgar, dismissive and (importantly) misogynistic retort; her point of view here serves to offer a sceptical, masculine-coded denunciation of the women's practice that the spectator is invited to share. Two ironies are left unstated. Firstly, even though their class is an act of resistance, the lesbian couple are still reliant on modern science to have a child in the manner that they want to. Secondly, the lesbian couple's distrust of the masculine nature of the scientific treatment comes to be incredibly well-founded, even though they remain as jokey stock characters. Nonetheless, their emphasis on the natural and alternative is still presented as a feminine, inferior, overly-emotional and ultimately flaky alternative to the rational and scientific, even if in this case the scientific is destructive and hostile.

While the film presents IVF and genetic modification as technologies that can nominally offer infertile couples hope, it also acts as a cautionary tale about what might happen when cutting-edge technology isn't subject to proper oversight and scrutiny – although who 'should' provide this oversight is often left unstated. However, as in similar films, the genetic technology in the film has progressed as far as it has, for good or ill, *because* there has been no oversight. Dr Meyerling's scientific goals are explicitly eugenic, and his ability to operate without interruption has given him the freedom to create a technology that ostensibly helps couples who have exhausted their other options. However, helping patients is a side effect of Dr Meyerling's core research, which is to add chromosomes to the children's genetic code so as to fix nature's problems and make improved babies – children that are strong and hyper-intelligent, even if it results in the death of the mothers and others around them. He sees this as a step along an evolutionary pathway and off-handedly provides a vague motive: humans have damaged the world and these posthuman children might provide a way forward. However, he looks at the mothers as collateral damage, the material (*res extensa*) that will allow his creatures to grow, until he can find a more stable ectogenetic pathway. When confronted he apologises for the pain and trauma that he has caused Virginia, but deems it a necessary sacrifice. Beth's earlier warnings to Virginia are resonant: Beth identified Dr Meyerling as a *researcher*, not a doctor, with the implication that where a 'doctor' may have a duty of care towards his patients, a 'researcher' who is acting only in the pursuit of knowledge does not, and will happily breach ethical considerations in order to advance 'his' studies.

That said, it is interesting that *The Unborn* displays some ambivalence towards reproductive technology, so that science and its potential for positive change and opportunitistic, generative becomings isn't demonised altogether. Prior to Virginia's experiences under Dr Meyerling's care, she and Brad discuss the opportunities offered by genetic manipulation and screening. Their conversation explicitly invokes some of the debates surrounding eugenics, genetic screening and so-called designer babies, for despite wariness about reproductive science, "there is a demand for these techniques in a society characterized by individualism and the drive for self-realization" (Weingart, Muhl and Pansegrau 2003, 281) that embraces the notion of efficiency, industrialisation and personalisation in a process that is characterised by its 'risk'. Virginia says that she couldn't deal with a child with congenital abnormalities or deformities, or a child like their friends' son Bobby, who is cruelly described as retarded. When she brings up the issue of heredity and her family history of mental illness, Brad shrugs off her concerns and responds that her intermittent depressive episodes don't make her genetically 'deficient'. Their conversation alludes to the potential personal benefits of genetic screening, but Brad's emphasis upon deficiency certainly infers a form of genetic hierarchy. He implies a distinction between Virginia's depression and Bobby's intellectual disability, but the bounds of that distinction are not articulated further. The inclusion of this conversation, as later compared to Dr Meyerling's mega-lomaniacal posturing, offers up a sense of ethical uncertainty at the same time as suggesting that there is due cause to alter or eliminate that which is diagnostically, culturally and personally deemed to be unwanted or inferior.

Re-gendering mad science in *Splice*

The cinematic mad scientist is usually male: he 'does' masculine science, which challenges or alters (feminised) nature or the (passive) female body. Nonetheless, there are some female mad scientists: many feature in camp, low budget horror comedy films such as *Abbott & Costello Meet Frankenstein* (1948), *Blood of Dracula* (1957), *Jesse James meets Frankenstein's Daughter* (1966) and *Flesh Feast* (1970). These characters are played for comic value and sex appeal; for instance, Dr Myra in teensploitation B-movie *Teenage Zombies* (1961) sports a faux-Eastern European accent and wears heavy make-up and an evening gown, which she occasionally covers with a white lab coat. Even the character of Dr Susan McAlester in the monster action movie *Deep Blue Sea* (1999) harkens back to these earlier women. Certainly, she is ambitious: she is attempting to create super-intelligent sharks in the hope of using their genetic material in a cure for the type of Alzheimer's disease that is affecting her father, even if it means contravening international codes of ethics and cultural taboos surrounding the augmentation of human genetic material with that of non-human animals. At the same time, she is frequently objectified; there are extended scenes in which she is wearing little more than her underwear, and one of the film's theatrical release posters features her in the water, wearing a wetsuit, but with her cleavage exposed. These representations are less about the science itself, and rely more on the juxtaposition of an attractive, sexualised woman performing 'masculine' science (see Flicker 2012). As such, they are defined as much by normative, if not misogynistic representations of gender as they are by their profession.[1]

More recently reproductive technohorror films have shifted to consider mad science in a more complex manner, and in doing so they challenge some of the fundamental assumptions underlying the historic representations of the hyper-rational male and hypersexual female mad scientist. Canadian science fiction horror film *Splice* (2009) considers how reproductive horror and mad science can be articulated in terms of maternity and a lack of normative feminine affect, and its conclusion offers a teratological meditation on the embodied nature of pregnancy and reproduction, that decentres human claims of authority over bodies and becomings. *Splice* also acts as an interesting companion to the films discussed in this chapter as the mad scientists are not isolated individuals but a heterosexual couple: brilliant geneticists Clive and Elsa, who are named for actors Colin Clive (Dr Frankenstein in James Whale's *Frankenstein* and *Bride of Frankenstein*) and Elsa Lanchester (Mary Shelley and the monster's 'bride' in *Bride of Frankenstein*). The pair experiment with ways to splice together the DNA of various animals for a company, Nucleic Exchange Research and Development (or NERD), that wishes to use the proteins extracted from these new hybrids to develop pharmaceuticals. Although the pair work within a corporate, technocapitalist entity that is seeking new ways to commodify and industrialise non-human animal or genetic material, their notoriety means that they are largely left to themselves so long as they maintain production. They are driven by a desire for fame – or, perhaps, infamy – and they actively ignore the warnings of their employers so that they can pursue their own line of research.

As with the work of Dr Frankenstein, the pair's monomaniacal search for 'forbidden' knowledge is explicitly transgressive. Elsa's impatience leads her to include her own DNA into one of the experimental hybrids without her husband's consent or knowledge. The posthuman, trans-species 'specimen' initially appears to be aggressive and physiologically and emotionally unstable, but its multiple, dynamic capacities and configurations seem to settle into the form of a sweet, child-like, apparently female creature that they name Dren in an inversion of their employer's moniker. After Dren's 'birth' Clive expresses deep reservations about the nature of the experiment, but Elsa becomes increasingly obsessed with the project and insists that they let the hybrid live. As Dren rapidly develops from child to adolescent she outgrows her cute, playful femininity and begins to demonstrate the hallmarks of overt, almost aggressive female sexuality – something that Elsa chooses to ignore. Finally, Clive is seduced by the hybrid in a scene coloured by infidelity, alongside incestuous, perhaps paedophilic intent, but they are interrupted mid-coitus by Elsa; this blunt reference to Freud's 'primal scene' is influenced by an earlier scene in which Dren spies on Elsa and Clive's lovemaking. Dren starts to jealously turn on her mother-figure, but because of their escalating arguments Clive and Elsa fail to recognise that one of their earlier animal-hybrid speci- mens has spontaneously changed sex. The couple decide to terminate the experiment – language that invokes the idea of abortion – by killing Dren, but before they can do so Dren appears to sicken and die. Clive and Elsa do not realise that this is not a death, but a metamorphosis, a new phase, and after they bury Dren's seemingly dead body the creature returns having changed sex. This new, 'male' Dren is larger, more violent and aggressive, and explicitly predatory. He hunts down Elsa, mirrors his sexual relationship with Clive by violently raping her, then kills Clive with an enormous, phallic stinger before Elsa is able to finally stave in his skull with a rock in an act of filicide. In the film's final scene Elsa is seen in a meeting with her employers talking about the value of the chemical compounds found in Dren. Elsa has been paid a significant amount of money to assure her silence regarding the disastrous series of events and for 'volunteering' to advance the experiment, and as she leaves and her full body moves into the frame we see that she is heavily pregnant, presumably to Dren.

The mad science films discussed in this chapter display a fascination with the creation of life outside of the maternal body. Importantly, they challenge the mother–father dyad by either eliminating the need for one or both of the parents, or by introducing other individuals, such as geneticists, into the acts of conception and gestation. However, *Splice* reframes reproductive technol- ogies, and the creation of life outside of the body, as a conceptual site through which to explore the dissolution (or even the irrelevance) of the heterosexual family unit through the exploration of a toxic Oedipal script, and by revealing the static, fragile mother–father–child relationship to be only one in a diverse, dynamic array of potential relationships and connections, be they productive or toxic, open-ended or catastrophic. Early in the film Elsa tells Clive that she has no interest in bearing a child until men can do so too, eschewing socio- biological determinism and choosing instead to focus on their intellectual creations in the lab. Yet, Dren is very clearly framed as a child stand-in for Clive and Elsa and the quasi-parental pair celebrates the creature's 'birth' as their greatest success. Dren's role as child (subject), instead of science project (and object), soon becomes complicated. Elsa forms a strong maternal and normatively feminine bond with the creature, dressing her in little girls' clothes and jealously lording her relationship with Dren over Clive, who considers Dren to be a specimen (an it) to be contained as opposed to a person (a she). Their later arguments over Dren, and Clive's growing dis-ease, explicitly frame the couple as bickering parents who cannot agree upon the proper way to raise their child. Clive's discovery that Dren was created with Elsa's DNA is the inverse of a discovery that one's child was fathered through an affair, but it's not unreasonable to suggest that in this case Elsa, in her self-replication, is faithful only to herself. Later arguments, and Clive's sexual encounter with Dren, reframe the relationship as dysfunctional and on the brink of collapse. Elsa and Clive's relationship over the course of the film is an accelerated version of familial bonding and disintegration, mirroring Dren's accelerated childhood, puberty and adolescence. Clive accuses Elsa of propagating the experiment because she is too frightened of having a human child, and that creating a child in an experimental setting (allegedly) allows her a greater sense of control. Clearly, this backfires on Elsa – her unruly experimental child becomes an obsession, then rapes her, removes the family patriarch by killing her husband, and then colonises her body through the necessarily coextensive relationship that is formed between human mother and chimera-foetus.

At the film's conclusion, the revelation that Elsa is pregnant can be read as horrific in two distinct ways. Her initial transgression – over and above the taboo of experimenting with human genetic material – is that she secretly uses her *own* DNA instead of that of an anonymous donor, and then tries to raise the creature like her own child. This circumvents the need for pregnancy and birth and also ensures that Elsa, as subject, is autonomous and intact – until she is violently raped by Dren; the one-way flow of her genetic 'gift' is horrifically reversed. Her second, equally deliberate transgression is that she has chosen to continue the experiment by keeping her new, unborn child, which was conceived in an act that was equal parts incestuous and bestial given Dren's status as an animal hybrid. Although the pharmaceutical company she works for is complicit in the action, Elsa's incessant desire for knowledge and creation is coupled with a desire to somehow bear the child she has, perhaps, been denied, through the death of her partner and the death of her first 'creation' – but only within the context of what is erroneously thought of as a controlled experiment. Elsa's pregnancy also alludes to parthenogenesis, as she is both mother and father to the creature, which perhaps posits her as animal as her offspring. Given her disinterest in wanting to have a baby with Clive, this is the ultimate act of hubris, and in the final scene she seems perversely driven. Her monomaniacal choice is not the elimination of the woman's role in reproduction, as with *Frankenstein* or *The Island of Dr Moreau*, but in wilfully removing the need for a man.

Elsa's relationship with(in) her body plays upon the conceptual split between self and other that is so prevalent in gynaehorrific films. She is pregnant because of something that was done *to* her, not a consensual conjugation, and by treating her pregnancy and her reproductive body as another experiment she is explicitly distancing her physical, fleshy self (as corporeal environment) from her intellectual scientist-persona. However, this recursive relationship is not productive nor generative, but cancerous and (auto)cannibalistic. Pregnant Elsa looks wan and sickly; where philosopher Iris Marion Young (1990) contrasts her own (female) corporeality with her (masculine-coded) academic goals as a philosopher, the film suggests that no matter how hard Elsa tries to disavow or reframe her pregnancy, she cannot escape or transcend her embodied (human-animal, organic, singularly sexed) state. This ending likewise shifts reproductive horror back into its 'rightful' place: Elsa shares her body with another, so that her body, as space and site of inquiry, is now her laboratory. The gynaehorrific punchline is that her punishment for having used science to create life outside the body is to be a vessel and bear the next monster herself.

Dren, then, is a thrumming locus of desire, not in the psychoanalytic sense, nor even really in the sense that it is formed from an ambitious and industrialised abstraction of heterosexual coupling. Instead, it is a tangible, living, queer, techno-organic manifestation of the drive to make connections, over and over, expanding and collapsing kaleidoscopically through diverse permutations and genetic possibilities, exerting extraordinary capacities that coalesce, becoming dissolute, and restratify. In their creation of the chimera, Elsa and Clive have created life, but not necessarily in the sense that they intended, for as monster Dren is a marvel, offering the wonder and horror of becomings without end. There is nonetheless a degree of anthropocentrism at play – the winning 'secret ingredient', after all, is Elsa's own DNA – but the monstrous promise and threat of these becomings bleeds through the film's final moments, for there is no real sense that this new, incestuous hybrid will be any easier to control than its parent.

Brave new worlds: cyborg futures and female subjectivity

Given that the horror genre is deeply concerned with probing the physical and philosophical limits and capacities of the body and the self, I find it remarkable that so few films engage with the problems of sexual difference or gendered (or postgendered) subjectivity in a meaningful way by offering alternative ways of charting subjectivity or centralising the capacities of female sub-jectivity in a manner that doesn't frame the sexed, reproductive female body as a problem, a vessel, a weakness or an impediment. This posits the female as an obstacle to be erased instead of one of a multivalent set of potentialities: a point of departure, a springboard, a solution, a site of embodied identity, one snapshot of congruence in a broader block of becomings. Instead, the films about reproductive technologies discussed in this chapter, and those concerned with pregnancy in the chapter prior, express an extraordinary dis-ease about the potential permeability of the physical and conceptual boundaries that are constructed between the notions of 'self' and 'other'. For the most part they treat any ontological uncertainty *itself* as a site of horror and anxiety instead of potentially productive or subversive. Instead, these films work very hard to individuate the pregnant woman and the foetus or unborn, reifying and shoring up these distinctions so as to offset the abject 'I-and-not-I' relationship between the two, as opposed to seeing the embodied self as a dynamic entity-in-process. This happens narratively and aesthetically by distancing, abstracting or eliminating the pregnant subject in a manner that attacks rather than expands her capacity, or by positing either the foetus or the woman herself as a monstrous other, both of which set up an antagonistic conflict between woman and the unborn that reflects cultural and scientific discourses of pregnancy and embodiment. So, to close, I ask whether other explorations of the body and the self *vis-à-vis* technology might help overcome this anxiety over subjectivity and the 'indivisible' self, particularly with regards to women, reproductive technologies, and bodies in film. After all, the monstrous can be considered as a productive category, too, such that the troubling of the conceptual boundaries such as self and other, and human and monster, can be framed as a positive expansion of capacity and affect and an aggregation, not a destructive dissolution.

The intersection of technology and the organic is central to Donna Haraway's seminal article "A Cyborg Manifesto: Science, Technology, and Socialist-Feminism in the Late Twentieth Century" (1991), which offers one way of leaving behind this restrictive division between self and other while simultaneously celebrating the expansion or the augmentation of the concept of the subject. Although the concerns in this work have been taken up, expanded upon and, in some ways, superseded by alternative formations of posthuman hybridity, it remains canonical. Its emphases also speak to (and perhaps, respond to) the fetishisation of technology itself that is keenly expressed in much reproductive technohorror, and I would also posit that given the reciprocal relationship between philosophy and popular culture it has had its own influence within the genre. Because of these intersections, it offers a good point of departure.

Haraway notably defines the cyborg, or cybernetic organism, as both a social reality and a fictional creature (p. 149). Within Haraway's schema, the cyborg invokes a utopian socialist-feminist philosophy to challenge the notion of submission and domination that is found within mainstream feminist and Marxist engagements with science and technology. It looks to new and interesting combinations of the biological and the technological, and considers how these aspirational combinations and alliances might offer openness and new possibilities, not restrictions. This means that it is a productive, progressive entity, instead of a regressive one, and is a figure that has the potential to counter the conservatism at the heart of so many reproductive technohorror narratives. Haraway positions the cyborg as something we all are – "chimeras, theorized and fabricated hybrids of machine and organism" (p. 150) – so that the figure of the cyborg is as much an ontological position as it is a metaphor and a literal description of the human body within technology-saturated, late-capitalist culture. It is inherently non-androcentric and refutes majoritarian politics. Excitement and tension occur where the distinction between dualities such as organism and machine intersect, for the relationship between "organism and machine has been a border war. The stakes in the border war have been the territories of production, reproduction, and imagination" (p. 150).

Clearly, this tension between bodies, selves and technologies is at the fore in philosophical accounts of pregnant subjectivity, as well as cinematic explorations of reproduction. Instead of treating this border as a site of fear or disavowal, Haraway advocates for the pleasure that can be found in boundary confusion. This is a pleasure – and a sense of protest – that is aggressively and playfully present in early cyberfeminisms, such as the work of Australian avant-garde feminist art collective VNS Matrix, whose project very clearly addresses some of the spaces of inquiry raised in this chapter, including the problematic fetishisation of technology that informs the practice and representation of reproductive technology. The collective, which was active from 1991 to 1997 and thus contemporaneous with Haraway's manifesto, took Haraway's 'sheroic' (cf. heroic) work and explored its potential through the creation of art, video games, posters, billboards, installations, interactive works and other such interventions that existed in both cyberspace and the 'meatspace' – that is, the offline world. Their work is helpful and instructive because it highlights how the blank, flattened space of the digital and cybernetic – much like the space of science – has never been neutral at all, but is implicitly and insidiously gendered. As collective member Virginia Barrett states in a recent retrospective of the group's work, "The technological landscape was very dry, Cartesian, relevant" (Evans 2014b). It was – and is – a masculine space, an "exclusive boy zone", and the people who write the code "maintained control of the productions of technology" (Evans 2014b).

VNS Matrix's utopian, speculative work, like that of contemporaneous cyberfeminists, looked to 'corrupt' this androcentric technology by using it to playfully interrogate divisions of sex and gender (Evans 2014a) and insert women and bodies into digital space by unpicking mind–body distinctions and encouraging digital play. Their best known work, the multimedia project *All New Gen*,[2] incorporated their 1991 "Cyberfeminist Manifesto for the 21st Century", which combines the gleefully sexual, the abject, and the technological:

> we are the modern cunt
> positive anti reason
> unbounded unleashed unforgiving [...]
> we are the virus of the new world disorder
> rupturing the symbolic from within
> saboteurs of big daddy mainframe
> the clitoris is a direct line to the matrix [...]
> go down on the altar of abjection [...]

The manifesto's engagement with sex, technology, agency and disruption closes with the statement that "we are the future cunt". Alongside the deliciously monstrous figure of cyber-heroine All New Gen (accompanied – of course – by her posse of 'DNA Sluts') this moves past a self-descriptor to become a challenge, a threat and a strident assertion of space and identity that attacks implicit exclusion of non-men and sticky, wet embodiment from digital and technological spaces. This is especially powerful, given that the 'wild west' of the comparatively unstructured internet and first-wave net-culture of the early-1990s was giving way to spaces that were much more widely accessible by the public. VNS Matrix's work is representative of the broader cyberfeminist project of the 1990s in its insistence on engaging in an artistic and political techno-practice which is "not about boring toys for boring boys" (100 Anti-theses). Instead, it sought to 'un-man' the future and take back space from "technocowboys" (Evans 2014b) through a celebration of the disruptive powers of alternative femininities, queer bodies and desires. In the allegedly blank and open space of the digital, identity is asserted through the deliberate articulation of difference – here, specific difference from the supposedly neutral but ultimately gendered framework of big daddy mainframe, and all the political asymmetries that that implies. From the perspective of the norm – that which is challenged – this intrusion is, itself, horrific, and beautifully, productively so.

VNS Matrix's ground-breaking cyberfeminist work directly plays with some of the many ways gender, sex and power might operate in digital space, but other intersections of the body and technology are not as invested in the potential for explicitly gendered embodiments. Haraway notes that the cyborg is "a creature in a post-gender world" (1991, p. 150); that is, the cyborg is a potentially emancipatory and utopian construct precisely because it negates structures of patriarchal domination by rendering gender irrelevant or obsolete. For Haraway, this productive liminality is a necessary condition of being cyborg, and she asserts that "Late twentieth-century machines have made thoroughly ambiguous the difference between natural and artificial, mind and body... Our machines are disturbingly lively, and we find ourselves frighteningly inert" (1991, 152). And yet, an escape from the body does not necessarily mean an escape from the negative ways that sex and gender are leveraged.

Technology is ostensibly without inherent gender and may, instead, offer a fluidity of sex and gender roles. Yet, technologies are created by people and operate within social contexts, and their use and conceptualisation is shaped as such. As Claudia Springer demonstrates in great detail in her discussion of the intersection of technology, eroticism and sexuality in her 1996 book *Electronic Eros*, "technology has no sex, but representations of technology often do" (p. 8). She also highlights how some cyborg narratives about the creation and destruction of life, such as those found in the science fiction films *Demon Seed* (1977) and *Eve of Destruction* (1991), much like the False Maria of *Metropolis*, emphasise and even aggressively shore up sexual and gender difference (1996, 68; 119; 150–1).[3] Even in the representation of virtual or cerebral sex acts in science fiction literature, graphic novels and films, in which minds interact without bodies, "gender roles tend for the most part to remain stereotypical" (1996, 11). This is ironic, given that one of the potentially liberating outcomes of non-embodied sex (and the associated jettisoning of embodied identity), is a side-lining of the sociocultural, political and economic restrictions that apply disproportionally to women's bodies within social structures that idealise the heterosexual nuclear family and the woman's efface-ment of her own autonomy and subjectivity in the name of maintaining the private sphere (1996, 70).

Further, the call for such an emancipation from the lived, embodied body – from the 'meat space' of the lived world, with all the term's phallic insinuations – can be read as a suggestion that gender and sexual difference themselves are problems, instead of things that are made problematic through systems and histories of inequity and oppression. However, this also insinuates that, in doing so, women should give up their sexed bodies and identities – a call that certainly sits at odds with philosophies that explore sexual difference, such as the call by feminist philosopher Christine Battersby (1998) for an embodied, phenomenological philosophy that doesn't rest on the perceived or assumed subordinate place of the female body, or even Luce Irigaray's exploration of an ethics that is contingent on a mutual respect for sexual difference in *An Ethics of Sexual Difference* (1993). If sexual difference – that is, difference from men – limits women, this speaks to the failure of our ways of thinking about sex, gender, subjects and bodies, not a failure of those bodies and subjects themselves.

This is made even more complicated by the fact that within the relatively blank space of the digital, difference itself becomes an important part of articulation of identity. Inequity is built into the very absence of signifiers, for within these spaces there remains a presumption that the subject, by default, is normative: heterosexual, male, cis-gendered. Certainly, as Springer attests, pleasure may operate at the interface between the human and the technological, especially in the fusion of human flesh with electronic devices (1996, 58), but within the narratives discussed in this chapter these interactions are less ecstatic than they are bound up within asymmetric power structures that suppress the autonomy and subjectivity of embodied female subjects. These re-inscriptions of sexual and gendered norms are all the more powerful given that "popular culture represents a collapse of the boundary between human and technological as a sexual act" (1996, 61). Film, as a visual medium, expresses these erotic, sexual and sometimes abusive intersections within a cinematic language that embeds sexual inequality and the imbalances and anxieties about reproductive politics into its visual grammar, and in doing so naturalises some of the ways that we think about the relationships between bodies and technologies.

Within cyberfeminisms, cyborg narratives, and what we might think of as technohorror, the notion of gender and reproduction becomes fraught. Although the cyborg itself might be an ambivalent character, Springer suggests that anxiety regarding the (lack of) integrity of the body, in part influenced by post-nuclear, late 20th-century threats to the body, perhaps leads to a wish to abandon the body and to preserve human consciousness outside the body. The intersection of the human body and electronic technology, then, "represents a paradoxical desire to preserve human life by destroying it" (1996, 77). Springer discusses the recurrence of 'imaginary' and 'cerebral' sex in science fiction, cyberpunk and other cyborg discourses – "sex without physically touching another human" (1996, 70) – and the prevalence of narratives in which (physical, embodied) sexuality is feared, for "sexuality evokes the creation of life" (Springer 2005, 81). Within this schema, disembodied sex is for *recreational* stimulation, not for reproduction. In the context of sex, procreation, reproduction and the embodied nature of gender and sexuality, reproductive freedoms perhaps become the freedom *from* reproduction, or at least the network of restrictions that are placed upon the reproductive body. Likewise, digital reproduction – the self-reproduction of systems, selves, meanings and code – does just as much conceptually to displace the notion of biological reproduction, even if certain types of reproduction, like that of transmission and reproduction of viruses, comes to utilise a language that both denotes and connotes certain types of unruly biological processes. Springer indicates, then, that the cyborg is a new incarnation of the fascination and disgust that is associated with the limits of the corporeal body, in particular how technology paradoxically "represent[s] both escape from the physical body and the fulfilment of erotic desire" (Springer 2005, 71). It is telling that such a duality links together highly gendered notions of abjection, through the intertwining of attraction and repulsion, and a disavowal of embodiment as we understand it. This dual aim elides the nature of the fleshy, reproductive body itself, and digital reproduction – the reproduction of systems, selves, meanings and code – does just as much conceptually to displace the notion of biological reproduction.

Techno-bodies, be they physical or digital, also exist within as many webs and snares as fleshy ones. Haraway's position is explicitly utopian, a self-professed "effort to build an ironic political myth" (1991, 147), but in speaking of the promise of cyborg ontology and politics, she does not entirely address the use and abuse of power, be it technological, political, physical or otherwise. Haraway's enthusiasm for a promising, emancipatory cyborg future, does not overtly engage with the unfortunate practicalities that are a part of the pragmatics of the cyborg, including the intent behind and the application of science itself, or the conditions that may bring about or result from couplings of body and technology. Haraway certainly alludes to the position of reproductive bodies as they exist within power structures, noting that "women's bodies have boundaries that are permeable to both 'visualization' and 'intervention'. Of course, who controls the interpretation of bodily boundaries in medical hermeneutics is a major feminist issue" (p. 169). However, this statement is more an aside, and she does not return to this, even though the cyborg as a material construct is particularly bound to the female body.

Haraway's later considerations of post-gender utopia and dystopia in *Modest_Witness@Second_Millennium.FemaleMan_Meets_OncoMouse: Feminism and Technoscience* (1997) offer a powerful and nuanced account of the intersection of technologies with human-animal and non-human animal bodies, but they are distanced from and do not resolve the issues of pregnant subjectivity and the sexed body that are raised in this chapter.

After all, if technologies are reprodict-*ive*, what does that mean for reproduction and flesh? Canadian director David Cronenberg's corpus(!) of body horror speaks most directly to this, in its emphasis upon the literal and figurative (re)production and (re)births of bodies, information, violence and desire. Body horror films such as *The Brood* (1977), the uncanny gynaehorror *Dead Ringers* (1988), and his grotesque re-imaging of *The Fly* (1986) offer narratives that end with the apparent destruction of the key agent or expression of monstrosity, even if said monstrosity's seemingly inevitable return is suggested in a final repudiation of closure. Other films crescendo with a more triumphant sense of reproductive becomings that are both abject and surreal. *Videodrome* (1983) ends with its protagonist's fervent, perhaps suicidal acquiescence to 'the new flesh', an enigmatic calling that can be read, perhaps, as the apparently corporeally destructive but ultimately transcendent integration of flesh and technology, and all the productive and monstrous changes in affect, experiential capacity and eroticism that come with it.

Similarly, Cronenberg's *Scanners* (1981) ends with a new and unusual form of self-reproduction. During a violent and visceral psychic battle between two of the titular telepaths, the villainous Revok tells his brother, the powerful scanner Vale, that as he sucks his brain dry everything about Vale will be reproduced as a part of him. The brothers try to destroy one another but Vale, on the brink of corporeal dissolution, is incinerated (or perhaps incinerates himself), and throws his psychic self into Revok's body, thereby creating, or producing, a new self and a new form of being that may be even more powerful than before. His final declaration that "we" have won begs the question who "we" actually is, and what this means. This film, too, speaks to other sorts of expansive reproductive horrors: in a nod to the Thalidomide scandal of the 1960s, it is revealed that telepathy and telekinesis are specifically caused by a tranquiliser that is being given to pregnant women. Revok is secretly dosing pregnant women so that he may use the currently unborn as an army of 'scanners' when they become adults; as in the prenatal 'augmentations' in *The Unborn*, the illicit creation of scanners is a deliberate intersection of the technological and the human that uses women's bodies as incubators. In a key moment, another scanner working in opposition to Revok sits in a doctor's waiting room and realises that she is being scanned – not by the pregnant women sitting near her, but by the woman's telepathic foetus. In the worlds of each of these films the monstrous is an expansion of human capacity and a rerouting of desire, not something that counters the human (or even the humane).

These films are the exception rather than the rule in reproductive technohorror. In general, this skirting around – and, perhaps, this rejection of – the notion of sexed, reproductive bodies within this loose category of films can be problematic, and indicates how tricky it is to separate such bodies from the highly inequitable and insidiously embedded web of power structures that we exist within. The 'female problem' of sexual difference (that is, difference from the ideal male subject and his body, but difference that is necessary to its conceptual construction) remains profoundly prominent. Haraway asserts that the state of 'being' female is not enough to bind women together, especially as femaleness is in itself a sociosexual, political and scientific construct (1991, 155), but the constructed-ness of these categories does not mitigate their everyday, lived realities. As such, a tension remains in Springer's and Haraway's work between the conceptual and emancipatory possibilities offered by cyborg feminisms and the reality of the historically, socially and politically produced embodied and gendered body. Such fleshy bodies are certainly offered a little more purchase in the anarchic, slimy and gleefully profane space of VNS Matrix's installations and cyberfeminist manifesto, which reaches out to gender(s) and queer desire(s) and asserts itself (or gate-crashes, even) into cyberspace. Possibilities, too, exist in Cronenberg's work, although these reproductive becomings and technohorrors more often than not explore the expansion and reproductive possibilities of the male or male-coded body – although not to the exclusion of the female body, as in many Frankenstein narratives.

However, the limitations of such utopian thinking are echoed by VNS Matrix's Virginia Barratt, who suggests in a recent discussion of the legacy of cyberfeminist work in the 1990s that, "the narratives around liberation from racism, sexism and so on in the brave new virtual world were promises which were empty" (Evans 2014b). Her co-creator, Francesca da Rimini goes on to indicate that the anarchic, destabilising impulse that drove these cyberfeminisms is alive and well in other forms of media and activism, from female hacker groups and techno-savvy art collectives, to the utilisation of interesting computer-based technologies by female artists working with roller derby terms,[4] but that their own artistic work (like, perhaps, Haraway's initial formulation of the cyborg) fulfilled its purpose in its particular social and historical context and needs to be situated as such.[5]

Nonetheless, it is difficult to find ways of aligning conceptualisations of utopian feminist-socialist cyborg futures and pleasurable interfaces, at least as they are stated here, with the sorts of philosophical models of subjectivity that I discuss in the previous chapter, which allow for, rather than negate, expansive modes of female embodiment, the experience of pregnancy, and the flexibility of the notion of the allegedly 'individual' subject. The ability of entities and systems to replicate, produce and reproduce in digital or cybernetic spaces is not inherently an escape from physical reproduction, and even if sex, pleasure and eroticism are untethered from reproduction, this doesn't necessarily liberate the embodied, reproductive subject from systems of power and domination. This utopian figure of the technofeminist, queer cyborg also sits uncomfortably alongside cinematic representations of women and technology that posit 'female' cyborgs as alluring, servile and (sometimes) sexually available yet dangerous, and reproductive technologies as both dangerously unregulated and a convenient way of 'liberating' reproduction from the problematic bodies of equally problematic women. Within these films, technologies that offer both freedom *from* reproduction and freedom *to* reproduce do not co-exist well. The result is a tangled, gynaehorrific web that traps, victimises and eliminates the individual, no matter what she chooses to do, for an embodied subject position posited as 'female', let alone reproductive, sits perpetually as other-to the implicitly male metaphysical matrix which is deemed neutral and value-free.

A more productive way to address these contradictions might be found in Rosi Braidotti's (2002) account of the connections and disjunctures between Haraway's cyborg and Gilles Deleuze's rhizome. Braidotti highlights the importance of sexual difference (and other forms of minoritarian micro-politics) in the configuration of patterns of becoming, not to argue for a sort of sexual essentialism, but to acknowledge that the politics of such asymme-trical power structures and the "non-coincidence" of the masculine and the feminine inform and respond to the possibilities of said becomings (p. 214). As she reminds us, sexuality and sexual difference are "too structurally embedded in subjectivity to be merely laid aside as the obsolete properties of a cybernetic self" (p. 243). The Deleuzean subject offers an alternative: as a type of mobile, dynamic 'in-between', a "folding-in of external influences and a simultaneous unfolding outward of affects" (p. 230), which renders the inter-section of technology and flesh a series of perpetual snapshots of the now, a change-event that re-configures subjectivity outside of modes of fixity and is always its own centre. What is particularly helpful to this discussion is that Braidotti advocates for the materialism and the embodied-ness of this body-in-process, which sits as a challenge to the "eroticised fetishization of the technological" (p. 233): the feminisation of the unruly technologies of modernity, the masculinisation of technologies of corporeal colonisation, and the dupli-citous 'making-neutral' of gendered digital space, whose sexual indeterminacy nonetheless reinscribes phallocentric modes of knowing and being.

Deleuze and Guattari (2004) suggest, provactively and certainly con-tentiously, that all becomings begin with 'becoming-woman' (as an expression of disengagement with the molarity that is Man; see Grosz 1993) and lead to the immanence of becoming-imperceptible (pp. 307–8). It is worth remem-bering that becoming in this sense not to change into one thing nor to imitate it, but to form a molecular and mutual alliance between two 'organs' (or organised bodies), so that one becomes *with* another (p. 285). One enters into composition with another (p. 289) into its own rhizomatic haecceity, or this-ness, that is defined by its capacity to affect, to be affected, and its relations of movement and rest (p. 288). Braidotti looks, strategically, to the figure of the cyborg through the lens of meta(l)morphoses – techno-organic becomings that acknowledge the cultural coding of technology as gendered and that bear the marks of difference (gender, sexual, racial) (p. 235). A becoming-machine, then, implicitly includes expressions, politics and capacities of sex and gender, and evidences the tracing of the human/organic/social upon technology as much as technology enters into relations with the organic, the one tracing and producing the other.

Such a sense of reciprocal relations is present in the near-future British science fiction thriller *The Machine* (2014). This film sits somewhat outside of the horror genre but it speaks to the heady connection of the terms 'monster' and 'marvel', and is a lens of augury through which teratoscopy, or the divination through monsters, might productively occur. The film's explorations of gendered cyborgs and artificial intelligence are offered in a manner that suggests intersections between technologies and the notions of the human and the subject are productive and complementary, even if the conditions under which such encounters occur are dubious and unethical. Scientist Vincent McCarthy is working to develop new forms of artificial intelligence and cybernetic technologies, although his work is shaped by socio-political forces: Britain is mired in a Cold War with China, and his research funding comes from the Ministry of Defence with some significant strings attached. This includes his role in damaging and unethical work involving the cybernetic augmentation of a group of wounded and brain-damaged returned soldiers, an apparent fix that stitches them further into the military-industrial complex. These cyborgs continue to work on the military base as guards and though they appear to lose the capacity for human speech post-operation, they secretly develop their own language and social organisation, although McCarthy initially attempts to protect himself by remaining deliberately unaware of the extent of the cruelty of the experiments. McCarthy hires Ava, a similarly sympathetic and compassionate scientist who is perhaps named for computing pioneer Ada Lovelace. She has created a profoundly innovative and 'human' AI that can learn, and during their work the couple form a strong emotional bond. Ava's reactionary politics and her compassion for the soldiers who are acting as experimental subjects result in her being assassinated at the behest of one of her overseers. McCarthy, grief-stricken, installs Ava's perfected AI model into a streamlined cybernetic body based on her bodily form, creating what initially seems to be an avatar that expresses a sort of unimaginative apotheosis of technofemininity. The resulting gynoid creation is dubbed Machine. 'She' is a creation that the Ministry of Defence hope to turn into a perfect soldier, although McCarthy's interference means that she develops a strong sense of ethics that is a deliberate reaction against the previously 'grey' area of his research and the violent intentions of his superiors.

The film is a thoughtful rumination on the nature of technology, intelligence and identity, and it is unusual in the way that it posits a cyborg future not just as an inevitability, but as an interesting and productive one. We see early on that the augmented soldiers' new language is efficient, creative and functional. As they settle in to their newly expanded bodies, their experience of the world changes, alongside their consciousness. They remain silent, resentful and watchful, although they feign acquiescence, but their acknowledgement of Ava's interest in their wellbeing pre-disposes them towards later helping

McCarthy and Machine escape the base. This subplot involving the cyborg soldiers, in which the creations ultimately undermine and then overthrow their human Ministry of Defence masters, looks back explicitly to the Frankenstein model, whereby the nature of the creation and its 'humane' development shines a light on the inhumanity of the creator. However, their masters in this instance are warmongering politicians, and the soldiers are active in refusing their pre-determined role as weapons in a global war and revolt, pitting the 'new' world against the old and the subjugated against their masters. These issues are further emphasised through the ever-present electronic soundscape: it explicitly references progressive rock musician Vangelis's soundtrack to the neo-noir film *Blade Runner*, which is similarly interested in issues of artificial intelligence, cyborg subjectivity and corporeal obsolescence.

Beyond the issues of the development of new forms of experience and consciousness, the film offers a thoughtful engagement with issues of posthuman gender and embodiment. Throughout much of the film McCarthy is torn between the demands of his work and the wellbeing of his profoundly ill daughter Mary, each of which are coded as a form of fatherhood. He maps her brain using Ava's technology, thereby constructing an exquisitely intricate 'back up' or replication of her consciousness, but after her death this copy, the living, digital ghost of his daughter is used by his employers as leverage in another techno-industrial act of stratification and control. Ultimately, he realises that the safest way to 'save' his daughter is to unpick his assumptions about the nature of alternate forms of being and consciousness: he chooses to store Mary's within Machine's own mind until she can be moved elsewhere, combining his once living daughter and the newly-living creature in a manner that emphasises plasticity and hybridity. This decision embraces the complex social and historical web of reciprocal encounters between the technological and the organic instead of seeing the 'now' as a neutral, static site after which there is only difference. Importantly, it connects or combines the two while allowing each to retain their autonomy, refuting any concrete distinction between I and not-I by reconfiguring the notion of the in-divisible, individual subject. After their escape, and in the film's final moments, we see McCarthy interacting with Mary's AI through a tablet computer, but she asks if she can spend some time with her 'mother' – that is, Machine. In an earlier scene Machine, trapped inside the military base, wonders at a picture of a sunrise, and the film's resolution shows Machine standing before the rising sun at the dawning of a new day and a new era, her profile and posture distinctly non-human. She holds the tablet and communicates – plays! – with Mary in a way McCarthy cannot begin to parse, for the machines' language, their temporality and affectivity, and the configurations of their relationship are humanly incomprehensible, even if some of the language is familiar. It is a contemplative and hopeful ending, not a dystopian one, and one that works to find new forms of relationships, parenthood, birth, reproduction, intelligence and identity. As spectators we are aligned with McCarthy's point of view. We share his curiosity, even his bewilderment, at the events, but for him the prospect of artificial intelligence is a positive development and not something to be inherently feared, even if its uncertainty produces anxiety. It becomes apparent that by forcing himself to look at the consequences of his work, by challenging his own anthropocentrism and his understanding of what it means to be human(e) (or even alive), he has become a more ethical person. His realisation that humans in their current state will become obsolete or irrelevant frees him; the current expression or iteration of humanity is just a fleeting moment in a broader living history.

Certainly, the film draws from stereotypical constructions of masculinity and femininity: Machine is hyper-feminine in appearance and has a breathy, girlish mode of speech that oddly evokes that of Marilyn Monroe, even as it is juxtaposed against her fearsome physical capabilities. The sequence charting her birth collapses into the fetishisation of femininity and technology. Machine's raw, cybernetic skeleton curls up in a mock-foetal position, then uncoils and stretches out, offering a blunt echo of the scene in which *Metropolis*'s False Maria is brought to life. The body rises through a clear viscous substance, and as its opaque, firm but gelatinous computer-brain is inserted the portentous synthesised chords of the soundtrack find visual purchase in a neo-chiaroscuro emphasis upon metallic, reflective surfaces and the elegance of the process's industrial sleekness. The camera moves up the unfinished body as it is pumped full of a red fluid, and the image of the slick, transparent form containing and shaping the flow of the blood-substitute, especially as it flows down and into the shape of its breasts, is a powerful expression of the complex co-mingling of technology and the abject female body. Outside of these signifiers and expressions of techno-femininity, Machine also comes to adore McCarthy as a father-partner figure in a manner that sits strangely against his earlier, burgeoning relationship with Ava, and that reads as particularly gendered. And yet, despite this slip into normativity, the film posits monstrosity – that is, the breaching of normative boundaries, and the expansion of non-human capacity, the desirous production of connections – as productive and hopeful, and a way of surpassing the meagre limitations of human corporeality and intelligence. It is deliberately ambiguous, in that it does not seek to demonstrate hard answers to many of the moral questions it poses. *The Machine* also offers an interesting challenge to representations of female subjectivity in films about pregnancies and reproductive technohorror. It moves beyond a fleshy female body without rendering embodiment, femininity, maternity or affect obsolete, and in a manner that, unlike earlier representations of unruly technology, doesn't inherently conflate the feminine with destruction, weakness or expendability.

Notes

1 An oddly positive scientist – not quite mad, but certainly transgressive and a little odd – is Rosetta Stone, who creates three digital clones of herself in the unusual and gentle science fiction romance *Teknolust* (2002). This film ends positively, for

Rosetta is lovingly framed as both mother and sister, and each of her clones comes to experience the world in their own way and find connection outside of their digital confines; see Stacey (2010, 195–224) for a detailed reading of the film. A more recent example can be found in 2016 reboot of the 1985 comedy *Ghostbusters*, which replaces the originally male team of paranormal scientists with four women – three scientists and a transportation worker. Although none of the women are objectified or framed in terms of their sex appeal, it is notable that the team's 'mad' scientist, the delightfully zany Holtzmann (played by lesbian comedian Kate McKinnon), is explicitly coded as queer. The casting of the women was met with hostility and outright misogyny by a small but vocal subset of fans of the original, whose distaste for a female-centric film led them to launch online harassment campaigns against the film and its actors, and to accuse the film's makers of "reverse-sexism" and "PC ideology" (Sims 2016).

2   See *VNS Matrix: All New Gen* (Australian Centre for Contemporary Art) and *VNS Matrix: All New Gen* (Media Art Net) for images and documentation of the project and installation.

3   This is especially the case in the latter film: secret military project Eve VIII is a cyborg that has been made in the image of, and is endowed with the memories of, her creator Dr Eve Simmonds. The cyborg is described as hypersexualised and psychopathic, and in many ways 'she' is presented as Simmonds' violent, unruly id. Eve VIII's female-ness is a core part of both her character and her threat, especially as she is armed with a nuclear warhead that sits where her cervix and uterus should be, rendering her reproductivity and her feminine techno-embodiment quite literally lethal.

4   See the website *Bloodbath by BUMP in association with Sydney Roller Derby League* (2016) for information on and documentation of this interdisciplinary, multi-media project, in which artworks are created live during roller derby bouts based on data sent from the players to the artists, and are then projected during the game.

5   For the purposes of this discussion, it's notable that the "100 Anti-theses of Cyber-feminism", which were drafted at the Cyberfeminism International gathering in Berlin in 1997, include "cyberfeminism is not a horror movie" (#78) and "cyberfe-minism is not science fiction" (#79), thus attacking head-on a sort of marginalising set of definitions – as genre, as fiction, as containable and definable – and in doing so positing that cyberfeminist causes and practices are more slippery and robust than something that can be more easily co-opted (*100 Anti-theses*).

Bibliography

'100 Anti-theses' 1997, *Old Boys Network*, accessed September 11, 2016, from <http://www.obn.org/cfundef/100antitheses.html>.

Al-Gailani, S 2009, 'Magic, science and masculinity: marketing toy chemistry sets', *Studies in History and Philosophy of Science Part A*, 40(4), pp. 372–381.

Australian Centre for Contemporary Art 2013, 'VNS Matrix: All New Gen', *Australian Centre for Contemporary Art*, accessed September 11, 2016, from <https://www.accaonline.org.au/exhibition/vns-matrix-all-new-gen>.

Battersby, C 1998, *The phenomenal woman: feminist metaphysics and the patterns of identity*, Cambridge, UK: Polity Press.

'Bloodbath by BUMP in association with Sydney Roller Derby League' 2016, *bumpp. net*, accessed September 13, 2016, from <http://bumpp.net/>.

Bordo, S 1986, 'The Cartesian masculinization of thought', *Signs*, 11(3), pp. 439–456.

Braidotti, R 2002, *Metamorphoses: towards a materialist theory of becoming*, Cambridge, UK and Malden, MA: Polity Press in association with Blackwell Publishers.

Braidotti, R 2011, *Nomadic subjects: embodiment and sexual difference in contemporary feminist theory*, 2nd ed., New York: Columbia University Press.

Braidotti, R 2013, *The posthuman*, accessed December 16, 2016, from <http://www.123library.org/book_details/?id=105441>.

Broege, V 1988, 'Views on human reproduction and technology in science fiction', *Extrapolation*, 29(3), pp. 197–215.

Cook, J S 2016, 'From Siri to sexbots: Female AI reinforces a toxic desire for passive, agreeable and easily dominated women', *Salon*, accessed September 11, 2016, from <http://www.salon.com/2016/04/08/from_siri_to_sexbots_female_ai_reinforces_a_toxic_desire_for_passive_agreeable_and_easily_dominated_women/>.

Creed, B 2005, *Phallic panic: film, horror and the primal uncanny*, Melbourne: Melbourne University Publishing.

Davis-Floyd, R & Dumit, J (eds) 1998, *Cyborg babies: from techno-sex to techno-tots*, New York: Routledge.

Deleuze, G & Guattari, F 2004, *A thousand plateaus: capitalism and schizophrenia*, London: Continuum.

Ebenstein, J 2016, *The anatomical venus*, London: Thames & Hudson.

Edwards, R G 2001, 'The bumpy road to human in vitro fertilization', *Nature Medicine*, 7(10), pp. 1091–1094.

Ettorre, E 2002, *Reproductive genetics, gender, and the body*, London and New York: Routledge.

Evans, C L 2014a, '"We are the future cunt": cyberfeminism in the 90s', *Motherboard*, accessed September 11, 2016, from <http://motherboard.vice.com/read/we-are-the-future-cunt-cyberfeminism-in-the-90s>.

Evans, C L 2014b, 'An oral history of the first cyberfeminists', *Motherboard*, accessed September 11, 2016, from <http://motherboard.vice.com/read/an-oral-history-of-the-first-cyberfeminists-vns-matrix>.

Farquar, D 2000, '(M)other discourses', in G Kirkup (ed), *The gendered cyborg: a reader*, London and New York: Routledge in association with the Open University, , pp. 209–220.

Flicker, E 2012, 'Women scientists in mainstream film: social role models – a contribution to the public understanding of science from the perspective of film sociology', in P Weingart & B Huppauf (eds), *Science images and popular images of the sciences*, London and New York: Routledge, pp. 241–256.

Franklin, S 2006, 'The cyborg embryo: our path to transbiology', *Theory, Culture & Society*, 23(7–8), pp. 167–187.

Galton, F 1904, 'Eugenics: its definition, scope, and aims', *American Journal of Sociology*, 10(1), pp. 1–25.

Gaston, N 2015, *Why science is sexist*, Wellington, New Zealand: Bridget Williams Books Limited.

Griggs, B 2011, 'Why computer voices are mostly female', *CNN*, accessed September 11, 2016, from <http://www.cnn.com/2011/10/21/tech/innovation/female-computer-voices/index.html>.

Grosz, E 1993, 'A thousand tiny sexes: feminism and rhizomatics', *Topoi*, 12(2), pp. 167–179.

Halberstam, J 1995, *Skin shows: gothic horror and the technology of monsters*, Durham, NC: Duke University Press.

Halberstam, J & Livingston, I 1995, 'Introduction: posthuman bodies', in J Halberstam & I Livingston (eds), *Posthuman bodies*, Bloomington, IN: Indiana University Press.

Haraway, D J 1991, 'A cyborg manifesto: science, technology, and socialist-feminism in the late twentieth century' in Haraway, D J, *Simians, cyborgs and women: the reinvention of nature*, London: Free Association, pp. 149–181.

Haraway, D J 1997, *Modest_Witness@Second_Millennium.FemaleMan_Meets_Onco-Mouse: feminism and technoscience*, New York: Routledge.

Hoffmann, D E & Tarzian, A J 2001, 'The girl who cried pain: a bias against women in the treatment of pain', *The Journal of Law, Medicine & Ethics*, 28(s4), pp. 13–27.

Huxley, A 1946, *Brave new world*, New York: Perennial Library.

Huyssen, A 1981, 'The vamp and the machine: technology and sexuality in Fritz Lang's *Metropolis*', *New German Critique*, 24/25, pp. 221–237.

Irigaray, L 1993, *An ethics of sexual difference*, Ithaca, NY: Cornell University Press.

Jeffords, S 1994, *Hard bodies: Hollywood masculinity in the Reagan era*, New Brunswick, NJ: Rutgers University Press.

Kelly, A 1985, 'The construction of masculine science', *British Journal of Sociology of Education*, 6(2), pp. 133–154.

Kristeva, J 1982, *Powers of horror: an essay on abjection*, New York: Columbia University Press.

Lupton, D 1999, 'Risk and the ontology of pregnant embodiment', in D Lupton (ed), *Risk and sociocultural theory: new directions and perspectives*, Cambridge, UK: Cambridge University Press, pp. 59–85.

MacCormack, P 2012, *Posthuman ethics: embodiment and cultural theory*, Farnham, UK and Burlington, VT: Ashgate.

Martin, E 1991, 'The egg and the sperm: how science has constructed a romance based on stereotypical male–female roles', *Signs*, 16(3), pp. 485–501.

Media Art Net 2016, 'VNS Matrix: All New Gen', accessed September 11, 2016, from <http://medienkunstnetz.de/works/all-new-gen/>.

Mentor, S 1998, 'Witches, nurses, midwives and cyborgs', in R Davis-Floyd & J Dumit (eds), *Cyborg babies: from techno-sex to techno-tots*, New York: Routledge, pp. 67–89.

Merchant, C 2001, 'Dominion over nature', in M Lederman & I Bartsch (eds), *The gender and science reader*, London and New York: Routledge, pp. 68–81.

Moore, L J 2003, '"Billy, the sad sperm with no tail": representations of sperm in children's books', *Sexualities*, 6(3–4), pp. 277–300.

Moore, L J 2009, 'Killer sperm: masculinity and the essence of male hierarchies', in M C Inhorn, T Tjørnhøj-Thomsen, H Goldberg, & M la Cour Mosegaard (eds), *Reconceiving the second sex: men, masculinity, and reproduction*, Fertility, reproduction and sexuality, New York: Berghahn Books, pp. 45–71.

Mulkay, M 1996, 'Frankenstein and the debate over embryo research', *Science, technology & human values*, 21(2), pp. 157–176.

Nickelsberg, M 2016, 'Why is AI female? How our ideas about sex and service influence the personalities we give machines', *GeekWire*, accessed September 11, 2016, from <http://www.geekwire.com/2016/why-is-ai-female-how-our-ideas-about-sex-and-service-influence-the-personalities-we-give-machines/>.

Raymond, J G 1995, *Women as wombs: reproductive technologies and the battle over women's freedom*, North Melbourne, Vic.: Spinifex Press.

Shelley, M W 1988, *Frankenstein, or, the modern Prometheus: with supplementary essays and poems from the twentieth century*, Washington, DC: Orchises Press.

Sims, D 2016, 'The ongoing outcry against the *Ghostbusters* remake', *The Atlantic*, accessed September 11, 2016, from <http://www.theatlantic.com/entertainment/archive/2016/05/the-sexist-outcry-against-the-ghostbusters-remake-gets-louder/483270/>.

Skal, D J 1998, *Screams of reason: mad science and modern culture*, New York: W.W. Norton.

Springer, C 1996, *Electronic eros: bodies and desire in the postindustrial age*, Austin, TX: University of Texas Press.

Springer, C 2005, 'The pleasure of the interface', in A Utterson (ed), *Technology and culture, the film reader*, In focus–Routledge film readers, London and New York: Routledge, pp. 71–86.

Squier, S 1995, 'Reproducing the posthuman body: ectogenic fetus, surrogate mother, pregnant man', in J Halberstam and I Livingstone (eds), *Posthuman bodies*, Bloomington, IN: Indiana University Press, pp. 113–132.

Stacey, J 2010, *The cinematic life of the gene*, Durham, NC: Duke University Press.

Steiner, M & Born, L 2000, 'Advances in the diagnosis and treatment of premenstrual dysphoria', *CNS Drugs*, 13(4), pp. 287–304.

Toumey, C P 1992, 'The moral character of mad scientists: a cultural critique of science', *Science, Technology & Human Values*, 17(4), pp. 411–437.

Ussher, J M 2006, *Managing the monstrous feminine: regulating the reproductive body*, London and New York: Routledge.

VNS Matrix 1991, 'Cyberfeminist manifesto', *Sterneck.net*, accessed September 11, 2016, from <http://www.sterneck.net/cyber/vns-matrix/index.php>.

Wassarman, P M 1988, 'Fertilization in mammals', *Scientific American*, 259(6), pp. 78–84.

Weindling, P 2010, 'German eugenics and the wider world: beyond the racial state', in A Bashford & P Levine (eds), *The Oxford handbook of the history of eugenics*, Oxford and New York: Oxford University Press, pp. 315–331.

Weingart, P, Muhl, C & Pansegrau, P 2003, 'Of power maniacs and unethical geniuses: science and scientists in fiction film', *Public Understanding of Science*, 12(3), pp. 279–287.

Woliver, L R 2002, *The political geographies of pregnancy*, Urbana, IL: University of Illinois Press.

Young, I M 1990, 'Pregnant embodiment: subjectivity and alienation', in I M Young, *Throwing like a girl and other essays in feminist philosophy and social theory*, Bloomington, IN: Indiana University Press, pp. 160–176.

4   The monstrous-maternal
Negotiating discourses of motherhood

The Australian horror film *The Babadook* (2014) locates terror and monstrosity deep within the heart of a mother. Amelia, a widow who once had a career as a children's book illustrator, is trapped within a tangled cat's cradle of anxiety, loneliness, grief and resentment; her young son Samuel was born the night her husband, his father, was killed in a horrendous car accident. Amelia has never recovered from this trauma and seems to sleepwalk through life, working a low paid, demanding job and negotiating judgemental family members, at the same time as trying to care for her son in their gothic, decrepit home. Samuel is an intense and difficult but deeply loving child, and as his seventh birthday approaches – along with the anniversary of his father's death – the two are first haunted and then terrorised by an uncanny, monstrous black and white figure. The angular, expressionistic, Edward Gorey-esque Mister Babadook is a storybook monster who they simply can't get rid of, no matter how many times Amelia tries to throw away the mysterious red-bound book from which he apparently arises. This is no external manifestation, though; it is soon apparent that the horror is implicitly connected to Amelia. When she finally lets the monster in in a moment of weakness, and is then possessed and granted near-supernatural powers, we see the Babadook for what it is: an expression all of the hatred, sadness and loathing she has pent up for years, including the ill-will she bears her son, who lived when her beloved husband died. Samuel knows that Amelia doesn't love him, and tells her as much, but he fights the Babadook to save himself and his mother, hoping that his profound love for her is enough for them both. Amelia, then, is a monstrous mother in both the literal and the figurative senses. She certainly becomes the monstrous antagonist of the story, but the deeper monstrosity is much more insidious. She is a mother who does not love her child. She struggles to raise him. She cannot cope. She wishes him dead. She places him in the very danger from which she is meant to protect him; indeed, she is the greatest danger to her son. The repeated refrain that 'you can't get rid of the Babadook' highlights the indelibility of her maternal ambivalence. She cannot live up to the impossible ideals of motherhood, and she cannot do what is, supposedly, a natural and essential part of a woman's experience. Because of these failures she is always, and already, marked as a very particular type of gynaehorrific monster, even prior to the overt arrival of the Babadook. In this chapter I explore the way that these fundamental themes and ideological concerns are deeply embedded within horror films about mothers and motherhood.

In previous chapters I have explored the gynaehorrific underpinnings of horror films about the construction and dissolution of embodied reproductive female subjectivities through an appraisal of the manipulation of on-screen and diegetic space, the malleability of corporeality, the fragility of female subjectivity, and the reification of heteronormativity. In this chapter I continue the trajectory through a woman's normative, culturally sanctioned sexual life to consider the presentation of mothers and mothering in the horror film. This is an ideal site through which to consider women in / and horror, for as sociologist Tina Miller (2007) indicates, "the unrealistic assumptions embedded in gendered discourses that pattern women's lives ... [are] nowhere more apparent than in relation to reproduction, mothering and experiences of motherhood" (p. 337). Throughout this chapter I move away from previous discussions of embodied becomings to consider some of the contexts in which these connections emerge and operate, and instead focus on how historically-specific discourses of motherhood are articulated and interrogated in horror film. By this I mean the "sets of shared and often unconscious assumptions" about motherhood (Reid, Grieves and Poole 2008, 212) that, firstly, contribute to a popular and communal cultural understanding of what 'normal' motherhood is and should be, and that, secondly, work to subtly police and enforce this norm. I suggest that horror films can be considered not as static *representations* of motherhood, but as culturally and historically specific, dynamic *negotiations* with the expectations and pressures surrounding the fulfilment of normative motherhood. Such popular and cultural understandings both inform and are, in turn, shaped by women's shifting experiences of motherhood to provide a gynaehorrific account of motherhood that villainises and demonises even the 'best' of mothers, and that suggests that there is something specific about motherhood itself that is (and that makes women) monstrous.

This approach draws from the highly influential work of Michel Foucault (1994; 1995) on the way that bodies are surveilled, disciplined and managed – that is, made 'intelligible' through intersecting systems of power and meaning-making. Through this lens, culture can be understood as "as a set of (governmental and other) practices aimed at producing certain sorts of persons, not as a collection of phenomena which hold[s] meanings like a bank, from which people withdraw and to which they deposit" (Kendall and Wickham 1999, 139). Cultural objects – in this case, horror films – are "ragbags of knowledge, practices and programmes gradually put together, with new practices being invented and old practices revitalised and pressed into service for new tasks" (Kendall and Wickham 1999, 139). As such, horror films can be considered as cinematic art and popular entertainment as well as discursive artefacts and sites of discursive conflict, in that they both contribute to the circulation and enforcement of cultural norms while simultaneously challenging or countering them. Such an approach is deeply helpful when considering horror films as cultural artefacts, dynamic sites of cultural expressions, and the makers and bearers of culture. Within the context of power, discourse and sexuality, we can use them to interrogate what it means to be a 'normal' member of society (Gavey 2005, 7) by using them to appraise the sorts of patterns and flows of meaning, practice and normativity that serve to shape and constrain our understandings and assumptions about normative culture and society.

Although I do not engage in depth with the specific practice of Foucauldian discourse analysis throughout this chapter, the notion of culture-as-management is nonetheless salient: discourses of motherhood can be considered those linguistic and social practices (Gavey 2005, 84) that manage the way motherhood and the maternal are understood, disciplined, enforced and enacted. There are myriad ways that discourses of motherhood are negotiated, and how mother-subjects and motherhood are shaped and managed, but for the purposes of this discussion I also highlight how ideas about what motherhood 'should' be are naturalised through accounts of non-human animal motherhood, and how these so-called common sense ideas are then enforced in legal discourse, often in a punitive manner. Situating the mothers of horror film within this complex discursive network honours the role of popular film in creating, exploring and expressing complex dynamic systems of meanings and knowledge(s).

The anxieties, traumas and slippages inherent within horror as a genre also marks such films as sites of discursive instability, in which complex and often contradictory ideas about the nature of motherhood, femininity, subjectivity and what it means to mother 'properly' are negotiated and interrogated. This is fraught territory: on one hand, the notion of *essential* motherhood acts as a biological and cultural imperative that centres motherhood as an innate, desirable and inevitable part of a woman's life and experience (DiQuinzio 1999, viii). At the same time, there remains an extraordinarily powerful social imperative for women to conform to the figure of the '*ideal*' mother – that is, the fictional, aspirational figure of the self-sacrificing 'good' mother who performs her role in an ideologically-complicit fashion, whatever that might be. This dissonant contradiction indicates that the ability to mother well (or, perhaps, appropriately) is anything but natural, and must instead be learned, monitored and enforced. An understanding of motherhood in horror film can help interrogate what shifting meanings of and anxieties about motherhood are, without making any broad claims for what motherhood 'is' and 'should be'.

Throughout this chapter I also seek to problematise dominant readings of mothers in horror, which tend to emphasise the construction of 'good' and 'bad' mothers as, perhaps, essentialised categories or archetypes. Instead, I treat horror films as complicated sites of discursive and ideological negotiation, whose multivalent expressions cannot be easily distilled into clear categories of good and evil. Consider the following example: although the antagonist in most of the *Friday the 13th* series of slasher films is the hulking, hockey mask-wearing Jason Voorhees, the villain of the first film (1980) is revealed to be his mother, Pamela. A summer camp reopens after having been closed for two decades after a series of grisly murders. Despite this fresh start, the new camp counsellors are again picked off one by one by a mysterious figure who is eventually revealed to be Pamela, the camp's cook. She is trying to avenge the death of her young hydrocephalic son, Jason, who had drowned at the former camp because the teenagers who she had asked to mind him were more interested in having sex and getting stoned than they were in watching the boy. Pamela now hears voices compelling her to kill those she blames for the death, an impulse that is reflected in the film's unusual sound design: whispers of "ka-ka-ka-ka ma-ma-ma-ma" represent the dead Jason's commands to "kill them, mommy!"[1] such that Pamela's homicidal actions are shown to be motivated by both grief and maternal guilt.

Mrs Voorhees has been read as a violent and evil monstrous mother who is both overbearing and negligent (Arnold 2013, 68), but I suggest that she is a far more ambiguous figure who is shaped by both horror and redemption. Over the course of the franchise (at writing, 12 films), we learn that Mrs Voorhees became pregnant at 15 and was a fiercely protective mother to her son, in particular in her refusal to let him go far from her because of her concerns about his wellbeing. Mrs Voorhees exemplifies a particularly prominent type of mother of the horror film: she is so devoted to her child that she will do anything to save, protect or avenge him. At the same time, she was the one who put him in danger in the first place through the abdication of her parental responsibilities (in this case to irresponsible teenagers and by being a young solo working mother). Her importance as both a real person and a mythic mother-figure is confirmed in the first sequel: in *Friday the 13th Part 2* (1981), the mysteriously revived adult Jason acknowledges his mother's vengeful actions by taking her body and her head, which was severed at the end of the first film, and building a shrine around it in a cave in the woods, where he then leaves pieces of his victims as offerings. In this latter film's final confrontation the heroine convinces him to renege by instructing him to put down his knife, speaking to him as if she were a mother telling off a child. Jason, cowed by this replacement mother figure, is then wounded with the same machete that killed Pamela Voorhees and he disappears, leaving the shrine behind.

This dissonance and interplay between idealised and transgressive motherhood is emblematic of the way that discourses of motherhood are negotiated in the horror genre. Horror films are a space in which historically specific hopes and anxieties about the nature of motherhood and maternal affect are variously articulated, enforced and challenged, instead of bluntly represented as 'good' or 'bad'. Avoiding an emphasis on straight representation, and instead considering films in terms of the competing messages they express or articulate – that is, the aggregates or assemblages they form – allows for an exploration of what the nature and shape of dominant normative discourses of motherhood *are*, be they enduring or historically specific. For instance, how has psychoanalysis as popular discourse, rather than as interpretive practice, shaped the image of the mother? How does this once-dominant maternal discourse compare to millennial discourses of motherhood, which focus upon anxieties about the necessary impossibility of being the 'perfect mother'? And how do horror films, as complex sites of fear and wonder, participate in the (re)production of discourses of motherhood?

Throughout this discussion I consider this latter question through the lens of what I term the 'monstrous-maternal'. Through the use of this term I wish to acknowledge Barbara Creed's term 'monstrous-feminine', but I seek to apply the understanding of monstrosity in a manner that reflects the way that motherhood has been politically, culturally and historically framed and contested; that is, this is a gynaehorrific account of the nature of monstrous motherhood that seeks to deconstruct the monstrosity implicitly and culturally associated with the maternal, as opposed to a more archetypal identification of the way that reproductive functions and sexual otherness are framed as horrific and shocking (Creed 1993, 1). As with my discussions throughout this book, my use of 'monstrous' in this incarnation does not simply mean that which is literally horrific, ugly or frightful, but nor do I explore the productive, expansive possibilities of the monstrous that figure in the previous chapter on reproductive technologies in horror. Instead, here 'monstrous' refers to that which is deviant, transgressive or expressive of "antithetical moral values" (Weinstock 2012, 276). In particular, I wish to explore different territory than that of the psychoanalytically-informed formulation of maternal-as-abject in *The Monstrous-Feminine*. Instead, I refer to the contradiction whereby motherhood, as something that is coded as feminine, embodied and Other, serves to prop up patriarchal systems of knowledge and power – indeed, a system of thought that takes for granted the sorts of damaging and lop-sided dualisms that I have outlined in previous chapters.

Horror films about mothers and maternal relationships articulate a great sense of dis-ease about the discursive construction of motherhood. They suggest, insidiously, that there is something utterly and inescapably horrific about the psychological, emotional and cultural demands of motherhood that compels women in these narratives towards monstrosity and acts of evil. Such films suggest that the precarious balance between the needs of the self and the demands of motherhood can only ever end in destruction of the mother and/ or her child, and that this end comes about because of the inherent failings of the women themselves. In other words, these mothers try their best to fulfil the nebulous and shifting criteria of 'ideal' motherhood, but are doomed to fail. There is a tension here between two impulses: the idea that the specific demands of motherhood make one monstrous, but also the suggestion that somehow monstrosity is there, nascent and deeply embodied, stitched firmly into the very construction of 'essential' motherhood itself. In this sense, the evil in these figures is something rotten and insidious, an implied irrationality in the imperative 'to mother' and a fundamental failure of moral worth and nerve that both explores and articulates anxieties about what it is to mother appropriately. This monstrous-maternal is a troublesome double bind that frames the woman as always-already monstrous, and one that, perhaps, hides behind yet transcends more historically specific accounts of ideologically complicit or transgressive forms of motherhood.

Psychoanalytic discourses of motherhood

The analysis of mothers, motherhood and the maternal in cinema has been largely shaped by appraisals of the maternal melodrama, with a particular emphasis upon psychoanalytic film theories. This critical background is particularly important given the maternal melodrama's association with women and femininity, female spectatorship, sentiment and emotion, and – significantly – the centralisation of mother–child relationships; indeed, Lucy Fischer, in the introduction to her book *Cinematernity* (1996), suggests that the emphasis upon this genre in the study of mothers and motherhood in film has been "to the exclusion of other modes" (p. 6). E. Ann Kaplan's *Motherhood and Representation: the Mother in Popular Culture and Melodrama* (1992) remains the most lucid, extensive and authoritative of the work done on melodrama and the maternal, and it situates a variety of popular and melo-dramatic literary and film texts within competing modes of psychoanalytic interpretation. Kaplan's project explores how "fictional mother-representations are produced through the tensions between historical and psychoanalytic spheres" (p. 7) from 19th-century women's writing to the cinematic maternal melodrama and women's film. She considers how "prevailing cultural dis-course[s]" of an ideal 'angel' mother and a bad 'witch' mother have been developed and embodied in "myths, images and representations" (p.9), as opposed to actual lived experiences of mothers and families. Kaplan outlines in depth how motherhood is constructed and understood within patriarchal modes of representation, in particular, how cinematic and written texts may be variously complicit with or resistant to patriarchally constructed paradigms of womanhood and motherhood. She notes that:

> [i]t is on the level of what underlies the daily, conscious actions that representations exist and that we can uncover the mythic signifieds of a culture. These mythic signifiers are most evident in [the popular texts discussed and provide] "evidence" of myths being at work in the culture at any given time. (p. 16)

However, I posit that the consideration of motherhood should look beyond films and texts that are explicitly associated with forms of entertainment or representation, such as the 'weepie' or the woman's film, that are coded as feminine or seen as feminised. I certainly concur with Kaplan that "women, like everyone else, can function only within the linguistic, semiotic constraints of their historical moment – within that is the discourses available to them" (p. 16), but I would add that such discourses are not inherently confined within, nor necessarily best exemplified by, the melodrama, especially as that specific mode has arguably fallen out of favour within feature film-making.

Importantly, this emphasis upon melodrama is prominent in the study of motherhood in horror films. While some theoretical engagements with this theme have focused on areas such as the Oedipus complex (Williams 1996), unruly bodies (Paul 1994) and the relationship between Oedipality and classical myth (Greven 2011), or have conflated pregnancy with motherhood (Fischer 1992; Fischer 1996), this theoretical emphasis upon maternal melodrama is apparent in the only recent extensive study of horror and motherhood, Sarah Arnold's *Maternal Horror Film: Melodrama and Motherhood* (2013), which considers monstrous motherhood through the lens of psychoanalytic film theory. Arnold moves away from Barbara Creed's extensive discussion of the maternal-as-abject in *The Monstrous-Feminine*, and instead suggests that a comparison with melodrama is a key way of understanding how motherhood is represented not only in horror, but in film in general. Arnold argues that although "psychoanalytic theory researches the child's maturation by way of the mother, it also determines what kind of mothering is appropriate or inappropriate" (p. 6), and so through an acknowledgment of Kaplan's discussion of 'phallic' and self-sacrificing mothers in the melodrama, Arnold frames motherhood in the horror film with regards to what she terms the Good Mother and the Bad Mother. Given my interest in the discursive construction of motherhood (and, elsewhere, in the construction and dismantling of rigid binaries), this is a helpful place from which to depart.

This binary formulation of motherhood is explicitly couched within psychoanalytic discourses, and given its broad mythic significance it is worth unpacking. Drawing from the psychoanalytic work of Jacques Lacan, Arnold frames the Good Mother as the mother who sacrifices herself so that her child may move into the Symbolic realm. The transition of the child into the world of language and the rules of society, and the concomitant acknowledgement of and submission to the Law of the Father, involves a renunciation of the potentially dangerous, engulfing maternal body. The Good Mother conforms to the "popular discourse of motherhood that valorises self-sacrifice, selflessness and nurturance", which correlates "maternity and utter devotion to childcare" (p. 37). This construction that is, of course, in line with sociological studies of motherhood (see Miller 2007, 338), let alone other cultural myths, such as the way that the figure of the Virgin Mary has been culturally framed as the paragon of maternal abnegation (Kristeva 1985). However, given this Good Mother's sacrifice, she is determined in relation to and is often narratively overshadowed by the father, who is a figure who may either threaten or secure the family unit (Arnold 2013, 37). Conversely, Arnold indicates that the Bad Mother "identifies too extremely with the child" (p. 11) and refuses to fulfil the self-sacrificing paradigm of essential motherhood by not giving up her child to the Law of the Father (p. 79). This mother may be a villain, or overbearing, or narcissistic and selfish (p. 68), and she may pass her neuroses down to her child, as Arnold indicates happens in the films *Scream* (1996) and *Henry: Portrait of a Serial Killer* (1986) (p. 72). Arnold's exploration of the mother in horror cinema is extensive, but the categories of the idealised Good Mother and the monstrous Bad Mother can also function as restrictive paradigms, even though Arnold herself acknowledges that they are ambivalent and contested (p. 38). Instead, I posit that these categories are a tempting construct precisely *because* many of the horror films about motherhood that Arnold discusses draw from popular understandings of psychoanalysis and psychotherapy. This does not necessarily mean that psychoanalytic film theory is the only means through which to analyse such films robustly given that it, in turn, reinforces the discourses of motherhood that the films themselves are drawing from and recycling.

This example highlights how it is important to consider the way that psychoanalysis, as a discourse and an organising structure, not an interpretive practice, has been recirculated in the popular imagination, and in particular how it situates one's relationship with their mother as contributing to, if not acting as the cause of, psychological problems. The mainstream popularity of Freudian psychoanalysis in the United States from the mid-1940s and through into the 1960s has led to a widespread 'layperson's' understanding and normalisation of Freudian theories (Plant 2010, 48; Hendershot 2001, 93–4). These popular understandings of psychoanalysis have impacted upon the conceptualisation of family relations and how they may inform or influence one's mental health. Freudian models posited that the home and family were the crucible of both personal development and psychological pathology, at the same time as arguing that "the completion of women's [psychic] development, and women's experience of fulfilment, require[d] mothering" (DiQuinzio 1999, 176). Some practitioners of psychoanalysis wrongly blamed some psychiatric and developmental issues on maternal dysfunction; for instance, in 1943, the term 'refrigerator mother' was first applied to women whose perceived coldness towards their children allegedly resulted in conditions such as autism (Plant 2010, 13, 185). Similarly, in 1953, 'direct analysis' founder John N. Rosen infamously noted in his paper "The Perverse Mother" that "a schizophrenic is always one who is reared by a woman who suffers from a perversion of the maternal instinct" (p. 97).

Even though, as Kaplan (1992) notes, Freud rarely discussed the mother herself (p. 55), the simplistic idea that the relationship with the mother could be the root of psychological problems is one of the most popular interpretations of Freud's theories; the tongue-in-cheek term "tell me about your mother" has gone on to be an often comic shorthand for Freud's therapeutic practice in general. It is such a popular (cf. clinical or academic) and broad-stroke account that informs much of the North American cinematic representation of psychoanalysis – and, given the historic global dominance of the American film industry and the increasingly transnational model embraced by Hollywood, its representation more broadly within Anglophone cinema. The psychoanalytic stories and representations in films about horrific motherhood, particularly with regards to mental illness, can perhaps be read as a highly simplified product of popularly received and recycled psychoanalytic narratives more than they are indicative of a psychoanalytic 'truth' (Kaplan 1992, 110).[2]

The legacy of Mrs Bates: Norma, Thelma and Nola

This popular understanding of the construction of the mother within psycho-analytic discourses figures heavily in the depiction of motherhood in horror film. Perhaps the most famous presentation of the wicked mother figure is that in Alfred Hitchcock's 1960 film *Psycho*, a film whose influence remains remarkably pronounced within the genre more than fifty years later. *Psycho* lends itself beautifully to a psychoanalytic reading and is something of a touchstone in the study of contemporary horror. It has been considered within various psychoanalytic frameworks by numerous writers, including Barbara Creed (1993, 139–51), Lacanian researcher Robert Samuels (1998, 135–48), and Jungian psychiatrist Angela Connolly (2003, 420–2). This is also true of scholars who generally work outside of psychoanalytic paradigms, such as in film critic Raymond Durgnat's authoritative 2002 book *A Long Hard Look At 'Psycho'*, which provides an extensive explication of the film's formal features and textual themes, including its emphasis upon Freudian psychological causation. The film opens as office worker Marian Crane flees town after having stolen money from her employer. She stays at the quiet and remote Bates Motel, where she clearly piques the interest of the motel's owner, Norman, but as she showers she is murdered by someone who appears, to both her and the viewer, to be Norman's ageing mother. Marian's sister and a policeman come searching for her, and they eventually discover that years previously Norman had killed his mother, Norma, and Norma's lover, and that he now keeps Norma's mummified corpse in their family home. Norman had spent the ten years prior to the beginning of the film re-enacting and living out his dysfunctional, co-dependent, abusive relationship with the long-dead Norma by taking on the role of 'Mother' and then using 'her' to violently repudiate his own sexual desires. Thus, Norma(n) is a toxic, maternal figure about whom we know almost nothing, save for the psychological damage that she inflicted upon her son; it is only in later films and television series that the pair's relationship is explored in more depth.

Importantly, Norman Bates' imagined Mother – controlling, infantilising and abusive – has come, over time, to be a template for the popular representation of maternal overbearance in horror films (see Clover 1992, 49). This archetype is particularly apparent in a cluster of films from the mid-1970s to the early 1980s that are remarkable for their thematic similarities. *The Killing Kind* (1973), *The Exorcist* (1973), *Carrie* (1976), *Burnt Offerings* (1976), *The Brood* (1979) and *Maniac* (1980) all feature monstrous mother figures who in some way draw from or reinforce the narcissistic, dominating and hysterical 'phallic' mother paradigm that, although present in the melodrama and thrillers prior to 1960, was most obviously introduced into the modern horror genre by way of *Psycho*. The phallic mother is one who "satisfies needs for power [over her child] that her ideal function prohibits" (Kaplan 1992, 47). In *Maniac*, as in *Psycho*, the oppressive, controlling mother figure is a product of the killer's memory and imagination, and in *Burnt Offerings* the malevolent presence of the long dead matriarch Mrs Allardyce permeates the enormous mansion itself, and ultimately insinuates its way into the body of one of the house's new caretakers. In *Carrie* the eponymous character's mother, Margaret, is a disturbed and abusive religious fundamentalist with a twisted view of sex and sexuality, and she is ultimately killed by Carrie during Carrie's telekinetic rampage. In *The Exorcist*, it is heavily implied that young Regan's possession is facilitated by the independent lifestyle of her mother, Chris. Chris, a successful actor who is framed as a modern 'liberated' woman, is seeking a divorce and is tacitly blamed for removing a strong paternal presence from the home, which is then reinstated by the Catholic priests who are called for the exorcism.

The trope of the phallic mother is perhaps best ˏpresented in a knowing, tongue-in-cheek and exceptionally gory manner in the New Zealand horror-comedy *Braindead*, also known as *Dead Alive* (1992), which is set in 1957. Lionel lives with his overbearing mother, Vera, who is deeply upset when Lionel falls in love with a local shopkeeper's daughter. Vera is bitten by a plague-bearing 'Sumatran rat-monkey', which renders her undead and sets off a delightfully raucous zombie outbreak. In the film's climax Lionel confronts his mother, who is now an enormous and grotesque shambling creature with pendulous breasts (and yet is still wearing her string of pearls). At the beginning of the film he is a cowering mess, but here he confronts his mother, announcing that he is no longer afraid of her. In response, her bloated, abject stomach cracks open and he is drawn inside her as Vera tells him that no one will ever love him like her. Not to be stopped, and in defiance of his mother's quite literally smothering and lethal horrific maternal influence, Lionel hacks his way out of her monstrous womb with a crucifix. He is thus reborn, triumphant, in a torrent of viscera, ready to move out from his mother's literal and figurative control and into a healthy romantic adult relationship. This comic appraisal of the archetype serves to make plainly visible the core features of the phallic mother paradigm, and the way that such a mother must be destroyed for the sake and safety of her damaged child.

The psychological horror *The Killing Kind* and David Cronenberg's widely-studied body horror *The Brood* likewise draw from this paradigm, and here I wish to consider both of these films in greater detail. Where each film acknowledges the archetype of the domineering mother – the former film in particular wears its adherence to pop-psychological interpretations of monstrous motherhood clearly on its sleeve – a consideration of both films demonstrates how helpful it is to consider psychoanalysis as one of a number of competing discourses of motherhood, rather than as the key to the films' interpretation. At first glance *The Killing Kind* appears to fulfil the dominant paradigm of the overbearing 'bad' mother in that it aligns the simple-minded and troubled teenage protagonist Terry's psychopathy and sexual dysfunction with his mother Thelma's smothering, overbearing care. At the opening of the film Terry is involved in a pack rape. The other men try to goad him into physically participating, but he is stand-offish and unable to get an erection. Terry appears to be morbidly fascinated by the crime itself, but when his associates force him down onto the woman, Tina, his horror at both the prospect of sex and the confronting sight of the victim's naked body is shown through a freeze frame of his face, which is contorted in a rictus of fear and disgust.

This scene is both provocative and deeply problematic. The rape is filmed so that the camera, and thus the spectator's gaze, lingers upon Tina's body in an appreciative, suggestive fashion, which explicitly asks us to take a voyeuristic pleasure in the proceedings and suggests that the woman's normative attractiveness may have contributed to her attack. This frames Terry's transgression not as his participation in the rape, but his inability to be aroused by such an overtly sexual display. Instead, his failure to conform to a domineering form of violent masculine heterosexuality as framed its own sort of victimhood, thus privileging his apparent 'suffering' over that of the victim. This is exacerbated by the choice of actress; Tina is played by Playboy Playmate Susan Bernard, whose best known work prior to the film was as Linda, the underaged girlfriend of hot-rodder Tommy in Russ Meyer's 1965 sexploitation film *Faster, Pussycat! Kill! Kill!*, whose role as victim was to be kidnapped and trussed up at the hands of a trio of large-breasted, violent go-go dancers.

The rape acts as a form of inciting incident, for it both establishes the film's sexual politics and emphasises that Terry's somehow 'impaired' sexuality – within the film's unsettled logic, at least – sits at the centre of much of the film's action. After the incident Tina names Terry as one of her rapists and he is sent to jail, although Terry considers this to have been a false accusation. After some years he is released into the care of his mother, Thelma, an expansive and enthusiastic woman who runs a boarding house. Thelma is obsessed with her son and their relationship veers between an intimate family bond and something more erotic and transgressive. She fusses and frets over him as if he were a child, kissing him, peeking at him appreciatively as he showers, and bringing him glasses of chocolate milk. She takes scores of photographs of him to frame and place around the house; as she tells him, there are never enough. Soon, Terry begins to kill animals and women at the unwitting behest of his mother, for each time she complains about someone or something, Terry takes extreme measures to eliminate the problem so as to grant what he infers to be her wishes. Further, as with Norman Bates' murders, each crime is preceded by a moment of arousal and is associated with the cognitive dissonance he experiences as the result of disavowing his sexual impulses. This relationship between sexual dysfunction and violence becomes clear during a dream sequence in which Terry sits in a baby's crib with the rape victim, as Thelma and her friends point babies' bottles at him and chant "shame!" These anxieties burst forth when, in a moment of anger and frustration, he begins to choke Thelma as he is giving her a shoulder massage, before suddenly changing his mind and walking away.

This mother–son relationship clearly has the hallmarks of the 'bad' or 'phallic' motherhood paradigm, given Thelma's need to exert power over Terry in a manner that is considered transgressive or at odds with the construction of ideal motherhood. However, the relationship between the two is more complex, especially as Thelma herself is a clearly-drawn, nuanced and sympathetic character, not a stock figure or a psychotic harridan. When Terry, deeply upset, calls her a whore and tells her that she smothers him, she responds by telling him how hard it was to raise a bastard son – a statement that clearly marks her socially subordinate position as a single mother in a time when solo motherhood was rare and treated with overt disdain. Her infantilisation of her son and the cloying attention that she heaps upon him are not framed as cruel, but as a misguided attempt to protect him from the outside world and to guard their unconventional two-person family unit. Where Terry sees her as controlling, she sees her actions as a life of self-sacrifice for the only person she loves and the only person who loves her. Indeed, when Thelma discovers that Terry has been killing 'for' her, she is distraught. She wants to save him from returning to prison, where she knows he will be unable to fend for himself, so she kills him by lacing his chocolate milk with poison – an act that is certainly a symbol of her own inadvertently toxic mothering. They sit together on the couch as he dies, and she strokes his head, telling him about the various milestones of his life, before taking one last photo of him and waiting for the police. This ending is framed as an enormous act of sacrifice: despite devoting her life to her son and repeatedly telling him how much she needs him, Thelma chooses to give him up so that she may protect those around them from his murderous impulses, while also, perhaps, putting him out of his own misery. *The Killing Kind* appears to conform to standard narratives about terrible mothers and victimised sons within horror film, but it also demonstrates how hard it is to mark a firm distinction between 'good' and 'bad' mothering. Instead it shows a complicated relationship between mother and child that is largely shaped by Thelma's struggle to reconcile her love for her damaged son with her social position and her (in)ability to mother in an appropriate way.

These limitations are borne out through a reconsideration of David Cronenberg's *The Brood*, a widely studied film (Humm 1997; Beard 2006; Arnold 2013, 79–91; T. Connolly 2010) that has, perhaps, been most notably analysed by Barbara Creed in her discussion of the grotesque 'monstrous womb' and its abject generative powers in *The Monstrous-Feminine* (1993, 43–58). Nola is a troubled woman with a history of psychological issues, and she is receiving long-term, live-in treatment at the Somafree Institute of Psychoplasmics, a cutting-edge but contentious psychiatric treatment centre. Her husband Frank, who is not allowed to see her as a part of her treatment, raises their young daughter Candice alone; ironically, he owns a business that restores homes as his own marriage and home life crumbles. Nola's psychiatrist, Dr Hal Raglan, has developed a means of therapy that allows a patient's inner rage to manifest itself as a somatoform disorder. One patient is covered in lesions related to his issues with his father, and another, who has left the Institute, claims that his lymphosarcoma is as a result of his own externalised self-hatred. Nola, though, is Raglan's favourite and most 'successful' patient, therapeutically speaking, and her rage manifests itself as short-lived hare-lipped childlike creatures – her brood – which she births parthenogeneti-cally from an external womb. These creatures carry out Nola's subconscious wishes by finding and killing people who Nola feels are threatening her, including her parents and then Candice's school teacher, who has a brief flirtation with Frank.

The film's best-known image comes during the horrific finale when Nola proudly unveils her womb-sac to Frank. Frank is appalled and then strangles Nola in an overt act of hostility, which contributes to Creed's suggestion that Nola's rage has been caused by or is in reaction to her "husband's disgust at her maternal, mothering functions" and her reproductive role (1993, 45). The film suggests that Nola has always been disturbed, even in childhood, but I offer an alternative reading of this climactic scene that posits that this act of violence can also be read as Frank's final rejection of Dr Raglan's therapeutic practices and the damage they have wrought upon the family. Despite Dr Raglan's assurances that he was helping Nola, it is apparent that he is interested in her only insofar as she furthers his research. He calls her his Queen Bee and deserts his other patients (with tragic results) so that he can give her his full attention. Even the film's opening points to this skewed relationship: Raglan's preferred method of presenting his work to the public is through demonstra-tions in front of an audience in a small theatre, which frames the therapy as performance art. Dr Raglan positions himself as analyst-as-father, both eroticised and lauded, and when he succeeds in re-routing transference from patient-to-analyst to patient-to-body he capitalises on his discovery without providing any further care. Psychoplasmics, as he calls it, is shown to be a treatment that is far more destructive than the initial disease; it is not the illness that is horrific, it is the effect of the therapeutic model, which physically articulates and re-energises disease through somatic transformation instead of eliminating or mitigating it. When Dr Raglan is unable to maintain Nola or her id-children, to situate them within, again, a pop-psychoanalytic mode, the brood destroys him.

The Brood, then, can be read as taking a dim view of these sorts of extreme psychodynamic practices for it frames them as predatory, while also situating them within the context of broader discourses of motherhood. At the clinic Nola is further from her 'natural' family than she ever was, to the extent that she would happily preside over her bestial, parthenogenetic clutch of children rather than re-joining Frank and Candice. Although she is a 'good' animal mother to her brood, even licking one clean after she has bitten through its amniotic sac, she is an ineffectual mother to her human child, not only because of accusations that she has hurt Candice during some of the girl's visits to the facility (although no hard evidence is presented that Nola, person-ally, did anything), but because of her history of absenteeism. In turn, Nola accuses her mother Juliana of being abusive and neglectful – bad and 'fucked up' – although again, there is little specific evidence for this beyond Nola's allegations. Juliana indicates that she also had trouble with her own mother, which establishes a matrilineal line of mother–daughter conflict (see Arnold

2013, 72), but that this trauma is subjective; as she says to Frank, one's ability to lie to oneself about their past is as ingrained as the ability to experience itself. In short, there is a great deal of anxiety regarding how to be an effective, loving mother (as well as a loving daughter), but this anxiety is manipulated by Raglan for his own selfish ends. Nola is no longer capable of looking after her human daughter, but refuses to let anyone else do so, something that is borne out by her brood's attack on Candice's kindergarten teacher. The categories of essential motherhood – the innate, instinctual and perhaps *animal* ability to mother – and ideal motherhood – the ability to do so in a socially and culturally appropriate manner – are both complicated and critiqued. The insinuation that it is motherhood *itself* that is inherently unstable comes unstuck; instead, I suggest it is how motherhood is negotiated that is interrogated.

Essential and ideal motherhood

What *The Killing Kind* and *The Brood* demonstrate is that an interpretive emphasis on the archetypes of the 'good' and 'bad' mother does not necessarily account for the complexity and ambiguity that is inherent in the exploration and articulation of motherhood in the horror film. Instead, I offer that it is fruitful to consider dominant and conflicting messages about the nature of ideal motherhood, and to let these messages – these popular discourses – act as historically-specific indications as to what a mother should be and do. For example, the Bad Mother is one who "threatens to keep the child from entering the Symbolic" (Arnold 2013, 75) and who tries to control the child through oppressive maternal authority either through direct, physical means, or by asserting her dominance, even after death, perhaps by "'haunt[ing]' from afar" in the case of supernatural horror (Arnold 2013, 93). Yet, this perhaps presumes a certain type of strict, heteronormative nuclear structure, so that the relationship between the child and so-called non-traditional families, queer families or cultures and groups that share child-raising duties among the extended family or across multiple partners are unaccounted for within a highly restrictive paradigm. It is important to find ways to consider this shifting nature of motherhood (and parenthood in general) in a manner that is flexible as well as fruitful, and to acknowledge some of the biases, such as those towards heteronormativity (or even misogyny), that exist within theoretical frameworks.

Even in the case of so-called traditional heteronormative nuclear families that *do* conform to such a framework, ideas about whether or not a mother 'should' give up her child, and how this should happen, have changed over time. In one such example from the Western world, feminist historian Rebecca Jo Plant outlines such cultural shifts in her account of motherhood in the United States, *Mom: the Transformation of Motherhood in Modern America* (2010). In the 20th century alone the construction of ideal motherhood shifted from Victorian 'mother love' – the veneration of the mother as the moral core of the household, with the associated expectation that maternal influence should be of paramount importance in the adult son's life (pp. 89–91) – to a more distanced, so-called scientific type of mothering in the decades following World War II. This latter framework was heavily influenced by the popularisation of Freudian psychoanalysis as well as the anti-maternalist stance of Betty Friedan's seminal 1963 book *The Feminine Mystique*, and this shift "facilitated white, middle-class women's gradual incorporation into the political and economic order as individuals rather than as wives and mothers" (Plant 2010, 2). Likewise, opinions on how to 'successfully' mother are wildly divergent, even within tight-knit or specific communities (Lancaster 2003, 186–7), and can vary as much between individuals as between broader groups structured around location, class or ethnicity. As a cursory and recent example, both 'attachment parenting', an intensive framework that emphasises the development of strong emotional connections between the child and caregiver (usually the biological mother) through extensive emotional and physical availability (API's Eight Principles of Parenting), and 'free-range parenting', a looser attitude that emphasises a child's independence and works to counteract overparenting or 'helicopter' parenting,[3] have achieved prominence in recent mainstream American debates about mothering (see also Medina and Magnuson 2009, 91).

These shifts and swings indicate the importance of considering popular and cultural texts – in this case, horror films – as sites of discursive tension, for they articulate anxieties about the nature of motherhood at the same time as contributing their own 'worst case scenarios' to a broader public vernacular. From here, then, I consider some of the key assumptions about the nature(s) of ideal and essential motherhood that inform the construction of mothers in the horror genre by considering how seemingly simple but ultimately complex and contradictory taken-for-granted ideas about motherhood are both naturalised and policed.

Socially and culturally sanctioned models of motherhood have changed over time, but the notion of essential motherhood – the core assumption that motherhood is necessarily conflated with nurturance – has not. Even in its core definition, the term 'maternal' as 'mother-ness' implies a sense of nurturing care and emotional attachment that is not as present in the understanding of paternalism. 'Maternal' indicates a degree of closeness that 'paternal' does not; for instance, the term 'paternalism' refers to a relationship between a father and a child whereby the father imposes his authority over the child for the child's own good. Paternalism refers to actions, such as the creation of laws, that are interventionist, coercive and that may inhibit liberty (Dworkin 2010), but which are put forth with good intentions for the safety of the individual and the community. Comparatively, maternalism refers to "ideologies and discourses which exalted women's capacity to mother and applied to society as a whole the values they attached to that role: care, nurturance and morality" (Koven and Michel 1993, 4). It has been used to refer to a variety of social, welfare and public policies such as pro-natalism, state-supplied income for mothers (Orloff 1996, 57) or "family wages" for working fathers

(Orloff 1996, 61), and the suggestion that women should be encouraged to stay at home to care for their child full-time instead of returning to work (Orloff 2006). Both paternalism and maternalism are associated with benevolence and seek to benefit communities and societies at large, but, as is reflected by the psychoanalytic framework of family dynamics, law is constructed as coming from the father and nurture from the mother. So, before further considering the expressions of competing modes of motherhood in horror film, here I touch upon one of the fundamental imperatives and contradictions of ideologically complicit motherhood so as to establish one of the core tensions at the heart of the construction of discourses of ideal motherhood: whether or not the ability and willingness to mother is innate and a key aspect of what it means to be a woman.

In the introduction to *The Impossibility of Motherhood: Feminism, Individualism and the Problem of Mothering* (1999), feminist philosopher Patrice DiQuinzio highlights the ideological formation of motherhood as a cultural and biological imperative by framing essential motherhood as the construction that motherhood is both inevitable and natural. This is a function of "woman's essentially female nature" which "requires women's exclusive and selfless attention to and care of children based on women's psychological and emotional capacities for empathy, awareness of the needs of others, and self-sacrifice" (p. xiii). This set of assumptions suggests that women are 'made' to be mothers not just in a biological, reproductive sense, but that women's emotional and psychological selves are as they are so as to facilitate women's capacity for motherhood. Thus, essential motherhood is an integral part of the construction of normative femininity, dictating that "all women want to be and should be mothers [clearly implying] that women who do not manifest the qualities required by mothering and/or refuse mothering are deviant or deficient as women" (p. xiii). Such a construction challenges the autonomy and subjectivity of women and presumes a necessary duality, implying that they only way that a woman may be complete is to gestate, birth, nurture and guide their child. As with discourses of pregnancy, this implies that the mother must defer to the child's subjectivity in that they must look to themselves *or* their children (Featherstone 1997, 11; Ussher 2011, 192). This in turn frames women who do not have children (by choice, accident, necessity and so on) as selfish, for they are unable to fulfil their culturally-demanded abnegatory function. Discourses of ideal motherhood also frame motherhood as something that women can (and must) find enjoyable and enriching, but in doing so, offers a set of criteria that cannot possibly be fulfilled. As E. Ann Kaplan (1992) indicates, the ideal mother is "pure and unsullied, heroic in her undying loyalty and often ultimate forgiveness" (p. 99) – that is, she is a fiction.

Motherhood as instinct and imperative

The popular myth of ideal motherhood is reflected in, produced and reinforced by anthropomorphised accounts of animal mothering and reproduction. Such selective accounts of maternal behaviours and mother–child relationships are implicitly offered up as allegedly neutral, objective events and behaviours that are simply *recorded* by human beings, not as acts that are *interpreted* through a set of ideological lenses. These interpretations of non-human animal behaviours have a particularly important set of discursive functions in terms of the ways that (human) bodies and behaviours are framed, naturalised and managed. They are also important in considering how taken-for-granted ideas about motherhood are represented and interrogated in other forms of popular media, such as in the way that Nola's 'animalistic' maternal behaviour is framed in *The Brood,* for they form points in a broader cultural constellation of meaning-making. Narrative and descriptive voiceovers and story editing in nature documentaries and news stories about non-human animal behaviour draw from socially constructed assumptions about how men and women should act, and such assumptions and so-called common sense interpretations are used in turn to inform, naturalise and justify certain types of human behaviour (Coward 1984, 212; see also Crowther and Leith 1995; Sealey and Oakley 2013). Journalist and academic Rosalind Coward (1984) suggests that such programmes *"assume* as much as they *explain"* (author's emphasis), drawing upon normative, heterosexist narratives of male dominance and aggression, female submissiveness, "women's nesting instincts" (p. 213) and so on, "assuming that human meanings of 'mother', 'father', 'property' or 'home' can just be transferred on to the animals" (p. 213). The persistence of these embedded attitudes is similarly present in the allegedly objective but deeply gendered descriptions of the behaviours of ova and sperm that I discuss in Chapter Three.

Such narratives are invoked particularly strongly in discussions of cross-species friendships and fostering. As a representative example, consider a news story from American television network CBS entitled "Mother of the Year: Dog Nurses Kittens", which was broadcast to coincide with Mother's Day in 2008.[4] It features a Labrador named Lily nursing a litter of orphaned kittens, and these scenes are accompanied by archival footage of a cat nursing a wounded fawn, a foal being 'raised' by a goat, and a leopard 'mothering' the offspring of a baboon she had just killed. After asking why an animal like Lily would demonstrate such "grace" (a word steeped with Judeo-Christian inferences), the news item continues:

> Why – other than the obvious? ... For most mothers, it's just what they do. An instinct so deeply wired into them, that often all they know is to love and care for life. Understanding it completely will take scientists many more years, but feel free to appreciate it this weekend. (Mother of the year? 2008)

Although this piece is certainly framed as something light-hearted and sentimental, and a sweetly frothy fable through which to think about our own family relationships, the common sense, 'obvious' implication is that motherhood, framed here as the overwhelming impulse to nurture wounded or needy young, is an instinct so strong that it transcends species boundaries and, in the case of the leopard, the desire to kill its prey. Never mind, though, that in the latter example the baboon in question was only orphaned because the leopard attacked its mother,[5] or that dogs sometimes crush or step onto their puppies, or that maternal infanticide is common in a wide variety of species (Hrdy 1979; see also Lancaster 2003, 186). Indeed, what is considered here as 'normal' and innate human monogamous heterosexual coupling is far from the norm in amongst non-human animals (Bagemihl 1999). Instead, this nurturing behaviour is framed as universal, all-encompassing and inherently gendered, although somehow beyond the ken of scientists, and the news clip's final sentence actively encourages the viewer to take the anthropomorphised interpretation of the dog's behaviour and apply it, warmly, to their presumptions about ideal human motherhood.

Where the invocation of 'good' – indeed, ideologically complicit – animal motherhood is used to encourage sentiment and to ratify ideas about the supposed universal nature of positive maternal affect, the same animal comparisons draw a markedly different result in the discussion of destructive, violent, protective or visceral motherhood. Motherhood is also conflated with primal instinct in a way that implies that a mother's natural (animal) bond with her children is so strong that she will stop at nothing to protect or retrieve her children. Here, allegedly monstrous motherhood draws its horror from the extreme lengths that mothers will (allegedly) go to protect their offspring. This Mama Bear[6] trope posits that a mother will become dangerous when something comes between her and her 'cub', but is rarely articulated in terms of 'animal' representations of fatherhood – an association that, again, reinforces the alignment of women with nature and men with culture.

This is explicitly referenced in Quentin Tarantino's ultra-violent revenge action films *Kill Bill vols. 1 & 2* (2003 and 2004), and although they certainly can't be considered horror films per se, they are so explicitly aware of their aesthetic and narrative pedigree – in particular, B-films, episodic serials, grindhouse schlock, martial arts films, westerns and so on – that they make for a clear example of the way that such fare leverages taken-for-granted ideas about gender and violence for the benefit of a genre-savvy audience. A primal maternal urge drives the narrative: the assassin protagonist, known throughout much of the films as "The Bride", sets out to wreak bloody vengeance upon her former boss and former lover, Bill, who attempted to kill her on the day she was to get married to another man and, to the best of her knowledge, killed her unborn child. The films are made up of interconnected episodes, presented in a variety of genres and aesthetic modes, that show The Bride tracking down and killing her former (mostly female) assassin colleagues, and outlining her background and extensive martial arts training. The Bride's discovery that her daughter was actually born when she was in a coma, is still alive, and has been raised by Bill all this time drives the second volume. Near the end of this latter film The Bride's real name is revealed to be Beatrix

Kiddo, which strips her of her impersonal moniker and reframes her in an almost infantilising fashion. However, as she drives away, having reclaimed her daughter and finally killed Bill, an old fashioned title card reads "The lioness has rejoined her cub, and all is right in the jungle". Kiddo shifts from thwarted bride to wronged mother, and her ferocity is framed as an animalistic instinct to first avenge and then protect her young. Only once these goals are achieved may she take on a more docile maternal persona.

This construction of the mother as innately wired to defend her young is a common trope in horror cinema and monster movies, combining common sense understandings of maternal nature with the spectacle of female ferocity. Horror movie mother monsters such as the deformed mother bear in eco-horror *Prophecy* (1979), which is discussed in Chapter Two of this book, as well as Grendel's mother (*Beowulf and Grendel* (2005), *Beowulf* (2007), and other cinematic adaptations of the epic poem), and the titular monster in Larry Cohen's film *Q: The Winged Serpent* (1982), and the giant moth *kaiju*, Mothra, in the Japanese Godzilla films, are framed as all the more terrifying because they are driven by maternal wrath. These creatures undermine the passivity and submissiveness valued by conventional femininity, and they are willing to sacrifice their own lives to save or seek vengeance for their children.

This is exemplified in the climax of the science fiction horror film *Aliens* (1986): hero Ellen Ripley, wearing an enormous mechanical powered exoskeleton that is designed for industrial heavy lifting, rescues a young girl called Newt from the hulking, fecund, vicious Alien Queen, whose multitudinous eggs Ripley has just destroyed. Ripley's maternal affect is linked to her own thwarted motherhood: when she wakes from stasis at the beginning of *Aliens* she learns that she has been 'asleep' for nearly 60 years since the conclusion of *Alien* (1979), and during this time her own daughter has led a full life and since died. Ripley's maternal grief and her role as a mother-sans-child is framed as integral to her ability to connect with and comfort the traumatised Newt – who, incidentally, had done a far better job of evading the teeming alien horde than any adult – and this bond forms the emotional core of the film. Earlier in the film, a soldier describes the Alien Queen as a big, bad-ass momma, but this description is just as true of the furious Ripley in her mechanised power suit. Ripley's now iconic cry of "leave her alone, you bitch!", the image of the film's original poster – Ripley brandishing a gun and carrying a clearly terrified Newt – and the fury of the thwarted Queen all imply that both Ripley and the Queen are all the more dangerous for being slighted mother-figures. This well-known image was replaced by a simpler image for the film's theatrical release poster, yet the image of Ripley carrying Newt featured extensively on other advertising material, including the film's original DVD and VHS covers. It is significant that the art director of this poster, Mike Salisbury, calls this image "Classic Joan d'Arc [sic] protecting child from danger. [...] It is not the almost-Catholic image of the messianic egg in the sky of *Alien*, but ours is in the tradition of the indelible image of the Madonna protecting the child" (Salisbury 2010).

The legal implications of transgressive motherhood

I have outlined how essential motherhood is discursively constructed as a moral and biological imperative, and how this is stitched into cinematic accounts of motherhood, but there are significant negative consequences for women who fail to fulfil these ideals. These consequences are evident in social and legal discourses of motherhood, which similarly inform and are informed by pop culture and fictional accounts of what it means to mother in an appropriate or inappropriate manner. Transgressive mothers and forms of motherhood that fail to conform to ideologically complicit modes of maternal and feminine behaviour have received a great deal of attention from scholars, and such 'real world' accounts are deeply important in the way that motherhood is discursively constructed and negotiated, for they come to form their own sorts of social narratives. Work in this area in recent years has focused on issues as diverse as the prominence of discourses of 'bad' and 'thwarted' motherhood used by Canadian mothers with substance abuse problems (Reid, Greaves and Poole 2008), the mother-blaming of British and American women whose children are medicated for attention deficit and hyperactivity disorder (Singh 2004), the guilt and frustration felt by Australian mothers receiving contradictory advice on how to breastfeed successfully (Hauck and Irurita 2003), the way that discourses of class and ethnicity are integral to dominant constructions of victimhood and transgressive motherhood in cases of domestic abuse in New Zealand (Elizabeth 2004), and the legal implications for battered women in the United States who are charged with failing to protect their children from abusive fathers (Dunlap 2004). Each of these studies indicates how women may be implicitly or explicitly held to account, by themselves, others, or the state, for failing to conform to normative ideas of what a 'good' mother is, even if those ideas are impossibly contradictory. A clear account of this dissonance is cited in Justine A. Dunlap's legal appraisal of motherhood and domestic violence (2004), in which an anonymous respondent who grew up in an abusive household argues that the designation of a battered mother as a 'bad' mother who should have her children removed ignores that many of the mother's self-sacrificing behaviours, such as putting herself in harm's way to save her child, would otherwise be considered hallmarks of a 'good' mother (p. 565). These contradictions are deep-seated and deeply damaging.

An extreme example of these issues is outlined by Australian law professor Emma Cunliffe, who refers to the insidious nature of the ideology of motherhood as it pertains to cases of infanticide in her book *Murder, Medicine and Motherhood* (2011). She notes that although:

> Academic commentary of child homicide often remarks that it is difficult to persuade sceptical judges and jurors that a mother has killed her children ... a number of recent wrongful convictions of mothers suggests that prosecutors and courts may, for a period of time, have been too ready to accept allegations of homicide. (p. 2)

Cunliffe discusses two high profile cases of infanticide from Australia: that of Kathleen Folbigg, who in 2003 was convicted with regards to the deaths of her four infant children between 1989 and 1999, but who still protests her innocence, and that of Lindy Chamberlain, who in 1982 was convicted of killing her infant daughter while camping, but who was later exonerated when sufficient evidence was found to back up her claim that a dingo had taken the child.

Trials such as these can be considered a part of a wider hegemonic process and, in these instances, dominant ideological notions of both essential and ideal motherhood were perpetuated through the conflation of so-called 'common sense' understandings of motherhood with actual, hard evidence. As such, Cunliffe illustrates how, in each case, the taken-for-granted notion of what it is to be a 'good' mother permeated the cases of both the defence and the prosecution. Cunliffe suggests that Folbigg's "guilt was ascertained through a web of medical and social knowledge about motherhood and infant death" rather than through evidential proof beyond all reasonable doubt (p. 2), in particular value judgements over whether or not Folbigg's insistence on taking on paid work outside the home contravened "privatised, gendered ordering of childcare responsibilities within the heterosexual nuclear family" as they related to Folbigg's aptitude as a mother (pp. 98–9). Similarly, in the Chamberlain case, such notions "operate[d] as an implicit comparator by which a particular mother's behaviour can be judged", which extended from the charge of murder to "other aspects of [Chamberlain's] behaviour, especially her caregiving" (p. 101). Chamberlain was also deemed to have failed to fulfil constructions of ideal motherhood because of her blank affect throughout her trial, especially in contrast to her husband's openly emotional state, such that "her failure to grieve in a prescribed manner was considered strong evidence of her guilt" (Doka and Martin 2010, 151).

What these brief and selected 'real world' examples demonstrate is that monstrous motherhood is that which contravenes or fails to conform to the construction of essential motherhood, which is broadly deemed to be an innate capability to mother (and to want to mother) in a socially and culturally appropriate (that is, an 'ideal') manner, as opposed to a more prescriptive psychoanalytic construction that indicates that the woman's maternal self-sacrifice is necessitated by the child's shift into the Symbolic. Given that horror films are a form of popular culture that explicitly explore social anxieties, these circulating meanings are of significant importance to the way that such films are positioned within broader discursive shifts and flows. However, this way of thinking about motherhood highlights a significant tension, and one that will remain central to my argument over the remainder of this chapter. Both 'essential' and 'ideal' motherhood are fictions whose methods and criteria change over time, yet deviation from them is deemed monstrous and punishable. As such, I would like to offer the notion that the monstrous-maternal, is not simply not a way of thinking about a specific type of 'bad mother', but instead operates as a way of articulating the necessary and fundamental inability of mothers to be able to adequately comply with the socially, culturally and historically specific construction of the ideal mother.

Millennial mothering and the horror of the single mother

From here I move away from the archetypal model of the 'bad' mother of the maternal melodrama, and the way that this stock figure has been articulated, knowingly, in horror films. Instead, for the rest of this chapter I consider horror films from the late 1990s and into the 21st century that focus on single mothers and mothers who parent apart from the child's father. It's notable that these films delve quite self-consciously into lingering anxieties about the dissolution of the hegemonic formation of the nuclear family and the roles of women within heteronormative social structures, especially as there are few comparable horror films about the pressures on men who parent alone. Here I suggest that these 'millennial mothers' are fraught figures who are marked by instability and ambiguity. When they are presented as trying to be 'good' mothers – that is, conforming to essential and ideal motherhood – they are nonetheless the ones who pose the greatest threat to their children, often by being the first to expose her child to danger; indeed, in a film like *The Babadook*, it is truly the mother *herself* who is the greatest threat to her child. I close with an analysis of the 2009 film *Grace* (2009), which interrogates the self-sacrificing mother role at the same time as presenting a generational conflict between maternal ideals. These films demonstrate clearly that, despite changes in discourses of motherhood over time, the mother figure is always-already monstrous, for despite her best efforts she can never fulfil the criteria of ideal motherhood or conform to the needs, desires and capacities implied by essential motherhood. Instead, these films engage with the monstrous-maternal narratively and thematically by delving into issues surrounding maternal ambivalence and guilt, and in doing so they open up space in which to highlight and cut away at the impossible web of expectations within which women are bound.

The films from the 1970s that I have discussed earlier in this chapter feature women whose maternal functions and identities are explicitly informed by dominant pop-psychoanalytic models of motherhood, but films in the late 1990s and the first decade of the 21st century look more to mothers who try their utmost to fulfil the criteria of the ideal mother, but who seem doomed to fail. I do not wish to make broad generalised claims for transformations in the cultural and representational zeitgeist, for the changes in social and cultural conditions between the two periods of time cannot be easily nor helpfully simplified, although it is nonetheless reasonable to situate such dynamic changes within the shifting matrices of discourses of and surrounding motherhood. Such changes are informed by social, cultural and political shifts as diverse as the social and economic implications of the shift of more mothers into the workforce (Vincent, Ball and Pietikainen 2004), the impact of the so-called 'War on Terror' upon public discourses of fear and risk

(Altheide 2006), and – importantly – the influence of the internet and other communication and mobile technologies upon modern mothers and mothering practices (Madge and O'Connor 2006). However, there is one obvious difference between some of the horror films from the 1970s I discuss earlier – including *The Brood, Maniac* and *Carrie* – and horror films about motherhood in the 1990s and through into the beginning of the 21st century that directly pertains to the way that discourses of motherhood are expressed and negotiated. These more recent films are far more likely to have mothers as their protagonists and to emphasise the mother's subjective experience, and in doing so they offer a significantly different insight into the way that dissonant, conflicting cultural expectations work to shape, manage, police and punish the individual.

This emphasis on the individual mother necessarily shifts the focus from the child-centric parent–child relationship to an exploration of the pressures of and competing messages about motherhood and how best to mother. The mother is presented less as the psychological root of an individual's problems and more as a type of inefficient gatekeeper who is unable to fend off the horrors of the outside world.[7] I suggest that these mother-centric narratives are influenced by the contradictions and anxieties that result from escalating standards of mothering (Medina and Magnuson 2009, 90) and the popular (and wholly impossible) notion that the hard-won victories of second wave feminism mean that women can (and, perhaps, owe it to their feminist forebears) to 'have it all'. This dictum suggests that women can achieve a perfect, fulfilling and guilt-free balance between essential and ideal motherhood and employment outside the home even though, as psychologists and counsellors Sondra Medina and Sandy Magnuson outline in their excellent 2009 article "Motherhood in the 21st Century: Implications for Counselors", working outside the home inherently contravenes the lofty standards expected by modern hegemonic ideologies of mothering. Further, a devotion to home and family can impact upon the woman's ability to fulfil the expectations of her employer (p. 91)[8] – all of which can result in guilt, judgement (from both self and others) and a feeling of failure. As they state, "Either way, mothers in professional careers are not meeting social expectations" (p. 92), let alone those mothers who are working outside of white collar 'professions', or who hold down multiple jobs. This is a tension that is framed as a zero-sum game, in which a mythical balance can only be found by those women who simply try hard enough. This sort of a 'bootstraps' argument, of course, dumps responsibility at the feet of the struggling individual instead of situating relationships within broader systems of power and inequality.

This imperative to conform to the normative construction of ideal motherhood is made apparent through the prominent visibility of single mothers in recent horror films that emphasise mothers and motherhood. Single mothers, or those who parent apart from the child's biological father out of choice or necessity, have been prominent in horror films at least since *Psycho*, but films in the first decade of the 21st century have shown a particular fascination with solo motherhood and the changes to the 'traditional' (white, middle-class, heterosexual) nuclear family. Anglophone supernatural and gothic horrors *The Sixth Sense* (1999), *The Others* (2001), *The Babadook, The Ring* (2002) and *Dark Water* (2005), as well as the film adaptation of the survival horror video game *Silent Hill* (2006) and the psychological horror *Triangle* (2009), are critical of single mothers, positioning them as a source of danger, either explicitly or implicitly, even if the narrative itself centres on the woman's quest to save her child(ren) from a larger threat. As film scholar John Lewis (2005) wryly suggests, these films imply that the so-called "life choices" made by the mothers in each film "can be interpreted as catalysts for horror ... by presenting the viewer with the 'horror' of the ineffectual or monstrous single parent". Here, the neoliberal and individualistic rhetoric of 'choice' tidily erases all manner of systemic social and economic inequalities through the act of mother-blaming. This marks the mothers as inherently culpable and dangerous to their children in a way that the fathers, present or absent, are not, in large part because of their transgressive deviation from strictures of historically specific, ideologically complicit ideal motherhood.[9]

This emphasis on maternal choices drives the 2002 English language remake of Japanese horror film *The Ring*. Rachel, an ambitious, competitive and hardnosed journalist, begins investigating a cursed video tape after the mysterious death of her niece; watching the tape, a short film containing disjointed and sometimes nightmarish images, sentences the viewer to die seven days later at the hands of the vengeful ghost of a young girl, Samara. Rachel's role as a single, working mother is integral to the story. Her young son, a withdrawn and serious boy called Aidan, is almost painfully self-sufficient, something attributed to his mother's frequent absences. The fact that he calls her by her first name, not 'Mom', further marks their relationship as distanced and unconventional. Even though Rachel is still on good terms with Aidan's father, a video analyst with whom she still occasionally works, it is implied that it was her decision to keep and raise the boy alone, thus choosing to blatantly defy the hegemonic ideological prerogative to raise children within a normative nuclear family structure. Aidan never finds out his father's identity and when the father succumbs to the tape's curse there is an overwhelming yet unspoken sense of loss, especially at the relationships that might have been had Rachel been less focused on advancing her career and finding fulfilment through work rather than relationships.[10] Indeed, this feeling of melancholy permeates the film, and is exacerbated through the frequent presence of shadows, rain and water,[11] as well as pronounced colour correction that imbues the film's images with blues, greens and greys. Rachel's obsession with her work leads her to bring the cursed tape home, where Aidan watches it, and the remainder of the film is about her attempts to solve the mystery of the tape's origins, save both herself and her son from death, and atone for her maternal negligence. Rachel's wish to 'have it all' and keep her career as well as her son is implied to have deprived her son of a father and a warm relationship with his mother, as well as possibly dooming them all to a horrific death.

Although Rachel is presented unsympathetically as a self-centred and ineffective mother, she is not the only transgressive maternal figure of the film. The tape's ghost, Samara, is revealed to have been a disturbed and poisonous young girl with apparently supernatural and psychic powers. The family's doctor tells Rachel that Samara's mother, Anna, was unable to bear children, and that Samara herself had cryptic origins, having been adopted as a baby and brought back by the couple from an unknown place after her biological mother had allegedly died of mysterious complications. However, Samara would make those around her see horrendous things, and after a series of terrible events, Anna pushed the child down the well and left her to die before killing herself. Rachel remarks upon that fact that given that Anna had wanted a child more than anything, she cannot understand how Anna could do such a thing – but the film's irony is that this accusation is just as applicable to Rachel herself. Like Rachel's choice to raise a child by herself at the same time as working in a demanding professional job, Anna's choice to have and keep a child at any cost, despite her infertility, is framed as her downfall; as Anna's husband later tells Rachel, Anna subverted the natural order as she was not 'supposed' to have had a child. *The Ring*'s attitude towards both mothers is deeply cynical: both are punished for trying to conform to essential motherhood, specifically the notion that they should be mothers, and for both women motherhood is deeply challenging and far from an innate skill.[12] It is bleakly funny, then, that the way that Rachel evades the horrific outcomes of the curse is through an act of reproduction: by making a copy of the tape and passing it on.

In 2006's *Silent Hill*, as in *The Ring,* it is the mother who puts her child in danger – however, in this case essential motherhood is marked as irrational, and instead of featuring a single mother, we are shown a woman who decides to ignore her husband's wishes. Christopher and Rose's adopted daughter Sharon experiences night terrors during which she shouts "Silent Hill", the name of a foreboding and mysterious ghost town where a coal seam fire has been raging for decades. They are a warm and loving family unit, and Christopher insists that they can work through things together. He wishes to deal with their daughter's problems scientifically and rationally, through psychiatry and medication. Conversely, Rose instead decides to abscond with the girl and take her back to Silent Hill to confront the root of her trauma, something she sees as her maternal duty and, perhaps, as proof that she is a real mother to Sharon, despite their lack of blood relation.

As sociologist Barbara Katz Rothman (1989) suggests, there is a contradiction between the fact that where "patriarchal kinship is the core of patriarchy" (p. 89) and an agnatic view of kinship is *de rigueur* in many western societies, the mother has a disproportionally privileged emotional and psychological access to the child. In *Silent Hill* this access, and Rose's decision to prove her maternal worth to her adopted child in violation of her husband's wishes, are shown to have terrible consequences. Rose crashes her car just outside of

Silent Hill and when she regains consciousness the town is desolate, shrouded by fog and falling ash, and her daughter is gone. The film charts both Rose's dangerous quest to rescue her daughter from monsters and an evil cult, and Christopher's frantic attempts to find them, although we soon realise that 'his' abandoned, quotidian Silent Hill and their dream-like, monstrous one exist in parallel universes. When Rose and Sharon finally return home, they are no longer in the same brightly-lit world as Christopher; they all inhabit the same house, but they cannot communicate with or see one another, and instead exist at different frequencies, or different registers, that appear at least to centre on the same shared now. The film emphasises the strength of love between a mother and her child, including the repeated suggestion that a mother is like God to her child, but Rose demonstrates how quickly the idealised self-sacrifice of the 'good' mother becomes framed as dangerous, irrational and rash. Despite having saved her adoptive daughter and solved the mystery of Silent Hill, by acting apart from the rational father figure outside of a cooperative family unit and challenging his paternal authority she has condemned herself to a misty purgatory and irrevocably torn apart their previously happy, normative nuclear family.[13]

Where the exploration of what it is to mother well and appropriately is important to both *Silent Hill* and *The Ring,* the 2009 psychological horror film *Triangle* offers a far more blatantly pointed engagement with questions of what it is to be an ideal mother, particularly as it relates to single mothers, through a story that invokes a cycle of domestic abuse, maternal guilt and atonement. It is convoluted but tightly plotted, and given its intricacies, it is worth unpacking in detail. Jess, a waitress and a single mother to a young autistic boy, Tommy, is shown to be doing the best she can under challenging circumstances. She accepts an invitation to a trip on a private yacht by one of her customers, Greg, who is perhaps romantically interested in her, along with some of his friends. Nonetheless, Jess appears to feel immense guilt at the prospect of leaving her son behind. The yacht capsizes during a freak storm and they manage to escape onto an eerily deserted passing cruise liner. However, Jess experiences profound *déjà vu.* Soon the group are terrorised by a masked killer, and only Jess evades death. After a series of altercations the figure tells Jess to kill any people that board, and after Jess pushes the killer over the side of the ship she turns to see her own upturned yacht approaching the ship. She is in a möbius strip-like time loop, there are three iterations of her running around the ship – recalling the name of Greg's yacht, the *Triangle –* and everything that has happened to her has happened before and will continue to happen, over and over again. The only way she can get home to Tommy is if she can do things differently and break the cycle.

Jess's increasingly desperate actions are futile and, when she realises that the time loop resets each time all her companions die, she becomes the killer she has been trying to evade. Each piece of violence is framed as an act of extreme sacrifice: for instance, after butchering her remaining two companions so as to make the upturned yacht reappear, she mutters that she's sorry but she loves her son. Finally, she is pushed off the side of the ship by her earlier self and washes ashore. She makes her way home where the opening domestic scenes of the film are revisited, but we are privy to further details: far from being a patient and gentle mother, Jess is frustrated, overburdened and cruel. After she sees herself hitting and swearing at her son she violently bludgeons her abusive self to death in the bedroom – her own private space – in a cathartic rage of self-loathing. She plans to steal Tommy away from her 'bad' self, but he sees her crime. Instead, she stuffs her own body into the car's boot, coaxes the terrified boy into the car and drives off, promising that things are going to be different and telling him that she won't lose her temper, even if he does things wrong. However, when she hits a seagull, then throws its body into a pile of identical dead gulls, she realises that she is still trapped in the loop. Tommy's distraught screaming at the blood on the windscreen distracts her and she loses her temper then crashes her car, killing her son. Determined to do better and save Tommy from death, she stumbles away from the accident, reboards Greg's yacht, falls asleep, and wakes up, having forgotten everything. The punishing loop begins again, fixing her in a bounded and persistent past-present-future in which violence is always-already a key mode of expression.

The first way of interpreting this loop is optimistic: that a mother, confronted with her own failures and driven by both love for her son and the will to do better, can and will do whatever she can to make things right. Here Jess tries to live up to the impossible expectations of being an ideal mother. Like Rachel in *The Ring*, her identity as a single mother is frequently highlighted. Her situation is precarious: she works full time in a low-paying and tiring job at the same time as caring for her demanding autistic son, who attends an expensive specialist school. Further, she is struggling; 'bad' Jess lashes out and tells Tommy he is an 'asshole', just like his absent father. Tommy is her life, for better or worse, and even her decision to accept Greg's invitation is significant. When she tells Greg that she feels guilty for not being with her son, he tells her that that's because she's a good mother, but that she doesn't need to be a good mother, or even 'on the clock', all the time. However, it is quickly apparent how fickle the construct of the 'good mother' is: when they are on board the liner, he implies that her sense of confusion and shock is because of her guilt and he accuses her of being irrational and lost in her own Tommy-centric world. This criticism of her all-encompassing devotion to her son paradoxically suggests that where a 'good' mother makes extraordinary sacrifices, a 'bad' mother's sacrifice result in a loss of her sense of self.[14]

The line between the 'good' and 'bad' mother is increasingly indistinct, and this is made apparent through doubling in the camerawork, the *mise-en-scène*, and the sound design. The cruise liner's layout is confusing and dreamlike; hallways form a repetitive maze, which decentres any suggestion of a fixed or logical partitioning of space.[15] Jess's image, as well as the others', is often fragmented, distorted or repeated in the mirrors that line the ship's immense Art Deco dining room and that appear in each of the identical cabins. At key moments she confronts either images of herself, reflected in cracked surfaces, or other actual iterations of herself, as if she is trying to understand both who she was and who she might be. A reflection of Jess butchering one of her companions is repeated in triplicate in the mirrors of one of the cabins, alluding to the three Jesses that are circulating on board the cruise liner and the eventual death of the 'bad' Jess at the close of the film. These rhythmic visual repetitions are teased out through the film's queasy temporal shifts. Scenes repeat from different angles, emphasising Jess's alternative perspectives on events, and at key points the camera travels through a mirror to place the viewer in the subjective position of the mirror-Jess. When Jess finally realises what is happening a record she is playing skips, and this startling aural reiteration is supported visually through a sequence of repetitive and jarring jump cuts. In one obvious metaphor, her voice echoes around the ship, warning her companions (and herself) against her other selves. At several points Jess nearly kills one of her doubles, but each time the double's protestation that she has a son is enough to disrupt the killing blow, although when Jess kills her abusive self at home, it is just as *that* Jess has sat down in front of her bedroom mirror. Jess is the node through which all the film's trauma and action passes, and it is her desperation to reject the monstrous-maternal that drives the action. The more committed she is to her goal of getting off the ship and back to Tommy, the more callous and violent she becomes, even as the person she fights is, increasingly, herself.

The second, more cynical and fatalistic way of interpreting the time loop is that the cycle of abuse, regret and atonement will just continue and Jess, as an always-already monstrous mother, is destined to fail. The story's tension is that of a woman at odds with herself, for although she is a mother who loves her child she is also potentially unfit to raise him. It is not stated whether or not Jess behaves violently specifically because of the stress of raising a demanding special needs child without any visible means of support while earning a meagre wage, or if it is that she is someone who is already inclined towards anger and abuse, but it is clear that 'our' Jess sees herself as a good, even redemptive mother, and wishes things could be different. She tells Tommy (and herself) that she is his mommy, his nice mother, and that the woman who hurt him isn't mommy – a distinction that is also articulated by Nola in *The Brood*. However, every time Jess drives away with Tommy she passes a sign that reads "Goodbye – Please Return". This gruelling cycle is alluded to elsewhere. As the yacht departs, Jess tells Greg that with Tommy every day is the same and that if she does anything differently she loses him, although this statement is framed initially, and misleadingly, as a comment about Tommy's particular needs as a child with autism. As Jess makes her way around the ship she stumbles across disturbing artefacts of her previous selves: hundreds of pieces of notepaper that she has left behind, hundreds of necklaces that she has dropped in the same place, and – most ghoulishly – hundreds of iterations of one of her companions, dead, all of whom have dragged themselves to a far corner of the ship to escape Jess's rampage before dying. More subtly, a picture of seagulls on the wall of Jess's home is echoed by the way that seagulls seem to follow Jess from the land, to the yacht, to the liner (where they feast on the bodies of the dead) and back again.

Most tellingly, the empty cruise liner is named for Aeolus, the king of the winds and the father to Sisyphus, a man who was condemned to an eternity of rolling a boulder up a hill only to have it roll back down again at the last moment because, as one of Greg's friends summarises, he broke a promise he made to death.[16] This circular punishment can be read as any sort of guilty penance, but Jess breaks two promises that frame her Tartarean hell as explicitly couched in her role (and failings) as a mother. The first is that after promising Tommy she won't lose her temper any more she shouts desperately at him to calm down. In this manner the timing of the car accident is significant; Jess's distraction is caused both by her panic at realising she is still in the time loop and by her failure to mediate between being a kind yet firm nice mommy and falling back on her compulsion to yell at Tommy when he starts shrieking. The inference is that there was never really a nice mommy to begin with.

The second promise is more metaphysical. After the crash, the way that the bodies are lying in the road suggests that the 'real' Jess was killed in the accident, and that everything after is a torturous loop that requires her to pay guilty penance for her maternal transgressions, suffering through the sacrifice she was unable to make as a living person. 'Our' Jess, bathed in a flat, portentous light, looks out across the accident and is approached by a taxi driver, who tells her that there's nothing anyone can do to bring her son back. The driver is framed as a Charon-like figure, a supernatural ferryman, but Jess chooses, as she always has, to be taken back to the harbour to try to find a way to bring her dead son back to life. She promises him that she'll return, and, pointedly, he assures her that he will keep the taxi's meter running. The implication is that it is specifically her choice to perpetuate her torment, and that only by returning to the taxi, thus accepting her failures as a mother and her role in her son's death, might she find peace. This choice, perhaps, is false – an illusion. Instead, Jess is caught, forever, between her desire to be a good mother and her inability to fulfil this desire, and her punishment is to experience her son die over and over again.

Together, *The Ring, Silent Hill* and *Triangle* point to a system of conflicting, contradictory and impossible expectations that police a particular type of nurturing, intensive motherhood, while on the other leave the sense that no matter what a mother does, it is inadequate. Each of these mothers is challenged or punished for her desires, be they maternal or personal, and each is framed as at fault or culpable for the harm wrought upon their children and those around them. Further, each is shown to be unable to atone for her transgressions: Jess continues in her looping, Sisyphean torture; Rose is trapped with her adoptive daughter in a melancholy purgatory away from her husband; Rachel loses the father of her son and must pass the cursed tape on to an unsuspecting party or both she and her son will die. For each of these mothers the tensions and ambivalences between ideal, essential and trans-gressive motherhood are unable to be resolved. Overall, these millennial films indicate a great deal of anxiety over what it is to be an ideal mother and how one can mother appropriately given that, in the case of both *Silent Hill* and *Triangle*, extraordinary self-sacrifice, as befits the psychoanalytic and melodramatic models of 'good' motherhood, is never enough.

States of *Grace*: competing discourses of motherhood

It is clear enough to read a film like *Triangle* as an expression of anxiety about mothering in a specific time and place, and to position it within contemporary discourses of ideal and essential motherhood. However, the darkness that is implied within such expressions of the monstrous-maternal is not just that individuals may never measure up to personal or societal ideals, or that their failings will punish their children, but rather that there is something inherent to motherhood *itself* that is monstrous – something that cuts across generations and that distorts women in a fundamental way. Clearly, this is profoundly troubling, but the horror film, as a site of anxiety, also works to expose these ideas and to interrogate them, working them towards their horrific conclusions and exposing their misogynistic underpinnings, and not just simply recycling them. This tension is expressed and explored in the 2009 film *Grace*, which considers in great detail the nature of maternal self-sacrifice that is idealised in the melodramatic and psychoanalytic models of 'good' motherhood. *Grace* is unusual because it highlights the generational differences between two mothers. It also focuses on the dissonance between competing discourses and philosophies of motherhood by showing these discourses to be culturally and historically specific constructs. However, in doing so, the film shows both mothers to be inadequate and inappropriate, thus demonstrating that where monstrous mothers may fail to mother properly, the monstrous-maternal is not just an expression of maternal monstrosity; indeed, it is also the inability – of any mother – to conform to the rigid (and monstrous) demands of ideal motherhood.

Grace offers a nuanced exploration of grief and maternal need. It focuses on Madeline, an upper middle-class woman who is obsessed with organics, veganism, alternative medicine and clean living. She and her husband Michael have been desperately trying for a baby and they finally conceive; however, the couple are in a car accident that kills both Michael and the unborn child. Against all advice Madeline insists on carrying the baby to term and, miraculously, in the birthing tub the baby – Grace – revives and starts suckling. This moment of maternal bliss is short-lived. Grace, whose face is rarely shown, is not quite human: she smells unpleasant, her hair falls out when brushed, she bleeds mysteriously and she attracts flies. Grace won't digest breast milk, instead preferring the taste of her mother's blood. Madeline goes to extreme lengths to feed her unique baby. She deviates from her vegan diet to offer the child the juice from raw (organic, free range) meat, which gives the baby seizures, and then by regularly bleeding herself so much that she is left a sickly, anaemic wreck. Madeline's incredibly controlling mother-in-law, Vivian, starts trying to access the baby; she is a judge and moves to find Madeline incompetent so that she may take custody and fill the cavernous emotional hole left by the death of her son. As Madeline refuses to see her, Vivian sends her doctor to check on the baby, but in desperation Madeline kills him and tries to feed Grace with his blood, without success. Vivian arrives at the house to abduct the child but she and Madeleine fight and Vivian is killed. Madeline flees with Grace and in the company of her midwife and old friend Patricia they take to the road, like a latter-day Thelma and Louise. However, the film ends with Madeline, even more pallid than before, announcing that Grace is teething, and revealing her breast to be bloody and gnawed through.

As I discuss in Chapter Two, gynaehorror films about pregnancy, such as *Rosemary's Baby* (1968), frequently work to undermine the bodily and psychological integrity of the mother-to-be by framing her subjectivity as subject-to the needs of the unborn. Conversely, *Grace* is unusual in that it grants Madeline near total agency over the conditions of her pregnancy and birth, despite the half-hearted protestations of her husband. Further, Madeline is framed, at first, as the ideal 21st-century mother: she is white, educated, middle-class, married and financially unencumbered, and she actively chooses to have a child. However, the agency that Madeline exhibits is not framed as entirely empowering, and instead is undermined by the sardonic presentation of her and her husband's vegan lifestyle as narcissistic and self-indulgent, facilitated and enabled by their privilege and not a legitimate concern for animals or the environment. Their affluence and the breadth of choices they have stands in stark, grimly ironic contrast to the fact that Madeline is incapable of providing for her child without in turn killing herself. Despite this privilege, as with the mothers in *Triangle, Silent Hill* and *The Ring*, Madeline is the agent of her own demise: she insists on carrying the dead baby to term and seems to bring it back into life through strength of will, but her wish comes at a cost and she is doomed from the outset.

Madeline and Vivian are connected clearly in that they are both strong-willed women with a great deal of agency, and as such I suggest they come to reflect a generational conflict between the maternal ideals espoused in the films discussed earlier in this chapter. This is indicative of the complicated, mutable and conflicted nature of discourses surrounding how to successfully mother. On one hand, Vivian's controlling nature, her high-powered job as a judge and her overbearing interference appear old fashioned, recalling both the appeal to authority encapsulated in the 'scientific' model of mothering and childbirth between World Wars I and II (Plant 2010, 11–12), and the complicated mother–child relationships that were at the centre of popular understandings of psychoanalytic discourses in the 1950s and 1960s. This is emphasised through Vivian's choice of doctor, Dr Sohn. He is an old-fashioned stereotype, a traditionalist who carries a vintage Gladstone doctor's bag, and when he collects breast milk samples – for his own secret consumption – it is with an antique metal breast pump, an outdated, uncomfortable and invasive piece of machinery. On the other hand, Madeline is insistent that she is treated by Patricia, an old friend and former Women's Studies professor, with whom she once had a very close, intimate, live-in relationship that is strongly implied to have been sexual. Madeline represents both a backlash against scientific mothering and an embodiment of a 21st-century model that positions the pregnant woman as an informed consumer who is free to choose her medical provider – in this case, a provider whose holistic woman-centric methodology draws from radical feminist critiques of the medicalisation of pregnancy, birth and motherhood, and who attempts to aggressively negotiate the inter-professional tensions that result from the way that obstetrics and midwifery may be positioned as Other to one another in both discourse and practice.

This ideological tension between holistic and scientifically mediated practices recurs throughout the film; scenes in which these tensions spill over explicitly invoke modern debates over the provision of maternity care, and situate Madeline's body as a corporeal battleground between competing discourses (see Reiger 2008). An early scene, prior to the accident, establishes this hostility. Michael – who is less enamoured with the idea of alternative midwifery than his wife – asks Patricia for her credentials, emphasising his own need to see her as a qualified, authoritative figure that has been endorsed in a (Western, scientific) manner he deems acceptable. She states she has a PhD in holistic obstetrics and extensive training in eastern therapeutic modalities, but Michael is only satisfied when she reveals, stonily, that she also has an MD from Colombia University. Michael notes that he doesn't see any degrees hanging on the walls; Patricia responds that it's better that her clinic doesn't look like a hospital, as there is no need to medicalise a process that is already 'perfect', invoking the dualistic distinction between the beauty of feminine nature and the hardness of masculine scientific rationality that I outline earlier in Chapter Three of book.

Further, Patricia's holistic practice is shown – at first – to be both more caring and more efficient than the more clinical alternative. Madeline is taken to hospital with suspected eclampsia and Dr Sohn intercedes at Vivian's behest, demanding that the delivery be induced. When Patricia arrives she is furious at the hospital staff for allowing his intrusion, and she triumphantly finds that Madeline is only suffering from a gallstone, thus 'rescuing' her from an unnecessary procedure and putting Madeline-and-baby, as opposed to just the baby, back at the centre of care. However, later the film undermines this by showing Grace to be a child whose needs far outstrip the emotional and physical resources provided by Madeline and Patricia. At the film's conclusion Patricia indicates with enthusiasm and determination that together she and Madeline can keep both mother and baby healthy, before realising that Grace has already started eating into Madeleine's breast. The film closes as Madeline pronounces that the baby needs 'more' now – more than both mother and doctor can provide. Mainstream scientific intervention is shown as impersonal, callous and sometimes brutal, particularly as it is embodied by Dr Sohn, yet the holistic approach is nonetheless incapable of dealing with the demands of this 'special' child.

However, the tension between Madeline and Vivian's mothering philosophies moves from ideological to personal, so that it becomes a hostile and toxic competition between two individuals as to who can mother the best. Thus, I suggest that it is not that Madeline and Vivian are monstrous mothers; instead, motherhood *itself* is shown to be monstrous. In particular, Vivian becomes the cliché of the wicked mother-in-law, and her character draws from the filmic catalogue of villainous matriarchal figures, from *Psycho*'s Mrs Bates, to Joan Crawford in *Mommy Dearest* (1981), to *Now Voyager*'s (1942) Mrs Windle Dale; she is the phallic mother of the melodrama, threatening her son's masculinity and emasculating her husband. She attempts to police Madeline's body during the pregnancy, she is appalled at the idea that Madeline is using an alternative clinic and she greatly disapproves of Madeline's veganism and the perceived effects it will have on the baby. Later, she shifts from passive-aggressive meddling to active, violent intervention: she spies on Madeline's house, compels Dr Sohn to visit the baby and declare Madeline an unfit mother, and she finally tries to steal the child herself. She distances herself from her son's marriage to Madeline by denying Madeline's status as birth mother, stating that she won't have 'this woman' raising her grandchild, suggesting that her maternal right is stronger than that of Madeline. All the rationality that is implied through her job as a judge is undermined in her persistent pursuit of the child.

The pathologisation of motherhood is not just evident through the bitter competition over Grace. It is also a struggle over the emotional ownership of Michael's death, and it asks whether or not a mother's need for her child outweighs any other emotional, biological or legal claims. This is something that predates the car crash; it is revealed late in the film that Vivian has kept Michael's childhood bedroom, complete with his racing car bed, intact and untouched since he was small. We also learn that Vivian breastfed Michael until he was three years old – much longer than is considered 'normal' in the majority of western mothering discourses.[17] Her grief at the loss of Michael appears to affect her in a more profound way than it does her husband, so much so that her fixation on Grace comes to supplant her longing for Michael. She announces, early in the film, that women can continue expressing milk past menopause, so long as the nipples are kept stimulated, and in a scene that borders on the grotesque in its lingering fascination with her private grief she retrieves her old breast pump. She stares at herself in the mirror and pumps at her breast, and even though she is in her 50s and has not lactated for decades her milk eventually flows freely. When we see her being sexually intimate with her husband it is with an agenda: she asks him to suckle at her breasts not out of desire but to stimulate her nipples, an objective that she does not communicate to him. This mirrors one of the film's opening scenes, in which Madeline and Michael have sex: Madeline looks to the ceiling, only mechanically engaged, as she focuses on the act of conception rather than the act of lovemaking. Both husbands clearly love their wives, but in both instances the sexual and emotional bond of the woman with her husband comes secondary to that with the child, real or perceived.

Although *Grace* both pathologises Vivian's behaviour and shows Madeline to be incapable of living up to the visceral demands of the child, the film implies that essential motherhood – the notion that motherhood is a biological and emotional imperative that sits at the heart of the female experience – endures despite generational changes to discourses of motherhood, including the construction of ideal motherhood. It is significant that Patricia is also a parental figure, of sorts. When she is introduced she is looking at a photo of herself, Madeline and Madeline's cat, Jones, which had been taken years prior. She clearly aches for something for although she maintains an air of control and dignity, she has been anxiously worrying away at a spot on her desk with her thumbnail. When she visits Madeline and the baby at home, she plays with the cat and reminds Madeline that they were once seen as their own little family – Madeline, Patricia and Jones the cat as Ma, Pa and Baby J – but when she reaches out to stroke Madeline's cheek she is firmly rebuffed. Patricia's own longing – for Madeline, for the bond that they had had before, and perhaps for a child – makes her so far involved that she loses perspective and ceases to make professionally-appropriate decisions. In the film's epilogue Patricia seems to have finally found a place of happiness (and denial) as the three of them travel through empty country, until she discovers how terrible Grace's demands are. Patricia's longing for her own family unit with Madeline by her side blinds her to the grisly reality that they both face. The implication is that this new alternative family unit, consisting of the two women and the child, is also unable to fulfil the idealistic hopes of either woman.

Monstrous motherhood

All these different facets of the monstrous-maternal combine to express a deeply gendered monstrosity that crosses generations, ideologies and even sexualities. The monstrous-maternal's gynaehorrific double bind is that it is the construction of essential motherhood – motherhood as innate, as natural, as desirable – and the compulsion to conform to ideal, ideologically complicit motherhood that firstly facilitates such horrendous actions. It also then, in turn, frames them as monstrous and transgressive. Sarah Arnold (2013) in her reading of *Grace*, suggests that the film "situate[s] 'essential motherhood' in terms of corruption. In other words, the ideology of essential motherhood becomes horrific when pregnancy and resulting offspring are represented as monstrous" (p. 167). However, I posit that this emphasis on monstrous off-spring does not attend to the wider issues in the film: instead, I offer the idea that *Grace* shows women becoming *necessarily* monstrous through the demands of ideal motherhood and through the compulsion to mother, such as in Madeline's choice to carry Grace to term. It is obvious that both Vivian and Madeline are strong-willed and exhibit a great deal of control over their lives, their surroundings and their husbands, yet it is these attributes that are debased and warped through the rigours and demands of motherhood, as well as the desire to be a mother at any cost.

The film's title offers a clue as to how to frame the women. As I suggest in Chapter Two, the title of *Rosemary's Baby* serves to illustrate that even though Rosemary is the film's protagonist, her position as subject is decentred, if not eradicated, by her child and by the idea that Rosemary herself is little more than a physical vessel. The title of Grace reflects something different; Madeline retains her status as subject, but Grace becomes the film's object of obsession. The title asks us to consider not the child, who is rarely in frame, but the frenzied lengths that each woman will go to so as to care for or possess the child. It positions both women as evocations of the monstrous-maternal – literally, by the extremity of their actions, and figuratively, because none of the women is able to fulfil the impossible nonpareil of ideal motherhood. Despite of, or even in light of, the competing discourses of motherhood, they are all ultimately inadequate.

The discourses of ideal and essential motherhood, no matter their finer points and no matter the will or wants of the mother, wholly fail to acknowledge that being a mother is emotionally and physically taxing and not always pleasant. Psychologist Jane M. Ussher (2006) is worth quoting at length:

> Not all women enjoy motherhood. Not all women find the changes that come with it bearable. The reality of motherhood, for many women, is stark; rage, despair and disappointment are not uncommon. But this is not the sign of monstrous femininity, and the body is not to blame. How many mothers can say, with all honesty, that they have not experienced despair in the months following the birth of a child? (p. 106)

Here, Madeleine's despair and the macabre and intensive relationship that she has with her inhuman child can also be read as a metaphor not just for post-natal depression, but for the necessary and perfectly reasonable pressures placed on any new mother. Perhaps, then, the monstrous-maternal can be reconfigured so that it is not that it stands for a mother's inability to conform to the socially and historically specific perfect mother that is invoked through the discourses of ideal and essential motherhood. Indeed, what is monstrous is the notion that a woman can and *should* be judged using a set of impossible criteria against which she will always be found wanting.

The discursive positioning of motherhood within horror films, and the way that horror films in turn articulate and recirculate discourses of motherhood, contributes to a broader management of the way that motherhood and the maternal are understood, disciplined, enforced and enacted. Although discourses of motherhood are culturally and historically specific, there is a pervading sense that mothers can never fulfil the implicit and explicit criteria against which they are judged. I find this profoundly troubling and insidious for, on one hand, the myth of essential motherhood implies that motherhood is at once innate, natural and desirable. On the other, the demands placed upon women through the struggle to fulfil the criteria of ideal motherhood suggests that women are nonetheless incapable of doing what allegedly comes 'naturally' and that they must instead conform to certain unattainable and ever-shifting standards of 'appropriate' motherhood, often through the intervention of third parties. Thus, the melodramatic model of the archetypal 'good' and 'bad' mother that is present through studies of motherhood in film in general – and in horror film in particular – fails to acknowledge that both mothers and motherhood are ambivalently framed as always-already monstrous. The allusion to Sisyphus's impossible task in *Triangle* is apt, for the message to mothers in horror film is clear: you must do better, but you can never do enough.

There is one film, though, that attempts to negotiate a way through this predicament: John Waters' camp horror satire *Serial Mom* (1994), which lampoons the ridiculous standards of ideal motherhood. Its titular character, Beverly Sutphin, is a seemingly perfect white middle-class suburban housewife who harasses and murders anyone who she deems to have slighted her or her family, but her murder trial turns into a media circus and after successfully defending herself she walks free. *Serial Mom*'s jaunty, irreverent tone sits in opposition to its macabre content, so as to satirise the apparent respectability of 'all-American' family values and the lengths to which individuals and communities will go to prop them up – a continuation of the gleeful emphasis upon transgression, (bad) taste and the grotesque that runs through director John Waters' oeuvre. The film opens in a similarly tongue-in-cheek manner to David Lynch's *Blue Velvet* (1986) and Mitchell Lichtenstein's *Teeth* (2007): the establishing shots are of blue sky and a kitsch, picture-perfect American suburban neighbourhood, images that exemplify a wholesome, imaginary Americana whilst acting as a visual foil to the psychological rot that is shown to exist beneath the surface.

As with Terry's violent acts in *The Killing Kind*, each of Beverly's murderous actions is instigated by a transgression against her family or her sense of respectability. Beverly, pathologically well-meaning, sees herself as an agent of change and someone who must right the behavioural deficiencies in others, be it chewing too much gum, being rude to her daughter or refusing to sort their recycling. The humour of the film derives from the juxtaposition of Beverly's homicidal acts with her overall demeanour, such that even as she rips a man's liver out with a fire poker she is just as concerned about the mess on her hands and the state of her shoes as she is about making sure she has actually finished him off. This dissonance also highlights how the enforcement of white middle-class respectability is inherently bound up within the construct of ideal motherhood; immediately following her acquittal she bludgeons to death a juror who, while wholly on her side, has made a fashion *faux pas* by wearing white shoes after Labor Day.

By the time of her high-profile trial, which presciently predated the highly publicised and media saturated O.J. Simpson murder trial in the United States by a year, Beverly's identity is constructed through competing discourses of motherhood and madness. In his closing statements the prosecuting attorney announces that she's not a woman but a monster, thus stripping her of her humanity and gender. Meanwhile, Beverly's family wonder if her 'problems' and her homicidal behaviours are down to Beverly reaching menopause;[18] nonetheless, as her nervous husband Eugene says, they will love her no matter what she is. However, the cultural script of the monstrous-maternal is re-written and Beverly defends herself successfully by drawing upon her aura of respectability and homeliness. In a brief cameo, actress Suzanne Somers, who has signed on to play Beverly in an upcoming film, announces to the gathered press that Beverly is simply a normal housewife implicated by circumstantial evidence who should, instead, be considered a feminist heroine[19] – an ordinary woman who, like wives and mothers everywhere, is subjected to enormous daily pressure. (One of the housewives gathered outside the courthouse comments that she feels like killing a couple of people herself.) *Serial Mom* manages to highlight the outlandish expectations of ideal motherhood in a way that is playful, absurd and palatable: the film indicates that perhaps the only way to adequately fulfil ideal motherhood is by whole-heartedly embracing monstrosity, because the construct of the ideal mother is, itself, monstrous.

Notes

1 This is demonstrated beautifully in the 2006 documentary *Going to Pieces: The Rise and Fall of the Slasher Film.*
2 This is perhaps a reflection of three things: how Freud's own interpretations have been conflated with constructions by his successors, how narrative in and of itself is utilised within the therapeutic setting as a maker of meaning, and the way in which narrative claims in psychoanalytic settings do not necessarily align with verifiable reality-based claims; see Roth 1991.
3 The Free-Range Kids website, started by American journalist Lenore Skenazy, humorously offers its mission statement as "Fighting the belief that our children are in constant danger from creeps, kidnapping, germs, grades, flashers, frustration, failure, baby snatchers, bugs, bullies, men, sleepovers and/or the perils of a non-organic grape" (Free Range Kids). Skenazy set up her website after she came to prominence (and was labelled "America's worst mom") after writing a column about letting her 9-year-old ride the New York subway by himself (McDermott 2008).
4 Thanks to the excellent sociology blog "Sociological Images", which offered a link to this news story as a part of a broader round-up of Mother's Day-themed stories (Wade 2011).
5 Dereck and Beverley Joubert's National Geographic photo essay, "Lessons of the Hunt" (Joubert and Joubert 2007), follows this particular leopard's development and relationship with her own mother, from infancy to independent adulthood. It is particularly instructive in terms of the way that culturally specific human value systems and discourses of motherhood are overlaid onto non-human animals. Beverley Joubert's images of the subadult leopard and the baby baboon, events which are stated to be "bizarre", are framed in such a way as to suggest that the

leopard has learned from her own 'good' mother and that she is approaching a time when she will need to be a 'good' mother to her own cub. The caption beneath an image of the leopard grooming and sleeping with the tiny infant baboon before it died from cold reads "Was Legadema [the leopard] feeling early maternal instincts?"

6 This rhetoric is also applied in interesting ways within political discourses. Sarah Palin, the Republican vice-presidential candidate in the United States' 2008 elections, frequently invoked primal motherhood as a political ideal, emphasising her own self-identification as a "Mama Grizzly" as a way of signalling her suitability for office, in comparison to the way that women in politics who are mothers are often condescended to or demeaned because of their family role in a manner than men tend not to be (Silver 2010; McCabe 2013).

7 In a recent example from the United States, non-normative motherhood is sometimes demonised in blatant ways; a Senate Bill written in 2011 and sponsored by Republican Senator Glenn Grothman from Wisconsin intended to emphasise "nonmarital parenthood as a contributing factor to child abuse and neglect", thus entrenching the demonisation of non-normative parenting, especially solo parenting by women, within law. The bill failed to pass (Senate Bill 507 2012).

8 Medina and Magnuson (2009) also indicate that such expectations of motherhood increasingly undermine steps towards gender equality, in particular, more active, invested parenting by men (p. 91).

9 It is important, though, to note that this mother-blaming is not a recent phenomenon, even over and above the Freudian emphasis on maternal pathology. In *Mom* (2010), Rebecca Jo Plant charts not only changes in mothering styles and ideologies in the 20th-century United States, but the way that such changes are if not driven by then at least accompanied by seemingly perpetual criticism of mothers and styles of motherhood. For example, in her discussions of the critique of suburban motherhood in Betty Friedan's *The Feminine Mystique,* Plant notes that in the "1960s, many middle-class mothers, regardless of their employment status, felt condemned by a culture that subjected them to unremitting criticism" so that even as more women were entering the workforce, "many of the working mothers who wrote to Friedan still felt marginalized by a culture that lauded homemaking as the ultimate source of feminine fulfillment [sic]" (p. 138).

10 All of this conveniently ignores the fact that, from the perspective of the shoring up or dissolution of the nuclear family unit, Aidan's own father seems rather philosophical about the status of his potential paternity.

11 This is also related to the original Japanese film's association of Sadako, the ghostly antagonist, with water, an alignment between spirits, memory and water that is also loosely present in the American versions of *Dark Water* and *The Grudge* (2004). However, the more nuanced and culturally specific aspects of the association between water and the underworld in Japanese ghost stories (*kaidan*) are not overtly articulated in the American films (Wierzbicki 2010).

12 Sarah Arnold (2013) offers a cogent comparative analysis of the discourses of motherhood operating in the Japanese and American versions of the film, as well as the Japanese and American versions of the film *Dark Water*, in chapter three of *Maternal Horror Film.* She notes that the Japanese films privilege a nuanced maternal perspective whereas the American films highlight maternal incompetence, so that mother blame is more common in the American films. Similarly, Valerie Wee, in her excellent comparative study of the aesthetics of the cursed videotape in the Japanese and American films "Visual Aesthetics and Ways of Seeing" (2011), also highlights how the origin of the vengeful spirit changes: in the Japanese original the girl, Sadako, received psychic powers from her birth mother, who later committed suicide, and it was the father, not the mother, who murdered the girl and put her down the well in a patriarchal suppression of feminine supernatural power.

It is worth noting that the *Ringu* series has numerous entries across various media and countries and a sprawling mythology that is not entirely reflected in the American remakes (Meikle 2005).

13 This is similar to J. A. Bayona's 2007 Spanish-Mexican film *The Orphanage (El orphanato)*. Laura, who has reopened an old orphanage, spends the majority of the film hunting for her sickly adopted son Simon while being terrorised by a ghostly masked child. Laura transcends the barrier between life and death to try to save her son; however, in the film's final scenes, it is revealed that she inadvertently trapped her son in a forgotten basement during a party, that his desiccated body has been lying under the house for months, and that the ghost child had been trying to alert her. Like Rose, Laura is not a single mother, but she becomes so single-minded in her supernatural quest that her more grounded and rational husband is unable to cope and he leaves for most of the second half of the film. Finally, Laura chooses to overdose on tranquilisers so as to stay in the orphanage and look after her dead son and the ghostly orphans. Although the final shots insinuate that she may somehow return to her husband from beyond the grave, her suicide is framed problematically as a form of self-sacrifice: it is not selfishness, but rather a demonstration of the strength of her maternal instincts.

14 It is worth noting that Greg is also a parent, of sorts: one of their travelling companions is a 19-year-old who Greg had taken in and steered away from a life of crime, thus framing him as a 'good' and generous father figure.

15 The faded glamour of the liner and its long confusing hallways bear more than a passing resemblance to those of the isolated, haunted Overlook Hotel in Stanley Kubrick's horror film *The Shining* (1980). This association is made concrete when Jess and Greg find a message written in blood left for them in room 237, a room of ominous significance in Kubrick's film, which is home to the ghost of a drowned woman. Later, Jess butchers another one of the passengers there, providing the blood with which to write the message for her previous self. Jess's house is also number 237, linking her home life with the horrors of the ship and hinting to the viewer that the loop is still in place, and the pattern of her home's wallpaper recalls the geometric pattern on the carpet of the Overlook.

16 Victor, one of the other passengers, declares this punishment to be "pretty shitty".

17 For instance, in a 2013 study of breastfeeding continuation in the United Kingdom, health researchers Sally Dowling and Amy Brown note that while the World Health Organisation recommends that mothers breast feed exclusively for six months and then in conjunction with other forms of nutrition until the baby is at least 24 months old, only a minority of women breastfeed for longer than a year, and those women who do so report that they are often alienated and ridiculed.

18 As Jane M. Ussher (2006) notes, "Moral insanity due to menopause" has been accepted as a legal defence in a number of cases, both in the late 19th century and more recently (p. 128).

19 John Waters stated in an interview in 1994, "I wish my own mother had done that, basically. But I think everybody wishes that their moms would come to the rescue. *Serial Mom* is a good mom. I don't think of her at all as a villain of this movie. She's the heroine" (Grant 2011, 128).

Bibliography

Altheide, D L 2006, 'Terrorism and the politics of fear', *Cultural Studies ↔ Critical Methodologies*, 6(4), pp. 415–439.

'API's eight principles of parenting' 2016, *Attachment Parenting International*, accessed January 13, 2014, from <http://www.attachmentparenting.org/principles/api>.

Arnold, S 2013, *Maternal horror film: melodrama and motherhood*, Basingstoke, UK and New York: Palgrave Macmillan,.

Bagemihl, B 1999, *Biological exuberance: animal homosexuality and natural diversity*, London: Profile.

Beard, W 2006, *The artist as monster: the cinema of David Cronenberg*, Toronto: University of Toronto Press.

Clover, C J 1992, *Men, women and chain saws: gender in the modern horror film*, Princeton, NJ: Princeton University.

Connolly, A 2003, 'Psychoanalytic theory in times of terror', *Journal of Analytical Psychology*, 48(4), pp. 407–431.

Connolly, T 2010, 'Strange births in the Canadian wilderness: Atwood's *Surfacing* and Cronenberg's *The Brood*', *Journal of American & Canadian Studies*, 28, pp. 69–90.

Coward, R 1984, *Female desire*, London: Paladin.

Creed, B 1993, *The monstrous-feminine: film, feminism, psychoanalysis*, London and New York: Routledge.

Crowther, B & Leith, D 1995, 'Feminism, language and the rhetoric of television wildlife programmes', in S Mills (ed), *Language and gender: interdisciplinary perspectives*, London and New York: Routledge, pp. 207–225.

Cunliffe, E 2011, *Murder, medicine and motherhood*, Oxford: Hart, accessed January 15, 2014, from <http://public.eblib.com/EBLPublic/PublicView.do?ptiID=807522>.

DiQuinzio, P 1999, *The impossibility of motherhood: feminism, individualism, and the problem of mothering*, London and New York: Routledge.

Doka, K J & Martin, T L 2010, *Grieving beyond gender: understanding the ways men and women mourn*, revised edition, Hoboken: Taylor & Francis.

Dowling, S & Brown, A 2013, 'An exploration of the experiences of mothers who breastfeed long-term: what are the issues and why does it matter?', *Breastfeeding Medicine*, 8(1), pp. 45–52.

Dunlap, J A 2004, 'Sometimes I feel like a motherless child: the error of pursuing battered mothers for failure to protect', *Loyola Law Review*, 50, pp. 565–622.

Durgnat, R 2002, *A long hard look at 'Psycho'*, London: BFI Publishing.

Dworkin, G 2010, 'Paternalism', in E N Zalta (ed), *The Stanford encyclopedia of philosophy*, accessed January 13, 2014, from <http://plato.stanford.edu/archives/sum2010/entries/paternalism/>.

Elizabeth, V 2004, 'Viewing mothering, violence and sexuality through the lens of ethnicity: mainstream media constructions of Tania Witika as transgressive mother', in A Potts, N Gavey & N Weatherall (eds), *Sex and the body*, Palmerston North: Dunmore Press, pp. 51–70.

Featherstone, B 1997, 'Introduction', in W Hollway & B Featherstone (eds), *Mothering and ambivalence*, London and New York: Routledge, pp. 1–16.

Fischer, L 1992, 'Birth traumas: parturition and horror in "Rosemary's Baby"', *Cinema Journal*, 31(3), pp. 3–18.

Fischer, L 1996, *Cinematernity: film, motherhood, genre*, Princeton, NJ: Princeton University Press.

Foucault, M 1994, *The order of things: an archaeology of the human sciences*, New York: Vintage Books.

Foucault, M 1995, *Discipline and punish: the birth of the prison*, 2nd Vintage Books ed., New York: Vintage Books.

nge kids: how to raise safe, self-reliant children (without going nuts with ..y)' 2014, *Free-range kids*, accessed February 26, 2014, from <http://www.freera ngekids.com/>.

Friedan, B 2013, *The feminine mystique: annotated text, contexts, scholarship*, K L Fermaglich & L Fine (eds), New York: Norton.

Gavey, N 2005, *Just sex?: the cultural scaffolding of rape*, London and New York: Routledge.

Grant, J 2011, 'He really can't help himself', in J Egan (ed), *John Waters: interviews*, Conversations with filmmakers series, Jackson, MS: University Press of Mississippi, pp. 125–134.

Greven, D 2011, *Representations of femininity in American genre cinema: the woman's film, film noir, and modern horror*, New York: Palgrave Macmillan.

Hauck, Y & Irurita, V 2003, 'Incompatible expectations: the dilemma of breastfeeding mothers', *Health Care for Women International*, 24(1), pp. 62–78.

Hendershot, C 2001, *I was a Cold War monster: horror films, eroticism, and the Cold War imagination*, Bowling Green, OH: Popular Press.

Hrdy, S B 1979, 'Infanticide among animals: a review, classification, and examination of the implications for the reproductive strategies of females', *Ethology and Sociobiology*, 1(1), pp. 13–40.

Humm, M 1997, *Feminism and film*, Edinburgh: Edinburgh University Press.

Joubert, D & Joubert, B 2007, 'Lessons of the hunt', *National Geographic*, accessed January 14, 2014, from <http://ngm.nationalgeographic.com/2007/04/leopard-les sons/joubert-photography>.

Kaplan, E A 1992, *Motherhood and representation: the mother in popular culture and melodrama*, London and New York: Routledge.

Kendall, G & Wickham, G 1999, *Using Foucault's methods*, London, Thousand Oaks, CA and New Delhi: SAGE.

Koven, S & Michel, S 1993, *Mothers of a new world: maternalist politics and the origins of welfare states*, London and New York: Routledge.

Kristeva, J 1985, 'Stabat Mater', *Poetics Today*, 6(1/2), pp. 133–152.

Lancaster, R N 2003, *The trouble with nature: sex in science and popular culture*, Berkeley, CA: University of California Press.

Lewis, J 2005, '"Mother oh god mother…": analyzing the "horror" of single mothers in contemporary Hollywood horror', *Scope: An Online Journal of Film Studies*, 2.

Madge, C & O'Connor, H 2006, 'Parenting gone wired: empowerment of new mothers on the internet?', *Social & Cultural Geography*, 7(2), pp. 199–220.

McCabe, J 2013, 'Tea with mother: Sarah Palin and the discourse of motherhood as a political ideal', *Imaginations: Journal of Cross-Cultural Image Studies*, 4(2), accessed January 14, 2014, from <http://imaginations.csj.ualberta.ca/?p=4772>.

McDermott, N 2008, '"I've been labelled the world's worst mom"', *Spiked*, accessed January 27, 2014, from <http://www.spiked-online.com/newsite/article/errant_moms/ 5043>.

Medina, S & Magnuson, S 2009, 'Motherhood in the 21st century: implications for counselors', *Journal of Counseling & Development*, 87(1), pp. 90–96.

Meikle, D 2005, *The Ring companion*, London: Titan.

Miller, T 2007, '"Is this what motherhood is all about?": weaving experiences and discourse through transition to first-time motherhood', *Gender and Society*, 21(3), pp. 337–358.

'Mother of the year? Dog nurses kittens' 2008, *CBS News*, accessed January 14, 2014, from <http://www.cbsnews.com/news/mother-of-the-year-dog-nurses-kittens/>.

Orloff, A 1996, 'Gender in the welfare state', *Annual Review of Sociology*, 22(1), pp. 51–78.

Orloff, A S 2006, 'From maternalism to "employment for all"', in J D Levy (ed), *The state after statism: new state activities in the age of liberalization*, Cambridge, MA: Harvard University Press, pp. 230–268.

Paul, W 1994, *Laughing, screaming: modern Hollywood horror and comedy*, New York: Columbia University Press.

Plant, R J 2010, *Mom*, Chicago: The University of Chicago Press, accessed January 17, 2014, from <http://www.VIU.eblib.com/EBLWeb/patron?target=patron&extendedid=P_496634_0&>.

Reid, C, Greaves, L & Poole, N 2008, 'Good, bad, thwarted or addicted? Discourses of substance-using mothers', *Critical Social Policy*, 28(2), pp. 211–234.

Reiger, K 2008, 'Domination or mutual recognition? professional subjectivity in midwifery and obstetrics', *Social Theory & Health*, 6(2), pp. 132–147.

Rosen, J N 1953, 'The perverse mother', in J N Rosen, *Direct analysis (selected papers)*, New York: Grune & Stratton, pp. 97–105.

Roth, P A 1991, 'Truth in interpretation: the case of psychoanalysis', *Philosophy of the Social Sciences*, 21(2), pp. 175–195.

Rothman, B K 1989, 'Women as fathers: motherhood and child care under a modified patriarchy', *Gender and Society*, 3(1), pp. 89–104.

Salisbury, M 2010, 'James Cameron bummed me out', *One hell of an eye: the official blog of Mike Salisbury*, accessed January 22, 2014, from <http://www.onehellofaneye.com/2010/07/08/james-cameron-bummed-me-out/>.

Samuels, R 1998, *Hitchcock's bi-textuality: Lacan, feminisms, and queer theory*, Albany, NY: SUNY Press.

Sealey, A & Oakley, L 2013, 'Anthropomorphic grammar? Some linguistic patterns in the wildlife documentary series *Life*', *Text & Talk*, 33(3), pp. 399–420.

'Senate Bill 507' 2012, Wisconsin State Legislature, accessed September 12, 2016, from <http://docs.legis.wisconsin.gov/2011/proposals/sb507>.

Silver, A 2010, 'Mama Grizzlies – the top 10 everything of 2010', *TIME*, accessed January 14, 2014, from <http://content.time.com/time/specials/packages/article/0,28804,2035319_2034745_2034739,00.html>.

Singh, I 2004, 'Doing their jobs: mothering with Ritalin in a culture of mother-blame', *Social Science & Medicine*, 59(6), pp. 1193–1205.

Ussher, J M 2006, *Managing the monstrous feminine: regulating the reproductive body*, London and New York: Routledge.

Ussher, J M 2011, *The madness of women: myth and experience*, London and New York: Routledge.

Vincent, C, Ball, S J & Pietikainen, S 2004, 'Metropolitan mothers: mothers, mothering and paid work', *Women's Studies International Forum*, 27(5–6), pp. 571–587.

Wade, L 2011, 'The social construction of the mothering instinct', Sociological Images, accessed September 12, 2016, from <https://thesocietypages.org/socimages/2011/05/08/the-social-construction-of-the-mothering-instinct-2/>.

Wee, V 2011, 'Visual aesthetics and ways of seeing: comparing *Ringu* and *The Ring*', *Cinema Journal*, 50(2), pp. 41–60.

Weinstock, J A 2012, 'Invisible monsters: vision, horror, and contemporary culture', in A S Mittman & P Dendle (eds), *The Ashgate research companion to monsters and the monstrous*, Farnham, UK and Burlington, VT: Ashgate, pp. 275–289.

Wierzbicki, J 2010, 'Lost in translation? Ghost music in recent Japanese Kaidan films and their Hollywood remakes', *Horror Studies*, 1(2), pp. 193–205.

Williams, T 1996, *Hearths of darkness: the family in the American horror film*, Madison, NJ: Fairleigh Dickinson University Press.

5 Living deaths, menstrual monsters and hagsploitation

Horror and/of the abject barren body[1]

The horror genre is fascinated with female sexuality, gender and reproduction, and with acts and processes such as sex, pregnancy, artificial reproductive technologies and motherhood. An enterprising horror fan can find films about toothed or otherwise cannibalistic vaginas, women cutting babies out of other women, demonic pregnancies, inseminations via rape, pre-natal possessions, bloodsucking babies, heroes of the virginal and quasi-virginal types, abortions gone wrong, supernatural appropriation of *in vitro* fertilisation, sexy succubi and a whole litany of examples of terrible mothering, ranging from baffled neglect, to psychotic overbearance, to infanticide. The rollcall of gynaehorror is comprehensive – and yet, in the reproductive and sexual trajectory that I have offered thus far from first sex onwards, there is something missing: menopause and the experience of ageing, non-reproductive woman in horror.

In this chapter I offer a framework that considers the role and function of the menopausal and post-menopausal woman in horror that connects her to other abject expressions of infertile reproductive horror – in particular, the figure of the menstruating woman, whose abject seepage is a visual and corporeal reminder of fecundity during a time when the body has a very low chance of becoming pregnant. I refer to these as abject barren bodies. Barren, colloquially, refers to female (but not male) infertility. It also has negative, gendered connotations that I wish to strategically draw from, for its association with (un)productivity, lifelessness, aridity, and sterility inherently refers to a sort of material or environment (*res extensa*) that *could* be productive, but refuses to be so; compare this emphasis to the term 'impotent', which instead implies a loss of male power. This could (and, perhaps, its implied *should*) is important, for as I have indicated elsewhere in this book, the association of the female body as a material, a medium, an environment, a vessel and a space in which things may grow or develop, is a key scaffolding principle through which the embodied female subject is structured, both conceptually and in terms of its aesthetic presentation within cinema. The body that cannot or does not do this, no matter its form or state, is inherently transgressive.

The abject barren body

I acknowledge, again, the work of Julia Kristeva in the construction and exploration of the notion of the abject in her 1982 book *Powers of Horror*. Kristeva particularly draws from anthropologist Mary Douglas's study of ritual and taboo in *Purity and Danger* (2013 [1966]), in which Douglas outlines how filth or pollution is not a quality that is inherent to a thing (such as dirt or blood). Instead, it is category that is applied to and is defined with regards to the boundary of the physical and social bodies, such that it is the thing that is jettisoned or excluded from this boundary. This exclusion reifies the boundary (see Kristeva 1982, 69); for instance, Douglas notes that the elimination of dirt in purification rituals acts as a way of organising the environment by eliminating disorder (p. 2), for dirt is "matter out of place" (p. 36) and it must be attended to for the pattern of social order to be maintained (p. 40). What is particularly relevant to this discussion is Douglas's important assertion that order within the social is symbolised through the sexual: "many ideas about sexual dangers are better interpreted as symbols of the relation between parts of society, as mirroring designs of hierarchy or symmetry which apply in the larger social system. What goes for sex pollution also goes for bodily pollution" (p. 3). This emphasises the stakes involved in the codification and management of the sexual, reproductive body.

As Kristeva attests, "Abjection is above all ambiguity" (p .11). The abject is easily identified as those things that might disrupt the integrity of the I-subject (the ego) – the mucky bodily indeterminacies, excretions, leakages, affects (such as strong emotion, tears), and bodily responses (such as disgust or revulsion) that challenge the conceptual coherence of the narcissistic construction of the clean and proper body, which is itself a fantasy. Yet, the abject comes from both without ("excrement and its equivalents", disease, decay) and within (Kristeva 1982, 71). The abject(ed), jettisoned, excluded thing then becomes a lightning rod for anxiety – a scapegoat into which trauma is displaced. Through a reaction of disgust or revulsion we are not responding to the thing itself, but instead the cultural meaning bound up within the object. To explore and illustrate this, Kristeva offers a notable reading of the Biblical book of Leviticus, which outlines ritual practices regarding cleanliness and the containment of defilement, and links the maternal body to systems of decay (p. 101) – a body that is not clean and proper. Beyond a literal understanding of 'clean'-ness, she applies this phrase in terms of the cultural separation of men and women, the application of law and authority upon the body of the (contained) individual (pp.100–1), and the removal of any lingering trace of the maternal (p. 102). Secretion, discharge and blood are thus impure (pp. 102–3) in a manner that is explicitly morally and legally codified. The abject, then, shows us what we exclude in order to live, and these indeterminate objects and categories reveal to us the tenuous border at which we exist – the border from which our expelled wastes drop (p. 3). This notion of cultural separation will remain important throughout this chapter.

The barren body also reaches into a variety of registers of abjection, for its corporeal unruliness and volatility (through menstruation, or the varied vaso-motor expressions of menopausal changes) as well as its conceptual boundary confusions evade a clear division between subject and object. The barren body refuses to 'behave' in a culturally-sanctioned manner, or to sit within the social categories that are made available to and that therefore construct the female body. The barren body, as a type of specifically *female* body, both signifies the potential capacity and refusal to reproduce. Consider this in relation to Luce Irigaray and Julia Kristeva's conceptualisations of the cult of the Virgin Mary, which I outline in Chapter One; where the Virgin's perpetual virginity is rendered a clean, closed and unproblematic mode of female subjectivity and (a)sexuality that facilitates the masculine divine without sullying the son of God with traces of copulation or the abject maternal, leaving her docile and definable body as the pre-condition for another, the barren body (perhaps like other female or feminine autoerotic bodies) is for itself. It refuses to be co-opted into a system that positions female bodies and subjectivities as for, subject-to, or as a necessary part of the creation of a male/masculine subject, and thus it sits outside of the phallocentric order. Therefore, the barren body both excludes *itself* from the dominant social order and is *excluded* because of its failure to comply to a reproductive imperative that positions self-sacrificing motherhood as the ideal form of ideologically complicit female subjectivity.

A strategic deployment or even an embrace of the term 'barren' that refuses the negative value judgements ascribed to the term therefore considers barren-ness in its various forms as another set of phases or modalities of a repro-ductive body-in-process. This acknowledges the fundamental importance of sexual difference, in all its complexities, to corporeal feminisms in its invest-ment in the ways that the sexual, embodied subject is constructed and how it, in turn, shapes power and meaning (see Braidotti 2002, 47; Grosz 1994, ix). However, while gesturing towards the role and process of reproductive in the formation of the female subject, it also highlights that non-reproductivity or infertility is not a repudiation nor an absence of the reproductive (in the sense of the asexual), nor a form of failure (as it may be framed in terms of repro-ductive technologies or the social construction of essential motherhood), but an alternative modality of reproductive capacity in which reproduction doesn't happen, for whatever reason. Absence, instead, is a not a negative category but another form of expression, or an alternate modality. The notion of the abject barren thus connects reproductive female bodies across different stages of their lives in ways that other gynaehorrific expressions, such as the monstrous-maternal, are not necessarily able to do. If we are to define bodies by their capacities and their affects, by what they *do* rather than what they *are*, and by how they enter into compositions with other bodies (see Deleuze and Guattari 2004, 284), then each of these abjectly barren bodies shares a related mode of (not) reproducing.

It's helpful, too, to acknowledge that if we were to trace a thread of repro-ductive capacity or fertility through the life of the normative female embodied subject, then overall this body is perhaps more frequently non-reproductive than it is fecund. This calls for a reappraisal of the centralisation of the successfully, ideally fecund reproductive subject within structures of reproductive subjectivity and sexual difference, let alone broader social, economic and political structures that are based on the supposition of women's ideologically-complicit reproductive industry. The abject barren, then, is first encountered and expressed through the female body's entry into fecundity at menarche and then through each period of menstruation and its rhythmic corporeal expression of infertility and renewal; through broader shifts in fertility through one's adult life; through (peri-)menopause; and finally to the post-menopausal permanent cessation of fecundity in middle-age or late middle-age onwards. The wombless body, too, falls into this category, as do other sorts of socially, culturally or medically non-conforming female bodies (such as those with chromosomal variations). When considered *en masse*, these different modes and states speak to the immense amount of time that the ideal female reproductive subject exists, instead, in its seemingly non-ideal state. Importantly, these barren bodies are not the binary 'other' to the actively or successfully reproductive, fecund body, but instead have different capacities and the ability to make desirous connections and interesting assemblages in ways that are perhaps denied to actively reproductive bodies. So, although culturally excluded, both ignored and forcibly jettisoned, the abject barren is a reconsideration of the inconvenient reality that the ideal mode of reproductive female-ness is instead precarious, and it offers us a way of highlighting and connecting those forms of embodied female-ness that are instead disavowed.

To explore these connections and congruences, and the simultaneous veneration of and revulsion at reproductive capacities, I begin by offering a brief account of menstrual horror. In particular, I am interested in how menarche, as an event-process that is associated within horror with a marked upswell in female power, might be connected to sociocultural constructions of menopause as a disease of loss and deficiency. As I will later demonstrate, this in turn shapes and informs the invisibility of menopause and the comparative absence of older women in horror, as well as the broader expression of abject barrenness, ageing and female subjectivity within the genre.

Menstrual horror

Menstruation offers a conceptual contradiction. Menstrual blood and the experience of menstruation are a tactile, embodied and visual reminder of the reproductive potential of the female body – that is, the maternal 'use value' of this body, at least as the sexed female body is positioned with regards to the figure of the 'virgin' and her nascent reproductive potential. Yet, by associating it with disgust and uncleanliness it is a biological (and cultural) truth that is recognised and then suppressed or jettisoned through social consensus (Tyler 2013, 23). This liminality results in the inclusion (or even quarantine) of menstruation in the dominant order through the very act of its expulsion, which in turn polices and reifies the boundaries of the body politic and the body-proper through the cultural construction of menstruation as something that provokes disgust (see Tyler 2013, 20; Douglas 2013 [1966]).

This interplay between the categories of the clean and the impure, the abject push-pull between the desire for and revulsion at the maternal body, and the way the female reproductive body may (or may not) be rendered knowable and controllable, intersect in the codification of menstrual blood and the menstruating body. Menstruating bodies are abject from within (through the generation and the sloughing of endometrial lining) and from without (through the presence of blood). They are also threatening in the way that they reject the reproductive. Menstruation allows for nominally procreative heterosex with a very low chance of conception; as I outline in Chapters One and Three in my discussions of the *vagina dentata* and the female cyborg, sex that is likely to be both non-procreative and pleasurable for women reconfigures that phallocentric script (and the associated male orgasmic imperative) that sex is for reproduction and for the benefit of the male partner. Menstruation also challenges the notion of the vagina as passive receptacle, as a site that can be penetrated. It may allow a penis in, but it actively ejects a substance that is a signifier of both fertility and infertility, rendering the penis bloodied; beyond blood's own sense of indeterminacy this fluid may allude to wound-edness or the capacity to wound. This substance is a viscous reminder that the body is not clean and proper, nor is it closed off; indeed, along with excrement Kristeva identifies menstrual blood as but one of the two types of polluting bodily substances (1982, 71). This also frames menstrual sex as taboo, as sex that is not 'clean', even though having sex while menstruating can be helpful for a woman because of the increased lubrication, the poor likelihood of possible pregnancy, and the fact that orgasm can sometimes help lessen menstrual cramps.

Gynaehorror's multivalence is articulated in the way that female reproductive capacities and affects are at once celebrated and reviled. Reproduction is deemed both necessary and disgusting. Its social management is a way of suppressing women's embodiment, experiences and knowledge(s) at the same time as insisting that such discipline is fundamentally necessary. In the contemporary Western world, ritual management of menstruation serves to eradicate its traces from the public and even the private realm through an intersection of personal embodiment, commodity capitalism, and the rhetoric of self-empowerment, wherein to be empowered is to disavow the dynamic traces of one's own biology. This is best expressed through the widespread association of menstrual management with the value-laden aspirational term 'discrete', which speaks to both an acknowledgement and a displacement, a making-hidden. This structures the use and marketing of expensive, environmentally damaging and even scented single-use menstrual products around a bright, white ideal that disavows the organic or the embodied, instead situating culturally-appropriate 'hygiene' and 'cleanliness' in opposition to a sense of messy, smelly leakiness (Houppert 2000).[2] The disavowal of blood as a signifier for the dirtiness of both the female body and menstruation itself reaches its near-comic apotheosis in the clear, blue, inorganic and decided un-viscous fluid that has often been used to demonstrate products' absorbency in advertisements. If one were to be cynical, then within the context of the persistent medicalisation of, commodification of and pharmaceutical intervention with nearly all forms of female reproductivity, the contemporary demonisation of menstruation might be just another way of opening up and controlling a market by creating a persistent problem and providing an increasing number of products (sanitary pads and liners, tampons, rinses and douches, sprays, wipes) to deal to it. This tension between the contained and the messy is also reflected in the perplexing dearth of broader feminist engagements with menstruation, which perhaps signals an indirect avoidance of such a quotidian issue through the prioritisation of more 'important' feminist issues (Bobel 2010, 29–30).

Certainly, these cultural scripts mark menstruation as something that expresses a form of symbolic pollution in the sense outlined by Kristeva above. Yet, the cyclical nature of menstruation also marks it as productive. Acknowledging the vitality of this means emphasising that women are not simply passive victims, unfortunately-female subjects who live at the 'mercy' of hormonal shifts (Grosz 1994, 204), for the expulsion of endometrial lining is not necessarily a loss, but something that marks a cycle of renewal and regeneration. In Chapter Three I note that the female reproductive cycle is one that is often discussed through the lens of deficit and faultiness: that a woman is born with only so many eggs; that these begin to degrade; that menstruation is a loss and a sign of eggs that have not been implanted; that menstruation "carries out the idea of production gone awry" (Martin 1987, 46) and so on. As Emily Martin suggests, this is markedly different to the way that the loss of sperm cells is framed in male ejaculation. These cells are productive and continually produced, numerous and 'spent', but certainly not 'wasted' like the woman's eggs, despite the orders of magnitudes' worth of disparity between the number of cells involved (Martin 1987, xxiv; Martin 1991). Thinking about menstruation *as* something productive, cyclical and generative, and even as a mode of refreshment instead of an act of defilement, is a powerful way of turning the script that the female body is one that is in a perpetual state of dissolution and decay and thus in need of purification and containment. It also situates the conceptually barren as a space of potential regeneration, and not simply as an expression of loss, a deadening, or an end.

Menstruation, then, troubles the notion of the closed, self-contained body, for it is both leaky and cyclical. The collapse of meaning that occurs in places of boundary confusion is often framed as a threat rather than a liberation from strict segregation of spaces and categories; as Elizabeth Grosz (1994) suggests, "women's corporeality is inscribed as a mode of seepage" (p. 203). Yet, this seepage, and this boundary confusion, is also associated with power. Anthropologists Thomas Buckley and Alma Gottlieb, in their introduction to *Blood Magic: The Anthropology of Menstruation* (1988), suggest that menstruation taboos are far from universally negative. Instead, many such taboos are not a means of guarding society from a feminine evil, but are about protecting the "perceived creative spirituality of menstruous women from the influence of others in a more neutral state, as well as protecting the latter in turn from the potent, positive spiritual force ascribed to such women" (p. 7). The menstruating woman, then, is not 'dirty' but powerful. In some cases, this offers women a means by which to assert their own "autonomy, influence and social control" (p. 7) and an enhancement of status (p. 13). They posit that the assumptions that such taboos are inherently negative and act as a suppression of the feminine are more representative of andro- and ethnocentric assumptions than they are of the intent behind myriad cultural practices (pp. 5, 9; Datan 1995, 454–5).[3] From here, I look to this connection between menstruation and power in horror.

The clearest expression of the competing effects and affects of menstural horror comes in narratives that centre on menarche – the onset of menses. Menarche is framed as an immensely significant event, and one that is traumatic both in terms of the horror that engenders and the abrupt shift in the capacities and affects of the reproductive body. First menstruation offers a complex, rich and sometimes contradictory matrix of signification and expression: the female body, bloodied for the first time, is wounded; the presence of blood threatens the potential wounding of another; the containment expressed in the figure of the virgin is disrupted and the body is instead dangerously, provocatively open (for both the self and an-other); the role of the body in identity formation opens up new modes of being; the nascent power that is consumed in the sacrifice of the virgin is unleashed; the (re)generative body disrupts the phallocentric order thorough its abject leakage and its sudden indeterminacy; and the body that is coded and structured by culture is reshaped by nature. This dynamic body does not exist within binary structures; menarche is not either/or but reproductive *and* sexual *and* barren *and* interior *and* exterior *and* adolescent *and* mature *and*.... It overflows with signification. Menarche marks a space within which the female reproductive body becomes its own centre of meaning; it does not work to constitute or oppose either the male subject or the foetal subject.

Menarche is doubly abject, for its fleshy locus is the female *adolescent* body. Beyond troubling and denaturalising the border between the culturally-specific and socially constructed states of 'child' and 'adult', the adolescent body is marked as abject most obviously because of the physical and affective shifts it dynamically experiences as it develops into a state of emotional and sexual maturation. The adolescent is excluded from the adult social order and denied agency, so that adolescent subjective agency is in turn only exerted through self-abjection – that is, by embracing that which is unsanctioned and choosing non-conformity and alienation (Stephens 2003, 124). The adolescent female subject is more troubling still, for she unsteadies the ideal adult male subject; her emergence into sexuality is also an emergence from the pre-sexual neutrality of childhood (as Other to the adult) and into the embodied sexual difference of the female sexual subject (as Other to man), which highlights the temporality of the sexed subject. Importantly, the adolescent girl marks becomings and alliances that are unavailable to the ideal (fixed male) subject; after all, as Deuleuze and Guattari (2004) note in their articulation of 'becoming-woman', the figure of 'girl' (cf. 'woman') expresses and performs an interstitial, 'intermezzo' thisness or haecceity that nimbly evades dualisms (p. 305). One of the clearest cinematic engagements with this interplay between menarche, abjection (bodily and social), and the multiplicitous blocks of becoming through which the adolescent female enters into alliance(s) with the world is Brian de Palma's 1976 adaptation of Stephen King's novel *Carrie*, which centres on a troubled high school senior with telekinesis, whose awe-inspiring, destructive powers are unleashed when she begins her first period. Carrie's immense powers and her abject body are explicitly connected to her social abjection, for her exclusion from the social order is manifold: she is 'weird' (in part due to her pathologically strict religious upbringing); she doesn't dress or behave like her classmates; she is bullied and excluded; she hasn't experienced puberty in a normative manner. She has her own affects and capacities, and her knowledge(s) and ways of being in the world are quite different to those around her.

Our introduction to Carrie is one that firmly centres on her body and her sexuality. It is significant that when we first see Carrie at the beginning of the film it is through an erotic, voyeuristic lens that explicitly recalls Marian Crane's death in the famous shower scene from *Psycho* (1960) (see Briefel 2005, 21–2). This eroticism becomes one of the film's key sites of abject, embodied and sexual tension. Carrie, naked, is shrouded in the thick steam of the school's communal shower, which serves to soften the image in a manner that evokes soft-core pornography and erotica; already her body (as in, her fleshy-water-vapour aesthetic body; the capacities of this more-than-flesh body) is indistinct, and difficult to account for or understand. Her image clarifies through close ups of her slowly and gently washing her breasts, mouth, legs and buttocks. She drops her bar of soap (clean) and blood (dirty) begins to run down her inner thigh. Carrie looks at the blood on her hand, her brow furrowing, and we see the pooling, diluted blood trickle through her fingers. Due to her mother's refusal to acknowledge her puberty she has no understanding of what menstruation is. She becomes distraught, running towards her classmates and wiping blood in their clothes as she screams for help, but they laugh and pelt her with tampons and sanitary pads as she cowers in the corner. Carrie's hysteria is broken by her teacher, who slaps her across the face, and this act of violence is accompanied by the explosion of the lightbulb above them. The clear implication is that Carrie has caused this surge in power, indeed *is* this surge in power, aligning menarche, and not simply the trauma of the girls' nasty bullying, with the explicit emergence of her own telekinetic powers.

This opening sequence perhaps offers Carrie up as subject-to and the subject of the voyeuristic, implicitly male gaze that works to interrogate and perhaps demystify her body in a manner that initially coheres beautifully with Laura

Mulvey's articulation of the gendered function of the cinematic apparatus in her iconic article "Visual Pleasure and Narrative Cinema" (2000 [1975]). This is supported by the opening music. The soundtrack begins with a peaceful, yearning adagio for strings and piano that is perhaps better suited to a light, sentimental drama, and as Carrie's body comes into frame she is accompanied by a dreamy, light-hearted theme on the flute. Once Carrie's hand is bloodied the music fades swiftly and we are left with the diegetic sound of the shower; her reverie – and ours – is interrupted.[4] The opening shots invite us to consume and appreciate Carrie's naked, adult female body, but the removal of this pleasant music is a challenge. Whereas Marian Crane's death in *Psycho* (1960) is a violent snuffing out of the visual source of erotic pleasure and the renunciation, or re-routing, of carnal desire, the abrupt onset of Carrie's menses marks a different sort of sudden and abject refusal of the male gaze. If the voyeuristic spectator attempts to demystify the potential threat of the woman's body, as Mulvey (2000 [1975], 42) suggests, then this horrific menarche shifts her body from object-to-be-consumed to a site of challenge and potential trauma – the viewer's trauma, as well as Carrie's. Her menstrual blood says 'this body is not for you'. Carrie, in her ignorance, thinks she is bleeding to death, although her classmates and teacher know better, but this is also a reminder that the female body is not docile. Instead, the viewer – coaxed, perhaps, into appreciation and potential arousal – is overtly challenged by the reminder of an interiority that cannot be seen and controlled. The rest of the women know how to manage the bloody evidence of this interiority through their own gender-specific knowledge, passed from girl to girl and from mother to daughter, in a set of relationships that Carrie is denied.

The blooming emergence of menstrual blood is expressed again in the film's conclusion. Carrie, now radiant and voted prom queen, has a bucket of pig's blood dumped on her head during her coronation by the nastiest of the high school bullies. Carrie's coronation is preceded by a dream-like two-minute long crane shot that manipulates space, time and perspective. It places Carrie (overwhelmed, weeping, accepted, beautiful, desirable) at the centre of the social and sexual order. Beyond the unsettling, almost grotesque manipulation of cinematic space caused by the prom's lurid coloured lights and the juxtaposition of wide shots with extreme close ups of faces and hands, the scene is marked by temporal shifts (between slow motion, real-time footage and jagged jump cuts), aural manipulation (the suppression of environmental diegetic sound, the emphasis upon the sound of the dribbling, shower-like blood), and the use of mobile split screens that express an immense violence and centralise Carrie's abject, unsettling subjective position. The horrific, humiliating prank sets off Carrie's telekinetic wrath in an explosive, immense and destructive wave of becoming-fury that kills hundreds and nearly levels the town. This defilement, and the ongoing association of Carrie with pigs, blood and filth (Creed 1993, 80) again acts a repudiation of a certain type of voyeurism and a controlling male gaze, by swiftly rendering her an object of fear, horror and disgust instead of an object of attraction. However, rather than thinking about this menstrual blood in terms of a wound, or even as evidence of the toothed vagina of what Creed calls the *femme castratrice*, there is a perverse power in this refusal. By re-centring power within the body of the woman, and centralising the abject subject position of Carrie within cinematic time and space, this refusal counters modes of objectification that try to constrain and control her, especially as blood's (monthly menstrual) return refuses to be suppressed.

The association of menarche and puberty with monstrosity is well-evidenced. In Canadian horror-comedy *Ginger Snaps* (2000) the menstrual cycle – 'the curse' – is linked with the lunar progression of lycanthropy: teenage goth outsider Ginger gets her first period (like Carrie, quite late), and is she attacked by a werewolf almost immediately after its onset, connecting girl-monster-moon-blood in a violently animalistic alliance of blood and flesh. Ginger is furious at the betrayal of her own body and the film drolly suggests that her period, not the attack, is the more traumatic event, comparing the mauling that she receives from the wolf with the internal mauling of cramps and the sloughing of fluid. Her emergent, rhythmic monstrosity is linked to her growing sexual autonomy and a cyclical explosion of abject desire that connects the ecstasy of her increasingly murderous impulses with the pleasures of masturbation and orgasm. Although the film's association of menstruation (and female-ness) with monstrosity can be read as repressive, the figure of the werewolf symbolically serves to boldly illustrate the restrictions placed upon women's bodies: it is, instead, the gynaehorrific discourses surrounding menstruation and the cultural expectation of docile femininity that render women monstrous (Miller 2005), perhaps more monstrous than an actual, literal monster. Similarly, in *Jennifer's Body* (2009), Jennifer must cater to the vicious, carnal needs of the succubus that possesses her by seducing and killing a different young man on a near-monthly schedule.

Just as Carrie's powers and Ginger's monstrosity emerge at menarche, in *The Exorcist* (1973) young Regan's violent, abject possession by the demon Pazuzu is explicitly aligned with puberty. One of Regan's most shocking acts comes when she repeatedly stabs her genitals with a crucifix, combining mutilation and masturbation, and the resultant blood conflates menstruation with perverse, sadomasochistic pleasure and the spurting forth of an abhorrent, obscene wound. Other possession narratives, such as *The Last Exorcism* (2010) and *The Conjuring 2* (2016), similarly connect the abject liminality of female pubescence with an openness or a sensitivity to the supernatural, juxta-posing the reproductive and the barren. Aviva Briefel (2005) notably suggests that such menstrual monsters are fundamentally sympathetic given their obvious pain and suffering (p. 16), and that they engage in acts of self-destruction or self-mutilation to curb their own (reproductive) monstrosity (p. 21). This sympathy, combined with what she argues is, in fact, the female monster's utter knowability and predictability (as opposed its status as an "ungraspable Other" (p. 24)), creates a connection between the monster-figure and the spectator that engenders a particular type of self-aware interrogation of the process of identification, for her pain becomes our own (p. 24). In either reading, whether the female body is sympathetic and familiar, or unknowable and Other, the connection between menarche, menstrual blood and monstrosity is assured.

Menstruation and the female reproductive system are also historically and mythologically linked to supernatural powers such as witchcraft (Creed 1993, 77). One of the most artful examples of this comes in the atmospheric, foreboding film *The Witch* (2015), a film set in 17th-century New England, in which a stubbornly pious man, Caleb, and his family are exiled (excluded, jettisoned) from their Puritan community because of the idiosyncrasies of Caleb's extreme religious beliefs. The socially abjected family is left to attempt to survive alone in a small, unproductive farm on the edge of a large, imposing forest, a liminal space that is neither unbounded, terrifying nature nor the walled site of the people's village. Immediately their youngest son, an un-baptised and thus spiritually indeterminate infant, is abducted and killed by a witch who lives in the forest. The film explores the hysteria, paranoia and religious mania of the family as they struggle with the increasing predations of the witch, the bitter hardships of their isolated life, and the potential demonic possessions of their children and the family's black billy goat, who the youngest children insist can talk.

More quietly threatening, though, is eldest daughter Thomasin's nascent, emergent sexuality. Her impending puberty, and the sense that she is on the cusp of sexual maturity, is an unspoken but outright source of mounting dread. The sense of increasingly claustrophobic horror that envelops the family is as aptly expressed in the manner that Thomasin's next-youngest brother furtively and incestuously glances at her growing breasts, the way that her parents fearfully threaten to send her back to the village to marry, and the horrendous swiftness with which they are all willing to believe that she is a witch, as it is by the encroaching horror of the unknown, threatening yet alluring dark-ness of the forest. The family is eventually driven mad and killed and the farm ruined. Thomasin is left alone and terrified, but in desperation she pleads with the family's goat, Black Philip, to speak with her. He reveals himself to be Satan in goat-form and offers her the chance to embrace her earthly desires. Her fearful, exhausted and furious acquiescence, alongside her willingness to write her name in Satan's book and join the witch in the forest, culminates in her participation in a witches' black Sabbath with a naked coven in the forest. Whether one reads the film's final scenes as literal, as allegorical, or as a subjective expression of Thomasin's broken, feminine madness, this final, carnal conflagration is a gleefully animalistic and utterly subversive renunciation of all the social, sexual and religious repressions placed upon women within an oppressive, misogynistic and controlling society. It is abject in every sense, and gloriously so. The film ends as Thomasin begins to fly, naked, both crying and cackling, her desires and fears pouring out together as she joins her new, female community. This community exists only for the gratification of its female/feminine members, and it does not centralise ideologically-complicit codes of reproduction and fecundity. The forest's witch and her sisters may have been tempted by the presence of an unbaptised infant, let alone the isolated family themselves and the quiet violence of their repressed desires, but it is Thomasin's puberty and the associated interstitial sense of emergent alteration, be it one associated with the dread of the feminine or a type of bated anticipation, that keeps this door wide open.

All these films, then, point to puberty generally and menarche specifically as a horrific *onset* – the passage of the female individual into reproductive maturity, and thus the hypothetical ability to bear children. This onset is posited as something that is significant or even traumatic for the individual in its abject breaching of boundaries, but it also marks a shift in embodied subjectivity and new modes of becoming that are characterised by new affects and capacities, new alliances and symbioses. These new boundary confusions are subject to their own rhythms, which marks the abject and reproductive-yet-barren menstrual body as other-to bodies that are conceptualised (accurately or not) as persisting in a state of static be-ing. This alters the way that the subject experiences and lives in their own body, and this body-in-process is excluded from static modes of 'being'. This may be framed as negative, through the association of menstruation with injury, wounds and the ejection or 'loss' of unnecessary, unused organic material that is associated with dirt and decay. It may be productive and monstrously generative, through the cyclical renewal or regeneration of the viscous tissue and mucus of the endo-metrium, and the implication of a fleshy maternal bond between woman and child, which conflates menses with a certain sort of feminine power that sits outside of patriarchal authority and meaning. The cyclical changes of the menstruating body, both psychological and physiological, are undoubtedly diffi-cult for many, but these natural (albeit challenging) shifts are compounded by the ways that menstruation is pathologised, in that normal premenstrual changes are posited as a form of psychiatric illness (see Ussher 2011, 153–84) and discursively constructed as a sort of dirty, inconvenient aberration that must be rendered clean, contained and well-managed.

The horror of menopause

It is from here that I move away from the abject barren menstrual body to the abject barren menopausal or postmenopausal ageing body. If this onset on menstruation – this opening up, or this beginning – is rendered as both a site of horror and a point at which a certain type of generatively monstrous and fleshy power begins, then menopause, as the process through which menstruation stops, can be negatively constructed as a sort of cessation, as opposed to a transition to a different life-stage and a different set of affective capacities and relations. Book-ending a cissexual woman's normative reproductive life in this way offers up some interesting questions with regards to gynaehorror films, for although menstrual monsters are both obviously and allegorically present, menopause itself is conspicuously absent in the horror genre.

Menopause – literally, the end of monthly cycles – is the period of a woman's life during which the ovaries stop producing oocytes (egg cells) and menstruation ceases. It is defined retrospectively once a woman has not experienced spontaneous periods for a year; perimenopause is the technical term for the period of menopausal transition, but given the popular usage of 'menopause' as a catch-all term for this process, I will use this latter term. While this process usually begins around the age of 50, it can present itself as early as one's 30s, and as late as one's 60s. Given the slow upwards creep of women's life expectancy, physicians Tracy A. Takahashi and Kay. M Johnson (2015) indicate that American woman will spend 40% of their lives in the post-menopause phase (p. 521). Physical changes associated with the change in the body's hormonal balance include vasomotor symptoms (symptoms related to the constriction or opening up of blood vessels) such as hot flashes, as well as changes to the vulva and vagina, including a decrease in lubrication and a thinning of the vaginal walls. These latter changes might be accompanied by pain, dryness, discomfort and changes in urinary function. Menopause can also be associated with psychological symptoms, such as anxiety or depression. However, it is necessary to highlight that the experience of perimenopause (the pre-menopausal period where periods may become erratic) and meno-pause, and the ways that subsequent and coetaneous physiological and psy-chological effects are framed, varies widely depending on race, ethnicity, health, diet and global location – but it is important that these variations are not framed with regards to one particular ideal body against which all others are judged. For example, anthropologist Margaret Lock's remarkable cross-cultural analysis of the experience of menopause in Japan and North America, *Encounters with Aging* (1993), highlights the extent to which American women are significantly more likely to experience these sorts of negative psy-chological and physiological symptoms that their Japanese counterparts. There is an enormous degree of cultural specificity in terms of its discursive construction and lived experience of changes in reproductive function as one ages, and such differences are certainly strongly connected to whether or not ageing is culturally framed as an advancement or a decline – and, conversely, the extent to which youth is valorised and held up as a feminine ideal (Elliott 2003, 283). For the purposes of my argument here, I refer to the experiences of menopause and post-menopause that are most widely felt, reported and theorised in the West.

At the end of the previous chapter on motherhood I gestured to two women who fit the categories of menopausal or post-menopausal women. Vivian, in *Grace* (2009), is an older woman struggling with the death of her adult son and who seeks to re-articulate her maternal function in various ways, including stimulating her breasts with a breast pump so as to resume lactation, and attempting to steal her granddaughter so that she may raise the infant herself and reconnect with her lost (re)productive role. The baffled family of Beverley Sutphin, in the cheerfully satirical *Serial Mom* (1994), wonder if her homicidal rages might be associated with menopause – a fitting accusation, given that menopause has been associated with moral insanity and, in some cases, used as a defence when women have committed crimes (Ussher 2006, 128). Nonetheless, these two rare examples do more to highlight the lack of extended, specific engagements with menopause and ageing; simply put, there do not seem to be any horror films that are specifically *about* menopause in the way that there are about menarche or menstruation (or pregnancy or abortion, and so on). Given the importance of gynaehorrific narratives and subjects to the representation of women in horror, I posit that this absence is, in itself, meaningful. After all, as I discuss below, for many women the experience of menopause can be exceptionally challenging, and beyond any issues of physiological and psychological distress, the period from middle-age through to post-menopause also marks a period of social and sexual transition for women that is no less important than those shifts discussed elsewhere in this book.

There is certainly some writing on individual archetypes and representations of older women: these include (but are not limited to) analyses of the crone-witch (Walter 2015) and her sister the wicked stepmother; the archaic, parthenogenetic mother, such as the absent hive-queen in *Alien* (1979), who is both origin and end (Creed 1993, 17); and the matron (Green 2011), who sits in opposition to the figures of the mother and the maiden to offer a tripartite account of the female lifecycle. Vivian Sobchack's semi-autobiographical account of the 'excessive' ageing woman in low-budget horror films from the late 1950s through to the mid-1960s, including *The Leech Woman* (1960), offers the most pronounced engagement with this issue; as she suggests, "the visibly aging body represents a challenge to the self-deluding fantasies of immortality that mark the dominant technoculture. Furthermore, in a sexist as well as ageist technoculture, the visibly aging body of a woman has been and still is especially terrifying" to both men and women (Sobchack 2000, 343; see also Sobchack 2009). The films discussed by Sobchack serve to alienate, denigrate and humiliate their ageing women, framing their very existence as something that evinces disgust and fear in men, such that these 'scary' women become associated with abjection and death (for men) and the fear of powerlessness and irrelevancy (for women).

I am not satisfied that the cultural and supernatural power that is present in menstrual, reproductive outbursts of feminine potency simply bleeds away(!) or quietly dries up, but it is important to consider some of the complexities of representation, bias and cultural specificity here. Nancy Datan (1995), in her discussion of ethnocentric and androcentric bias (including her own) in the anthropological study of menopause, fertility and taboo, suggests that assumptions regarding the level of privilege 'femininity' has within cultural groups, and whether or not child-bearing and fertility are concomitantly associated with said femininity, reflect more on the investigators' positions than they do about actual cultural practice. Although Datan's self-reflective work here looks to the roles of sociologists and anthropologists, and specifically her own work in a broad study of middle-aged women in various Israeli subcultures, I suggest that her overarching point is helpful here. Datan indicates that her own bias as a young, pregnant researcher, and her male colleagues' masculine bias, led them to over-value the importance of childbearing and fertility when considering the way that some groups, significantly more than others, presented with psychiatric conditions such as clinical depression during menopause. Significantly, she notes that "the women in our study welcomed the loss of fertility that menopause brought. And we did not believe them" (p. 452) – thus highlighting her own ageism through what she terms "the narcissism of the lifecycle" (p. 453).

I highlight Datan's article to complicate and enrich the way we might think about the representation of menopause in popular media, especially given that the writers and directors of horror films are overwhelmingly male. Firstly, there is no doubt that when female monstrosity is present it tends to be in gendered terms that often centre on the reproductive cycle (Creed 1993), but also that women in horror cinema tend to skew young. This is particularly apparent in my discussions of virginity and first sex, but it is not drawing a long bow to suggest that the women in films about pregnancy and mother-hood are generally not 'older' mothers, especially if we consider the industrial pressures of women in mainstream film to conform to certain ideals of youth and attractiveness. Secondly, given the overt pathologisation of menopause in Western society, it seems odd that something that is discursively (and unfairly) constructed as a specifically gendered disease is not accounted for specifically within the genre, especially if we think about horror as a conservative genre instead of a radical one. I suggest, then, that this concern is expressed in other, less explicit but more conceptual ways, for instance through narratives that mourn a 'loss' of youth or that denigrate older women. I couch the term 'loss' here carefully, as suggesting that female ageing is specifically a loss reaffirms this emphasis on the primacy of youth and the centrality of repro-ductive potential, and though this might be the case in many media repre-sentations of ageing, it would be utterly foolish to insinuate that this is the actual experience of ageing for all, or even most women. Instead I wish to situate 'loss' in one of many affective expressions of the barren, for this highlights, again, how the ageing body troubles dominant, phallocentric con-structions of embodied reproductive female subjectivity that serve to support and construct male subjectivity or facilitate other forms of masculine power.

My discussion from here works to fill in some of the gaps that exist between pre-existing engagements with older women in horror, but I also wish to reflect upon the absence of films that are *literally* about menopause, post-menopause, and the process and experience of ageing. This, of course, relates to broader issues of gendered representation, and I suggest that even if menopause itself isn't present as a specific narrative conceit, there are none-theless ways that horror films explore fears about and attitudes towards older women's sexual and social roles, especially in the ways that older women and their stories are socially and culturally side-lined. As with the other gynae-horrific narratives explored elsewhere in this book, I look to productive, perhaps radical forms of monstrosity as well as reductive or negative demonisations of women and their (un-)reproductive bodies. Horror films don't need to have murderers who are provoked by the irritations of vaginal discomfort or hot sweats to engage meaningfully with issues of female ageing and embodiment, just as horrific representations of ageing women might also offer spaces in which women can act in a raucous, unruly manner that defies the notion of what it means to behave in an 'age-appropriate' manner.

Further, I suggest such negative attitudes towards ageing women are widespread, and contribute to a social abjection that reveals a cultural sense of disgust at the older body. I found it both significant and peculiar that, as I approached this topic and began to think about the presence or absence of menopause in horror film, many of the people I sounded out, including scholars, fans and film professionals, wondered (after a moment of silence) whether a lack of representation of older women and their stories might be related to a lack of interest in the genre itself on the part of female viewers in middle-age and older. This suggests, fallaciously, that spectatorship is a core issue – that is, that older women aren't a key demographic market, and therefore that horror films 'about' older women might not find an audience. Although I understand the broad logic behind this reasoning, it is also spurious and, perhaps, a little unimaginative, for beyond some pretty broad-stroke and possibly sexist assumptions about women's tastes in film, horror is a genre in which just about anything goes. I argue, instead, that this response is direct evidence of the subtle forms of exclusion that are experienced by the older abject barren body. As I indicate later in this chapter, shifts in production and distribution in the last ten years have meant that the number and diversity of horror films has increased markedly, just as video-on-demand platforms have made such films even more accessible. It is easier than ever for films to be made, and for them to find an audience. I suggest, perhaps cheekily, that films that feature serial killing rubber tyres (*Rubber* (2010)), homicidal tomatoes (*Attack of the Killer Tomatoes* (1978)), and killer elevators (*The Shaft* (2001)), or that centre on the subjective experiences of teenaged girls as cannibals (*We Are What We Are* (2013)) and amateur surgeons (*Excision* (2012)), or men who spend nearly an entire film watching other films (*Sinister* (2012)) or listening to tapes (*Session 9* (2001)), do not require much more of a conceptual leap in terms of spectatorship and identification than do the experiences of older women, be they protagonists or villains. If it *is* harder to accept the presence of an older woman in horror than it is a group of extradimensional sadomasochists, as in *Hellraiser* (1987) and its sequels, then that certainly highlights one of the core issues in attitudes towards female representation and spectatorship by indicating that the figure of the older woman is so profoundly abject that it is not deemed to be reasonable for an audience to identify with her or want to watch her. Instead, narratives about older women are significantly devalued, and their invisibility goes largely unnoticed. The unspoken assumption is: why would anyone want to watch *that*? My question, instead, is why wouldn't we?

A key consideration in the construction of ageing women in horror film, and a point of connection to the other issues of sexuality and reproduction I have explored elsewhere in this book, is the fact that within Western society and traditional medical discourses menopause is pathologised. This biomedical model constructs menopause not as a natural process, a change in experience, and a collection of vasomotor effects, but as a disease; this is contrasted to a state of 'well'-ness and, by proxy, 'virtue' (Lock 1998, 36). Specifically, menopause-as-disease is structured as a *deficiency* in ovarian oestrogen (see Gannon and Stevens 1998), even though oestrogens are also secreted by other parts of the body, and menopause also consists of changes in levels of the sex hormone progesterone, which is involved in the menstrual cycle. This emphasis upon lowering levels of ovarian oestrogen positions the older woman as hormonally 'lacking' in comparison to a younger woman (Kwok 1996, 33), and this deficiency centres firmly on the functionality of the reproductive organs, as well as the hormone that is most conflated with femininity. This is even more pronounced given the fact that human females are the only mammals that reach "reproductive senescence" (Lock 1998, 41) – a sense of loss that sits opposed to the emergence and productivity associated with menarche. This point that is often leveraged to suggest not only that female bodies are wanting, but that *human* female bodies are, perhaps, particularly flawed in a specific manner that sits against the 'intention' of nature; they are always-already abject, although the mode of abjection shifts over time. This also situates reproduction as the central feature of female existence, and it particularly denigrates female, but not male, ageing (Lock 1998, 41), for the gendered notion of the 'barren', in its most negative sense, suggests an aridity that undermines the construction of the ideal(ly) reproductive female subject. With its focus on symptoms, management and pathology, the western bio-medical model of menopause posits that other concurrent effects of ageing (such as osteoporosis) can be lumped together to form a type of syndromic disease profile that situates the reproductive system and the time following the cessation of menstruation as its locus, while emphasising (and perhaps universalising) menopause's negative effects. It also suggests that the natural lowering of levels of oestrogen in mid-life requires potentially aggressive pharmaceutical intervention.

This sense of deficiency, and the idea that aspects of youthful vitality (and thus normative femininity) can be restored through such intervention, is exacerbated by the discourses circulated by those same medical companies that benefit from the demand created through advertising campaigns and product positioning (Fugh-Berman 2015; Kwok 1996, 34; Ussher 2006, 132). Physician Robert A. Wilson's best-selling 1966 book *Feminine Forever* brought such medical discussions into the mainstream. It framed menopause as a disease of deficiency, much like the insulin-deficiency of diabetes, which comes about due to an inadequate level of oestrogen. This deficiency, he suggested, resulted in a state of 'living decay', of gnarled ovaries and dried up, wizened sexual organs, a state of passively *existing* instead than actively *living* that robbed older women (and, presumably, their husbands) of femininity, youth, and rich, fulfilling sex lives. Indeed, the startling opening line of the book's precursor article argues that the "unpalatable truth must be faced that all post-menopausal women are castrates" (Wilson and Wilson 1963, 347). Like other pharmacological engagements with sex, the (hetero)sexually available and willing body is posited as not only the norm but the ideal (Vares *et al.* 2007), and youth and fertility are valorised; the emotive language used for various physiological changes during menopause, such as vaginal 'atrophy', further reinforces this. The solution to this (implied) trauma, according to Wilson, was oestrogen replacement therapy (ERT), a form of hormone replacement therapy (HRT). Importantly, this diagnostic model originates as a way of co-opting the reproductive body, of stratifying it as an aggregate of capacities and affects into structures of capital, industry and commodity, for the book was financially supported by the pharmaceutical company Wyeth, for whom Wilson worked as a consultant. Wyeth had first marketed their own ERT, Premarin (whose name derived from 'pregnant mares' urine'), in the United States and Canada in the early 1940s (Fritz and Speroff 2012, 751), and the book served as a blatant promotion for and justification of their product.

Certainly, like other reproductive technologies such as the oral contraceptive pill, such a technological intervention can offer women a greater degree of control and autonomy over their bodies, even though marketing such drugs as a type of "fountain of youth" is quite a stretch (Houck 2003, 115). Such technologies also invite a pervasive surveillance and management of the reproductive female body. However, in addition to its benefits ERT has been linked unequivocally to an increase in risk of diseases such as breast cancer, endometrial cancer, cardiovascular disease and strokes (Ussher 2006, 132–4; Beral and Million Women Study Collaborators 2003; Writing Group for the Women's Health Initiative Investigators 2002) – a link that was first proposed in the 1940s, well before the widespread marketing of the treatment to menopausal women in the 1960s and 1970s. Even significant risk is still framed within medicine as a 'reasonable' trade-off in the management of some of the more personally and immediately uncomfortable vasomotor effects associated with menopause, such as vaginal dryness and hot sweats (Ussher 2006, 134), let alone the maintenance of an 'acceptable' quality of skin (Houck 2003, 115). Judith A. Houck (2003), in her comprehensive account of feminist responses to *Feminine Forever* from 1963–1980, also points to research that suggests that for some (but certainly not all) women, demand for such treatments was clearly influenced by "dire depictions of menopause in the popular media" (p. 125; see also Gannon and Stevens 1998), although she also indicates that feminist engagements with menopause, its pathologisation and the pharmaceutical interventions available varied widely. Hoeck also suggests, helpfully, that the feminist movement and feminist critiques of menopause encouraged women to have higher expectations of patient care and to be more open about their varied experiences of menopause, which perhaps aligns women less as passive patients and more as active consumers, although the extent to which consent for treatment could be 'informed' is up for debate. Nonetheless, the positioning of HRT as a way of restoring a woman's 'natural' state handily ignores the varying levels of ovarian oestrogen that a woman experiences throughout her whole life, from childhood through to old age. In a particularly representative shell game, the rhythmic, generative nature of menstruation is marked as abject and unruly, yet later in life the 'ideal' level of oestrogen is that which is associated with a woman's most potentially fertile reproductive years.

It is here that menopause as a medical and social *construct,* as opposed to a process and a collection of potential vasomotor symptoms, is a helpful lens through which to consider ageing women and reproductive changes in horror film. Kwok Wei Leng, in her article "On Menopause and Cyborgs, Or, Towards a Feminist Cyborg Politics of Menopause" (1996) suggests that a (critical) feminist reading of the biomedical model of menopause emphasises that the pathologisation of menopause within medical discourses "is an assault to the autonomy and integrity of women's normal bodily existence" (p. 36), and that this is conceptually opposed by an equally restrictive paradigm that centralises the notion of 'natural-ness' through a privileging of "a bodily-centred and thus woman-centred perspective" (p. 38). I offer my account of the biomedical model not to suggest that it can only be countered by, perhaps, an equally blanket approach to the management of expectations surrounding embodied experiences of ageing that positions nature against culture, and the personal against the corporate or institutional. Instead, I wish to highlight that the sociocultural assumptions that underpin the biomedical model – assumptions about ageing, desire, vitality, youth, and what qualifies as a well-behaved and well-managed body – are the same assumptions that need to be interrogated as we look to the representation, or the absence, of menopause and post-menopause in popular media such as horror cinema. Menopause-as-construct thus draws from multiple expressions of interior, exterior and social abjection, at the same time as situating the 'barren' as an ambivalent and composite category that is not static nor fixed but that includes dynamic and sometimes unexpected shifts in fertility, levels of internal lubrication, the quality of skin, the feeling and appearance of the vagina, vasomotor symptoms (like hot flashes), affective capacities (such as emotions), and so on.

The social construction of normative femininity centralises ideal, mythic womanhood with youth, and a particular type of attractiveness and sexual availability that implicitly comes with it, in a manner that both overtly and subtly intermingles with the capacity to reproduce. Conversely, as Ussher (2006) contends,

> The regimes of knowledge produced by science and medicine which act to circulate 'truths' about women at the menopause and beyond – the fictions framed as facts that provide the context for women's understanding and experience of their ageing bodies – tell us that disease, decay, atrophy and senility are the inevitable outcome of the end of fecundity. (p. 127).

If menarche expresses a powerful entry into the reproductive order, then menopause, is marked as an end and a palpable *loss* in a manner that has no real male equivalent, and that treats a certain type of (cissexual, unproblematically reproductive) female body, within a particular window, as an ideal body – even when that allegedly ideal body is demonised or managed in myriad other ways. Margaret Lock (1998) suggests that in "contemporary Euro/America the end of menstruation has become a synecdoche for middle-aged women in all their variety, who appear in current discourse as an estrogen-starved population, at risk of hot flashes, future heart attacks and broken bones" (p. 40). Even in more recent representations of menopause in the mass media, it remains associated with decay, decrepitude and a need for medical intervention (Gannon and Stevens 1998). The post-menopausal body is similarly marked by lack, loss and decrepitude; instead, "the non-reproductive post-menopausal woman is a perambulating anomaly" (Lock 1998, 41), given that a cessation of reproductive capability becomes equated with a loss in social and cultural value. These tangled contradictions add to the litany of ways that women's bodies are treated as abject and divergent, both perpetually deficient and 'too much', rather than as a multivalent body-in-process.

Before addressing the place of older women in (horror) cinema, I suggest that Robert Wilson's aforementioned insulting and dismissive consideration of menopause as a sort of 'living decay' gestures provocatively to modern day engagements with the living dead. The figure of the zombie, which emerged in its secular form in George A. Romero's *Night of the Living Dead* (1968) and in its virophilic form in 2002's *28 Days Later*, has been a persistent and massively proliferating cultural presence since the turn of the 21st century (Bishop 2010; Comentale and Jaffe 2014; Dendle 2007). The zombie is the abject body *par excellence.* Like the interior abject (as signified by menstruation and excrement), the perpetual threat of one's own transformation (the notion, as in the graphic novel and television series *The Walking Dead*, that everyone is always-already infected) means that its threat comes from within. Similarly, the zombie's association with the corpse marks it as an exterior site and source of the abject, as the initially familiar becomes unfamiliar and threatening through the breakdown of boundaries that serve to shape and manage the social order. The zombie renders immaterial the divisions between us and them, the living and the dead, the clean and the unclean, insides and outsides, the rational and the irrational, civility and incivility, and so on. Its corporeal dissolution expresses the dissolution of the body politic, and its emphasis upon horrifying ambiguity and conceptual boundary play marks the figure of the zombie as a rich expression of all manner of anxieties and ills, from terrorism, xenophobia and disease, to conformity, hyperconsumerism and social isolation. Situating the older, menopausal body as a figure of living decay, as both generative and tainted, marks the female body as an abject site that is always-already lacking in restraint, for the terror of the zombie is that it has always been with us, ready to be released. Stephanie Boluk and Wylie Lenz (2011) helpfully point out that it is not that the zombie encapsulates specific anxieties (such as nuclear war, or a racial other, or economic collapse), but that the zombie itself *is* metaphor, and that its "utility as metaphor is virtually without limit" (p. 9). Invoking the immense metaphysical potential of the living dead as a lens through which to parse the menopausal body reveals the boundaries that are writ and enforced through the expulsion of the abject. The shift from fecundity to infertility is a persistent 'threat' from within, for this is a threat to the phallocentric order that centralises reproduction as the use-value of the female subject, which attempts (but fails) to exclude the reality that the rhythmic transition between the states of reproductive capacity always-already shapes the reproductive body from menarche to menopause. Post-fertility and menstrual sex, as non-procreative forms of sex, is perhaps a form of zombie pleasure, but only in that it is abjected from the dominant social order. If we are to reclaim the notion of the (abject) barren, then one could argue that the body is always in a site of living decay, in that the conceptually dead and the rotting (that is, the expulsion of menstrual blood, as well as the sloughing and regeneration of skin, and hair, and so on) is the material from which new growth occurs.

Ageing women in cinema

I offer these sociocultural and biomedical constructions of ageing and menopause, alongside my earlier discussion of menarche and menstrual horror, as a way of connecting the abject barren body across various ages and embodied states. This is a helpful scaffold through which to consider patterns of representation, aesthetics and thematic expression in horror films that feature older or ageing women, or that focus on later life and bodily changes as spaces of trauma. Indeed, as Jane M. Ussher (2006) notes, it is no small irony that menstruation is labelled as a woman's 'curse', yet its eventual cessation is equally as demonised and results in women, still, being framed as abject, moody and mad, in a state of bodily and psychological disarray (p. 128) – the perfect territory for gynaehorrific narratives and expression. These representations must also consider and sit within broader issues of representation, so an exploration of the presence (or absence) of menopause and ageing in horror film requires a acknowledgement of broader patterns of cinematic representation of 'older' women. Here I use the term 'older' in a deliberately loose fashion, as the notion of what counts as 'older' shifts over time and can be considered less as bounded by a specific age range and more as a subjective category of 'older-than' that sits in opposition to youthfulness: older is *not-young*.

To put it crassly, female actors in mainstream American film (as well as other cultural forms such as television and theatre) have a much shorter 'shelf life' than their male counterparts. Loss of youthful normative femininity (and its implied sense of fecundity, sexual availability and reproductively) results in an expulsion from cultural space. It is not unusual for male actors in their 50s, 60s and 70s to be romantically paired up with women decades younger than they are, which emphasises the persistence of a type of masculine virility.[5] At the same time, female actors the same age as these male leads, if not significantly younger, are deemed unsuitable as romantic interests – 'too old' to be believable and, by implication, desirable to the audience (Child 2015). Instead, with the exception of a few high-profile actors such as Meryl Streep or Judi Dench, those female actors who do find roles from middle-age onwards are more likely to be cast as supporting, one-dimensional characters that fulfil unflattering stereotypes (Bazzini *et al.* 1997). Two quantitative studies demonstrate this well. In their content analysis of 100 top-grossing Hollywood films from 2002, Martha M. Lauzen and David M. Dosier (2005) demonstrate that older female characters are less likely to have defined goals than their older male counterparts, who outnumber them nearly three-to-one, and that the men are more likely to hold occupational power or be seen in leadership roles. They conclude that the "intermingling of age and worth consigns women over 40 to limited exposure and character roles" (p. 443). Similarly, Elizabeth W. Markson and Carol A. Taylor (2000) highlight how roles for older women centre on unflattering caricatures of old(er) age: spinsters, matrons and mothers, or other women who might continue to wield power within a family context, but rarely further. Their study of Academy Award winning actors aged 60 and over indicates that "the vast majority of older women in films project images of decline" (p. 156), as opposed to male representations, which reflect "the social fiction that, with a few exceptions, men can stay physically young despite their age, belying the notion of uselessness or power-less disability" (p. 155). Older women, then, are both abject and socially and culturally abjected.

This exclusion of older women in narrative film is a consistent and reductive mode representation that expresses itself in various aesthetic ways, including through films' formal and technical features. When older women *are* present, and present as sexual agents, their bodies, as sites of cultural dissonance, may be hidden or erased through editing and costuming. E. Ann Kaplan (2011) suggests in a study of May to December relationships in narrative drama film, the way that older women's bodies are exposed or hidden through costuming and strategic framing is clearly related to their perceived desirability, for instance through the occlusion of moments of intimacy. It is perhaps unsurprising to note that in such films older women's desire, eroticism and interest in pleasurable non-reproductive sex is presented as something transgressive and abject, especially when the sexual partner is a younger man. The constrictive notion of what it means to behave in an 'age-appropriate' manner is expressed in terms of clothing choice and sexual practice(s), as well as dialogue and narrative. More often, sartorial signification marks 'good' or benevolent older women as 'motherly' or 'grandmotherly' (Markson 2003, 83), be they dowdy or chic (Markson 2003, 88), as opposed to the implied grotesqueries of wicked or malign older women (Markson 2003, 89).

In the last two decades there has certainly been a slow shift upwards in terms of the age at which the female actor crosses the invisible and reductive line from attractiveness and desirability and into asexuality.[6] This can, perhaps, be connected to what gerontologist Merryn Gott (2005) has termed the stereotype of the 'sexy oldie': a construction that sits in opposition to the stereotype of asexual old age and decrepitude, but that implies that life-long sexual function, particularly in terms of expressing one's sexuality through sexual intercourse, is a key component of ageing healthily (pp. 23–4). In its own circular sense, this emphasis upon the necessity of sex is a way of staving off the negative associations of 'old age' through the performance of a certain type of 'ideal' (and youthful) active sexuality, given the numerous messages present within contemporary social and medical discourses that having sex may ward off 'old age' and help one retain one's physical and emotional health (pp. 25–7), that medical intervention is required to maintain 'ideal' sexual function (pp. 30–2), and that a youthful standard of beauty is a requirement for sexual attractiveness (pp. 32–4).

Despite these broader cultural shifts, though, which are certainly driven by the increased medicalisation of sex and an emphasis upon the individual-as-consumer (Gott 2005, 34–40; see also Vares *et al.* 2007), representations of older women in narrative film remain constrained, especially when compared to the roles made available to older men. Overall, the paucity and narrowness of roles available for the older female actor implies a narrative unworthiness that directly corresponds to older women's perceived lack of desirability, which is broadly associated within Western culture with idealised traits that include (hetero)sexual availability, normative attractiveness, the performance of a certain type of youthful femininity, and reproductive potential. When women and their bodies are no longer deemed fit to be subject of and subjected to the male gaze, they both literally and figuratively disappear from the screen.

Psychobiddies, *grande dames* and horrific harridans

From here I consider with much more specificity some of the key modes of representation of older women in horror film. The relative invisibility of older women in narrative film, which includes a denial of sensuality and an association of ageing with the grotesque, plays out in conservative ways in the sorts of Hollywood films discussed by Markson and Taylor (2000) and the arthouse fare considered by Kaplan (2011), but I suggest that the horror genre is not necessarily as ideologically complicit. Instead I posit that horror presents a complex and sometimes unsanctioned cultural space in which the abject perils and pleasures of ageing can be found and explored, albeit in specific subgenres and characters as opposed to more broadly within the genre. I also suggest that the negative sociocultural traits associated with menopause and ageing, and the biomedical construction of the ageing female body as deficient, are contested in horror films, even if menopause and the more specifically medical constructions of ageing are not as specifically present as other forms of medicalised forms of gynaehorror, such as pregnancies and reproductive technologies. Instead, horror films about abject barren bodies and subjects are manifold in their expressions and affects. They offer complex sites of inquiry that may certainly subjugate women and the feminine, but they are also cinematic spaces of celebration, resistance and contestation: through an embrace of the monstrous and effusive capacities of the abject barren, they refuse to acquiesce to the strictures of the normatively, reproductively feminine and the imperative that the female body must be in service of an-other.

A point of intersection between these mainstream representations and the horror genre is Billy Wilder's celebrated 1950 film *Sunset Boulevard*, a noir-ish comedy drama about a faded actress who was once a silent film star and the struggling writer who becomes her live-in companion as he tries to bash a terrible script she has written into shape. This film is, perhaps, the exemplar Hollywood text for stories about women ageing, but it is wryly subversive in its gothic visual language, its skewering of the narcissism and self-serving ambition facilitated by Hollywood, and its meta-commentary on the way that female actors are treated and mistreated by both audiences and their industry. The film is not within the horror genre, per se, but it is nonetheless ghoulish, almost gleefully so, and its atmospheric chiaroscuro aesthetic remarks upon the connections between film noir and expressionist horror films.

The film centres on the outrageously melodramatic and larger than life 50-year-old Norma Desmond, played with campy, hyperbolic relish by Gloria Swanson (herself a one-time silent movie star). Norma, once a celebrated film star, is abjectly, affectively excessive – by turns proud, vain, obsessive, pathetic, infantilised, delusional, powerful and suicidal. Now well past what would be considered her 'prime', and faced with the ignominy of being out of work (and thus, by the logic of Hollywood, invisible), she is a woman faced with and driven mad by her own obsolescence – something that is signalled even as the film opens, when we see a street sign for Sunset Boulevard not high up on a pole, but stencilled in the gutter. She is joined in her house by Joe, a slippery hack of a screenwriter who desperately needs work, and when he is hired by Norma to work on an unfinished screenplay and act as her companion, he sees an opportunity to take advantage of her wealth and connections. His cynical, hardboiled narration offers us a jaded and often cruel account of Norma that is exacerbated by the gothic nature of her place of residence. Her sprawling Sunset Boulevard mansion, hidden from the road, is in a state of decrepitude and disarray, and he initially mistakes it for deserted. Joe's disgusted commentary upon the nature of this domestic space is easily read as an analogy for his attitude towards Norma; that is, we are offered Joe's snide interpretation on Norma throughout, just as we are asked to bear in mind his sexism, ageism and self-serving nature.

The film turns on the tension between Norma's construction as a mythic, youthful, feminine figure on screen – an image that is sealed in time and played out fetishistically every night in her own private cinema – and the grim reality that within the Hollywood framework (and, more broadly, society itself) she is nothing more than an absurd spectacle, more worthy of pity than desire, all hyperbolic sentimentality and an embarrassment to the studio that once celebrated her. It is notable that one of the only people who offers Norma any sort of dignity is noted director Cecil B. DeMille, playing himself, who had acted as her director during her hey-day. His respect for her – which is shaped by the critical and financial success she helped bring the studio – sits alongside his discomfort at her erratic, histrionic behaviour and his sadness at the way the was treated by her fans and the press as she aged. He offers her a rare sympathetic hand in his acknowledgement of both her talent and her legacy, as well as the quiet knowledge that Hollywood is a place where he can remain active and successful in later age, even as Norma is side-lined, discarded and replaced by younger versions of herself who have a greater capacity for industrial and erotic (re)productivity. The film's emphasis upon fabrication and repetition – through the viewing and making of films, the nature of rewrites, the re-telling and mythification of history, and the proliferation of images of Norma from her heyday – further high-lights Hollywood as a dangerously liminal, hyperreal space of shimmering dreams and shifting, fickle desires rather than a physical place fixed in space and time.

It is Norma's self-delusion and her frequently abject performance of norma-tive female sexuality, and not just her age, that marks her as monstrous. Beyond her erratic and sometimes violent behaviour, and her ham-fisted attempts to seduce the much younger Joe, this is evidenced in the film's famous final moments. Norma shoots and kills Joe as he finally tries to leave her, and police and reporters gather to feast, vulture-like, on the sordid news. Norma admires her reflection in the mirror, certain now that stars are 'ageless', before announcing herself to the gathered reporters. Seemingly mad, preparing for her 'scene' and now ready for her 'close up', she advances down the sweeping staircase and creeps towards the camera, hands clawed, head titled back, staring straight down the barrel of the camera towards the spectator. She is a vampiric figure intent on sucking decades' worth of desire from the audience in the dark and, perhaps, punishing us for our expulsion of her as star-commodity and as desirous, desiring older woman. The sequence's framing, and the interplay between light and shadow, connect Norma-as-monster to both the titular vampire of the German film *Nosferatu* (1922) and Bela Lugosi's portrayal of the rakish vampire in *Dracula* (1931). Beyond its playful engagement with the aesthetics and register of horror, this sequence simulta-neously implicates the audience and their acceptance of Hollywood's impossible standards of worth and beauty in Norma's descent into madness and obso-lescence. She threatens monstrous becomings: she offers both contagion and occupation that enters into alliance with us through our affective response to the screen image. The abject-as-category is created and reinforced through its own expulsion, specifically creating (not reclaiming) order by identifying and expelling the disordered, and revealing that what we abject is in fact a detestable 'not-I' part of ourselves. Norma's monstrosity, then, is created and not inherent, for her abjection is an expression of our own fear and revulsion, and her refusal to go away confronts us with that which we have tried, and failed, to exclude.

Sunset Boulevard's sly, satirical rumination on the role of ageing women on screen can be found in Robert Aldrich's *What Ever Happened To Baby Jane?* (1962), a film that playfully combines the aesthetic and narrative languages of the family melodrama with those of the gothic horror – two genres that are, of course, deeply connected to the exploration and representation of women and transgressive femininity through a fascination with the abject female body. The film focuses on two ageing sisters who share a deep-seated hatred for one another; the sisters are portrayed by Bette Davis and Joan Crawford, whose bitter real-life rivalry certainly enriches the film's impact at an extra-textual level. Baby Jane Hudson (Davis) had achieved widespread fame as a cutesy-pie vaudeville child star in the 1930s, whereas her more moderate sister Blanche (Crawford) found success later in life as a 'serious' actor. Like Norma Desmond, both have left showbiz behind them, although Jane clings to memories of her childhood fame. As the film opens both women are in their 50s, and they live together in what can only be described as an exceptionally delicate and hostile equilibrium. Jane is increasingly mentally unstable and Blanche is confined to a wheelchair because of a car accident that we are led to believe was caused by Jane's drunkenness, although at the film's conclusion we learn that Blanche had crashed the car when she tried to run Jane over but has let Jane think, for decades, that she was responsible. When Blanche threatens to sell their family home Jane cuts her off from the outside world and begins systematically terrorising her. Amongst other cruelties, Jane stops feeding her – except to offer her the body of her pet parakeet – and eventually beats her unconscious when Jane finds that she's managed to get to a telephone. While the two have a lifelong enmity they are nonetheless violently, destructively bound to one another. They each express multiple categories of social exclusion (as older women, as disabled, as mentally ill), and in forming and being formed by each other through a mutual tracing, both contagion and alliance, they each become the other's favourite enemy (see Deleuze and Guattari 2004, 269).

Certainly, the film's escalating sadism, as presented in sharply expressionistic black and white, plays with the aesthetic of horror. Most notably, the film frames the pair – but especially Jane – as grotesque through a slippage between acceptability and abjection that Lorena Russell (2004) terms a "queer[ing of] normative female sexuality" (p. 214). This is most evident in the way that the increasingly unstable Jane continues to slather herself in thick, garish stage make up and to dress in cute, frilly frocks that recall those she wore as a child. Jane places an ad in the newspaper for a piano player, for (like Norma Desmond) she wishes to find a way to return to showbiz, and when he arrives she preens coquettishly and flirts ostentatiously with him, much to his obvious discomfort. While facing a mirror she performs "I've Written A Letter To Daddy" – the sentimental, schmaltzy song most associated with her childhood star persona – and this provides a transgressive juxtaposition between Jane's overt performance of youth (in particular a parody of a sort of libidinous yet girlish sexuality and a sense of incestuous over-familiarity), the constructed nature of her theatrical display, her ageing non-reproductive body and sexuality, and the bizarreness of her haggard, messy appearance. All these features, in their odd dissonance, challenge implicit understandings of what sort of sexual and desirous behaviour is considered to be 'age appropriate'. They refuse the strictures of social conventions regarding what older, post-reproductive female bodies should and shouldn't do, at the same time as highlighting the awful constructed-ness of normative female sexuality and the veneration of pre-sexual youth. This seriocomic presentation, the film's macabre humour, and the stars' hammy, overblown acting serve to mark *Baby Jane* as an outstanding example of camp horror (Russell 2004) – a style that is explicitly predicated on the deliberately theatrical and the inversion of categories of taste and value.

Beyond its own cultural status as an Oscar-winning film, *Baby Jane* is important because it sparked what has been variously termed the 'hagsploitation', '*Grande Dame Guignol*', or 'psycho-biddy' subgenre (Shelley 2009, 1). The subgenre spans from 1962 to roughly the mid-1970s, and includes titles such as *Die! Die! My Darling* (1965), *What's the Matter with Helen* (1972), and *Frightmare* (1975). Despite shifts in tone, aesthetic and content over time, these films are nonetheless united in the way that they feature older female actors playing mentally unstable or psychotic villains, vulnerable 'women in peril', and – in some cases – a slippery combination of the two (Shelley 2009, 8–9), in a manner that plays with the spectator's allegiances and sympathies let alone their expectations of normative, well-contained femininity. Hagsploitation films are overtly female-centric: they tend to highlight festering domestic female relationships, such as those between sisters, mothers, cousins, daughters, long-time friends, and women and their maids. The films combine the formal and narrative elements (and excesses) of the gothic melodrama with the raucous and visceral pleasures of cheap, sensational exploitation films, framing their explicit, sometimes gory violence in a manner that draws from the sort of expressionistic, noir-ish palate favoured by *Sunset Boulevard* and the bright, flat colours of some of the horror and exploitation films of the 1970s. Most importantly to this discussion, and as I will shortly outline, they offer exquisite examples of abject barren bodies, including a mode of horror that is predicated on the explicitly female or feminine yet refuses many of the structuring categories enforced upon the embodied female (post-)reproductive subject.

Two early examples continue to focus on the glorious scenery chewing of Davis and Crawford, and along with *What Ever Happened to Baby Jane* they solidify some of the codes and conventions of hagsploitation. *Hush, Hush... Sweet Charlotte* (1964), also directed by Aldrich, features Bette Davis as the titular Charlotte, a woman who has presided over her family's immense, rambling antebellum Louisiana mansion for decades – a particularly resonant example of cultural and historical abjection and the simultaneous Romanticised embrace yet rejection of certain parts of Southern history. Forty years earlier, the young Charlotte was to elope with her married lover, but instead he is warned away by her father and breaks off the engagement. Shortly afterwards he is decapitated and dismembered by a mysterious killer. Charlotte's discovery of her lover's body opens the film, and the widely-held suspicion that she was the vindictive murderer has hung over her ever since. Beyond this historic trauma the film centres on Charlotte's wicked cousin Miriam, who is trying to con Charlotte out of her house and her fortune. The house is now in the way of a new proposed highway, with technology and modernity threatening to bowl over the dreamy gothic grandeur of the house and the associated family history. To achieve her goals Miriam attempts to drive sweet, grieving Charlotte mad. This ongoing deception reaches its crescendo when Charlotte, drugged, comes across a staged murder scene, and her distorted experience and her grief is expressed through a shimmering five-minute hallucination scene during which Charlotte revisits the night of her lover's murder and re-experiences the giddiness of her past, albeit in a body that is now socially excluded. However, Charlotte is cannier than most give her credit for – her servant Velma sums up the entire genre well when she suggests that Charlotte is perfectly sane, but acts crazy because most people expect it of her – and once she uncovers her cousin's deception she gets her own back by dropping a massive concrete planter on the heads of Miriam and her lover. As in *Baby Jane* the house becomes an uncanny, sometimes threatening, and sometimes comforting force in its own right. The theatrical, expressionistic interplay of light and shadow, and Charlotte's movement in and out of darkness and through various registers of social and cultural categories, imbue the film with a sense of sorrow and dread that extends beyond the film's initial trauma to express a sense mournful nostalgia and a profound, haunted loss of both youth and love.

Like *Hush, Hush… Sweet Charlotte, Strait-Jacket* (1964) engages with the modern day implications of past trauma upon individual women and their family relationships. Lucy, played by Joan Crawford, has spent 20 years in an asylum for murder of her husband and his lover with an axe. Upon her release she is welcomed home by her doting daughter Carol, a sculptor who had witnessed the crime as a child and who seems to be remarkably well-balanced considering the trauma. However, Lucy is certainly not stable and she struggles anxiously with her transition back into the real world. Shortly after her release the murders resume, and the extent to which Lucy has control of her faculties is key to the film's unfolding. The film's strength, beyond its atmospheric chiaroscuro *mise-en-scène*, is Crawford's alarmingly swift gear-shifting between affective registers, from soft, empathetic, melodramatic actor to unhinged horror harridan. The abject, liminal and unsettling interplay between age and youth is central to the narrative, and also the horror: Lucy emerges from the asylum as a gentle, doddery, grey-haired spinster, but at her daughter's outright insistence she dons a wig and undergoes a makeover, resulting in a sartorial recreation of her 'former' self. Sexuality, again, is at the fore, and as with the abject presentation of Baby Jane's lust, Lucy makes outlandish advances on Carol's boyfriend. These overtures are framed as a grotesque indicator of her growing instability while also suggesting that these sexual passions could be just as easily connected to the murderous impulses that are driving the killer. The film's gory decapitations, the increasingly unsettling relationship between mother and daughter and a hasty denouement that best recalls that of an Agatha Christie plot all contribute towards the film's gothic-melodramatic and occasionally comic tone. During the film's climax Lucy grapples with the killer, who is wearing Lucy's clothes and a mask that resembles Lucy's face; fighting against this uncanny image of herself, Lucy rips the mask away to reveal her own daughter, juxtaposing and conflating her murderous past and her murderous progeny. As Carol (her murderous past-present) is taken away, Lucy's demeanour switches abruptly to something that better conforms to the social construction of the ideologically complicit older woman. She becomes soft, passive and empathetic as she voices, with regret, that it was her own actions that drove her daughter mad, and she leaves to go care for her, finally fulfilling the role of 'good', caring mother.

These generic patterns continue with other films too, although the visual and narrative modes slide further from the gothic and maternal melodrama and into the arena of schlock horror, shifting the protagonist from ailing, sympathetic victim and to gleeful, gurning bloodthirsty villain. Even later films, presented in colour, retain this sense of camp, gothic stylisation, and articulate multiple expressions and registers of the abject barren. *Whatever Happened to Aunt Alice?* (1969) is set in rural Arizona and makes much of the juxtaposition of the browns and greens of the desert and the cluttered, shadowy nouveau-riche house at the centre of the story. After the death of her seemingly wealthy but destitute husband a greedy, arrogant, murderous widow, Claire (44-year-old Geraldine Page), kills her maids for their meagre savings. She uses the holes dug to plant pine trees as graves in which to bury the unconscious women. This use of older female bodies as fertiliser results in an impressive garden. This tiny plantation is a site of productive organic materiality that offsets the barrenness and aridity of the surrounding desert, and plays upon the abject, ambiguous slippage between doomed living bodies and the alive-ness of the rotting, dissolute corpse, between the animate and the dead. The film centres on the game of cat-and-mouse between Claire and her new housekeeper, Alice (Ruth Gordon, then aged 72, who had won an Academy Award the previous year for her role of Minnie Castavet in *Rosemary's Baby* (1968)). We soon learn that Alice won the job under false pretences to find out what happened to her own much-loved previous house-keeper, Edna, who disappeared when she was working for Claire. They negotiate their relationships and attempt to outwit one another in a competitive expression of canniness and agency that belies dominant representations of older women: Alice suspects that her housekeeper died of foul play but suffers through the abuse of her employer; Claire distrusts Alice but wants access to her money; Alice's detective work and manipulations require significant manoeuvring and sleight of hand. Claire's paranoia and violent disposition sees her actions becoming increasingly unstable, and she finally murders Alice and dumps her body, inside a car, into a nearby lake. Believing that Alice has tipped off her neighbours, a woman and her young son, Claire drugs the two then attempts to burn their house down, but they are roused by their dog – which Claire had also tried to poison.

Issues of vanity, ageing and cruelty, each of which are coded in relation to affective expressions of femininity, underpin the differences between Alice and Claire. Claire is avaricious and vain and unwilling to surrender her opulent lifestyle, or even accept the facts of her destitution. She is a bully to her staff, whereas Alice's moderation and empathy is evidenced when she gives an impassioned speech about the level of respect and companionship she shared with her housekeeper Edna. The planting of bodies beneath the pines, and Claire's attempt to maintain a climate-inappropriate garden in the middle of the parched desert, signals Claire's refusal to accept her lot and age 'gracefully', at the same time as acting as a metaphor for the manner in which she feeds off of others. Beyond her abject, near-comic performance of gurning, overly-dramatic histrionics, and her increasingly dishevelled hair, Claire's villainy is emphasised through stylised framing. When she drops her pretence of civilisation she moves in and out of frame or is cast in thick darkness, and her audacious acts of violence, such as clubbing a housekeeper over the head with a spade, are filmed from a low angle and in harsh bands of light and shadow, adding to the film's heightened, theatrical monstrosity and liminality.

The fact that the actors involved in hagsploitation films were or had been A-list celebrities or highly regarded actors in their own right, like Davis and Crawford, means that such titles can be considered as exploitation flicks twice over. As lurid, often low-budget films that exploit niche interests – and perhaps, economically, the audience (Watson 1997, 76) – they fit the generic sense of the term. However, they are also films that perhaps exploit the actors themselves. The actors often play snarling, abject parodies of their former iconic feminine selves (Russell 2004, 219), so that the films implicitly ask the viewer to compare one with the other: the glamorous feminine past and the horrific present, in which art imitates a highly skewed and misogynistic presentation of life. Although this is certainly embedded into the narrative of *Sunset Boulevard*, in Norma's compulsive viewing of her own earlier films and her collection of images of herself, it is also a notable inclusion in Bette Davis and Joan Crawford's films above. A key prop in *What Ever Happened to Baby Jane?* is a life-sized doll of Jane as child star, a static pre-sexual yet erotically fetishised character figure that is in its own manner implicitly fictionalised, against which we are asked, impossibly, to judge the older Jane – and against which she can never compete. Footage from both women's earlier films stands in for footage from the films shot by their characters. Joan Crawford's Lucy, in *Strait-Jacket*, is forced to take on a much younger appearance by her daughter and re-create her 'old' self through clothes, make-up and a wig. Similarly, Carol has 'immortalised' her mother's younger visage in a sculpture so that her idealised mother may be young and beautiful forever; this is the image from which she casts the mother-mask she wears during her murders. Bette

Davis's Charlotte, in *Hush, Hush... Sweet Charlotte* dreams, through the haze of a drug-induced hallucination, of the night of her lover's murder. As her older self she walks through the hazy, youthful couples, but it's also notable that in the flashback that opens the film we never actually see the younger Charlotte's face, which is always obscured by a shadow, so our image of her previous self is one that we must fabricate. And yet, in each of these films old images of Davis and Crawford as much younger women, such as publicity stills and head-shots, appear in newspapers and framed photographs. The overall effect is quite uncanny in the sense that it is *unheimlich*, or unhomely, shaping the cinematic image of each woman as both familiar and unfamiliar. The women, then, are never too far from images of their younger selves, and are in a manner haunted as much by their previous cinematic and public incarnations as they are, narratively, by past crimes and family trauma. We are persistently reminded of the boundary from which the present-day failure to conform to normative ideals of vital femininity is expelled, but we are also reminded of the fictionalised, constructed, never-real nature of this deadened youthfulness.

The past and present, and the fictional and allegedly real, interact in other ways, too. These productive, sometimes dissonant encounters and alliances begin to express how the abject barren body is a productive, persistently-returning cultural category and not simply a mode of exclusion or cultural expulsion. During the lengthy opening credits of *Hush, Hush... Sweet Charlotte* Bette Davis, while ostensibly staring after some young boys who have been taunting her, looks directly into the camera, weeping. She clutches a music box that plays the song "Hush, Hush... Sweet Charlotte", a song written for the film that, in terms of the story, was written for Charlotte by her lover; the song went on to have its own success as a single. This two and a half minute long sequence is a mode of leaky, abject femininity that certainly conforms with the seeping affect of the maternal melodrama, but its protracted length, alongside a fade from a mid-shot to a close up of Davis's face, insists that the spectator endure it with Charlotte. This certainly creates a tone of yearning sadness and nostalgia that relates to Charlotte herself, alongside the glamour of the 'lost' South implied by her antebellum mansion. However, this takes on extra resonance and ambivalence if we are to consider, as with Norma Desmond's vampiric close-up in *Sunset Boulevard*, that this is also a mode of uncomfortable confrontation. This is an expression not of barren deficiency, but of overly productive, abject, saturated femininity. Our inclusion as spectators in a deeply personal yet alienating moment, and in a protracted encounter with leakage, is as related to the past of the actor as it is the past of the character, alongside our own implicit abjection of that which troubles the borders of normative femininity. This is a sequence that is simultaneously inviting, intimate, grotesque and alienating.

This expressive, challenging and ambiguous over-production of the affectively, abundantly feminine is a characteristic of hagsploitation, which overlaps the seemingly barren and excluded with outright excess. Those things that are safely contained within the strict constructions of a youthful feminine ideal instead overflow. *Whatever Happened to Aunt Alice?* ends with a close up long take of Geraldine Page, as Claire, weeping over her lost past and the destruction of her beautiful (albeit macabrely fertilised) garden, rendering her an object of pity, if not fleeting empathy, despite her nastiness throughout the film. This pattern continues in other hagsploitation films, too; consider the confronting emphasis upon the terrified face of *grande dame* and child-kidnapper Auntie Roo (Shelley Winters) as she burns to death at the hands of two orphans in *Whoever Slew Auntie Roo?* (1972), a film that plays with the story of Hansel and Gretel and that casts Roo as a sort of smothering, overbearing witch-figure. This final, immensely destructive conflagration emphasises Roo's pathetic nature and her desire to replace her dead daughter (whose corpse she still cares for in a hidden nursery), as opposed to her own unhinged and criminal actions, again delving into the ambiguous space between the living and the dead, the maternal and the barren. This sense of pathos is exacerbated by an earlier scene in which middle-aged, overweight Roo, like Baby Jane, insists upon performing – grotesquely – numbers from her past as a sexy showgirl for the group of orphaned children she has invited for Christmas dinner. These films must also be read intertextually, with a knowledge of both the actors' past work and personal lives shaping the over-signification of the film image. The image of Bette Davis descending a sweeping staircase in *Hush, Hush… Sweet Charlotte* can only recall her makeover from ugly duckling to glamorous swan in Irvine Rapper's 1942 melodrama, *Now Voyager*, just as Peter Shelley (2009) suggests that the inference that Charlotte has been seen in London mirrors Davis's own trip there to flee from the obligations of her contract with Warner Bros. (p. 62), for she objected to the roles that the studio was giving her (Springer 2015, 9).

These narratives are obviously heightened in terms of their emphasis upon camp, melodrama and sometimes gothic horror, yet they nonetheless set the tone for the broader representation of older women in horror, and they offer clear context within which more recent films can be situated. Certainly, there is the suggestion that where these films celebrate their leading ladies they also denigrate and ritually humiliate them, rendering them grotesque and pathetic, in a form of backlash against second wave feminism (Fisiak 2014, 42–4). However, I suggest that this perspective is, perhaps, a little reductive. Fringe, genre and exploitation films and counter-cinema have an enormous capacity to be sites of contestation and resistance (Mathijs and Mendik 2008, 8–10; Watson 1997, 66–7), given the way that they operate outside of, and some-times in opposition to, the rules of mainstream cinema, be they guidelines surrounding of narrative, aesthetic or even taste. Instead, I suggest that the conceptual spaces of gendered representation, alongside modes of genre, that are offered up within hagsploitation films present a richly complicated site of contestation and resistance, where apparently common sense rules of narra-tive, form and representation are bent and broken. This marks the abject barren body as a site of generation and an alternate mode of (re)productive femininity, rather than an end or a loss, and these modes of expression are an expansion of capacity in terms of the spaces created and restricted for women and femininity in cinema. For all the films' excesses, within hagsploitation titles women are given complex, demanding roles that are routinely denied to them by the mainstream, which rarely features older female characters. Instead, these horror narratives offer a great degree of freedom, and they present a violent renunciation of the societal imperative to be young, fecund, beautiful and docile – that is, to be bound by a particular mode of complicit reproductive femininity that serv(ic)es the production of male subjectivity. I suspect that within these films the rage against gendered double standards of worth and attractiveness is both contained and expressed, and I suggest that these films can be read as a self-conscious critique of the role of older women in film that, perhaps, has things both ways by both celebrating and denigrating its leads. These films offer a carnivalesque space in which to act 'inappropriately', but they also centralise the importance of women, their experiences, their fears and their relationships at the centre of the story. It is notable that similarly schlocky films about men don't juxtapose the past and the present, or youthful attractiveness with the social effects of ageing (and implied decrepitude), in such a manner.

Although the hagspoitation subgenre was relatively short-lived, some of the assumptions underpinning its mode of representation remain prominent. The negative stereotypes surrounding the ageing female body, including the emphasis upon loss and decrepitude in the cultural construction of the menopausal and post-menopausal body, continue to inform the sorts of representations of older women in horror, and from here I wish to indicate the way that expressions of abject barren femininity contest boundaries and are marked as violently excluded, even if the presence of these expressions signals an unwillingness to acquiesce to invisibility. The horror genre excels at challenging boundaries, be they the boundaries of bodies, aesthetics, taste or narrative acceptability, yet while hagsploitation roles offer a degree of expansive freedom within their own parameters, I suggest that representations of older women within the genre appear to remain relatively narratively constrained. Witch-like crones, such as gypsy woman Mrs Ganush in *Drag Me To Hell* (2009) or even the coven of witches in Dario Argento's *Suspiria* (1977) offer a wicked, withered presentation of feminine evil that sits in opposition to the fresh-faced, fecund youth of their victims. This is particularly pronounced in the latter film, given director Dario Argento's stylised use of a lurid colour palate inspired by Disney's 1937 film *Snow White and the Seven Dwarfs* (see Powell 2005, 142), which similarly places the naïve youth and innocence of Snow White against the envious predations of the older witch-queen, Snow White's stepmother. Monstrous mothers, such as some of those discussed in the previous chapter including *Grace*'s Vivian are defined by an unhealthy connection to their children or their own sort of perverse monstrosity; Mother in the Troma film *Mother's Day* (1980), Mother in the splattery comedy-horror *Braindead* (1992), and Norman Bates' Mother in *Psycho* do not even need names of their own, only designations. In religious horror *Legion* (2010), the elderly

Gladys seems to be present in the film only because the shock value of her monstrous possession rests upon its abject, dissonant contrast to her prior appearance as a sweet, stereotypical 'little old lady'. Women designated 'spinsters', such as Annie Wilkes in the Stephen King adaptation *Misery* (1990), are framed as disturbed women looking for fulfilment at any cost. Nana, in the darkly comic found footage film *The Visit* (2015), is certainly deranged and violent. Part of the film's wry humour – and the mounting horror for the two children at the centre of the film, who have never met their grandparents in person and so don't realise that the elderly couple they are staying with have killed and are impersonating their relatives – is that she and that man who appears to be her husband have escaped from a psychiatric residential facility; they are desperate to spend time with 'their' grandkids, even if the kids in question don't actually 'belong' to them, and the initially pleasant family visits ends violently. Each of these representations mark bodies that are socially and culturally abjected, as well as being abject in the sense of their own boundary confusion and transgressive femininity.

Monstrosity emerges alongside age-related disease by way of the overt presentation of the abject, older, ill female body in the found footage film *The Taking of Deborah Logan* (2014), and I highlight it as a rare recent example of a film that gives prominence to an older woman and issues of ageing. Its outright emphasis upon female relationships and the dissolution of the ageing body connects it to its hagsploitation forebears in a manner that is far more pronounced than other recent films, and I include it to signal the extent to which the core features of narratives about older women endure, even given shifts in genre and subgenre. The film begins as a group of documentarians chart an elderly woman's shocking decline due to a severe and rare form of Alzheimer's, and her adult daughter Sarah's increasing struggles to act as her caregiver and 'save' her, or at least protect her, from the worst excesses of her deterioration. The interplay between age, life-cycles, female relationships and horror is pronounced. At the beginning of the film the tone is affecting, almost poignant, in a manner that almost alludes to the maternal melodrama. However, as Deborah's actions become bizarre and veer towards the super-natural, the film transitions into a possession narrative – but one that focuses on the body of an elderly woman, as opposed to a pubescent one. Deborah has become possessed by the spirit of a local doctor who had been attempting to make himself immortal by sacrificing young women who had just experienced menarche, connecting their 'first blood' to his own quest for the renewal of life. The doctor's demonic activities are accompanied by snake imagery, which itself suggests both renewal, through the sloughing of skin, and the infinite and cyclical, through the image of the ouroboros, or the snake that eats its own tail. The climax of Deborah's possession narrative occurs when she absconds from hospital with a young female cancer patient and the documentary crew discover her, in a warren of underground tunnels, attempted to ingest the girl whole with her horrifically extended jaw, much as a snake would devour its prey. Her abject barren body becomes a site of extreme slippage, evading the boundaries between distinct, molar binaries such as old/young, animal/ human, open/closed and living/dead.

Arguably more horrific, and much more grounded in reality, is Deborah's precipitous decline into dementia. We see her 'well', to a relative degree, at the outset of the film, and we learn that the mother and daughter's acquiescence to the camera crew is so that the payment they will receive for the filming means that they won't lose the house. Conversely, we learn that Deborah sacrificed an immense amount to be able to raise her daughter, so the strength of their relationship is the measure against which the subsequent dissolution of their family unit can be judged. However, Deborah's physical and mental deterioration is pronounced. The association of literal possession with the figurative possession of mental incapacitation grounds the horror in a manner that highlights that one's ability to be cognisant is a way of staying 'alive' and that loss of self is a form of death. When we see Deborah's naked body it highlights her fragility and her instability, and not her sexuality, especially as it is juxtaposed against her image, at the beginning of the film, well-dressed and made up, in a performance of 'age-appropriate' femininity. Yet, Deborah's mental and emotional instability, and the shocking changes to her body, mark disease (and in this case, a disease explicitly associated with ageing) as its own form of monster, for as the movie continues it is almost impossible to tell which of the horrific effects are as a result of the disease, which are manifestations of possession, and which are intersections of the two.

The films I have discussed here – *Sunset Boulevard*, those of the hagsploitation subgenre, the films that leverage the grotesque monstrosity of the older woman, and the horror of disease-as-possession in *The Taking of Deborah Logan* – are connected by more than the age of their female actors. Most importantly, these stories are coloured by loss and longing. This might be for themselves, for a past that cannot return, and for the loss of agency and relationships. They may express a fear of ageing. They present alternatives to normative, idealised, youthful femininity as horrific. As such, these representations of monstrous, ageing femininity act as both threat and cautionary tale, for if women's core source of strength and power is youthful femininity (with its implied reproductive potential), then age qualifies as a palpable loss. The surge of power that is expressed through menarche and menstruation in menstrual horrors is perhaps lost, despite the early promise of renewal, but this loss is railed against – or, perhaps more transgressively, this power is re-routed into a space that is unaccounted for within the normative construction of the female subject, especially in her operation as the negative mirror through which the male subject constructs itself. As such, these films offer ambivalent representations of ageing, for they expose, quite explicitly, the sorts of negative stereotypes of the ageing women that are present in the social and cultural discourses that inform attitudes towards the physiological and psychological changes that accompany the cessation of menstruation. They revel in the degradation of the female body, and in the dissolution of both actor and character. And yet, they offer a space of significant resistance, and a way of interrogating the fictions that underpin value-driven constructions of feminine worth by revealing the nature of the boundaries that are created and enforced through the act of abjection.

With the exception of 2014's *The Taking if Deborah Logan*, the films discussed in depth in this chapter pre-date significant shifts in the digital production and distribution of horror films. The relative accessibility of digital film and editing technology, the development and proliferation of video-on-demand platforms (to the detriment of DVD and BluRay sales) and other forms of distribution, the ability to produce films on a microbudget or crowdsource funding, and the popularity of low-budget independent horror films in Hollywood itself mean that larger numbers of horror films are made, distributed and seen every year (see Conrich 2009, 2; Lobato and Ryan 2011). Beyond the fact that small-scale and underground horror titles have always had a passionate audience, and the genre itself a sort of DIY auteurism (see Badley 2009), even the smallest of releases have the potential to be supported and promoted by a passionate online community of horror fans, giving these titles a 'bump' perhaps denied to other genres. Hypothetically, at least, this removes some barriers to the creation of more diverse and incredibly niche horror films, such as the aborted foetus slasher *Red Christmas* (2016), which is discussed in Chapter Three. And yet, despite these shifts, and despite my earlier indication that horror is nothing if not diverse in its sites of horror, there remains a dearth of older women in horror – an overall lack of *grande dames*, grannies run amok, and menopausal harridans. If we consider trends within the production of horror films not as a reflection of some social reality or the desires of the audience-consumer, nor even as a form of representational art, but instead as commodities that are deeply embedded within industrial and economic contexts such as production and distribution (Lobato and Ryan 2011, 191–2), then this points to broader ideological reasons for this absence. I suggest, instead, that this absence is not remarked upon or addressed because it is not noticed; that is, the seeming irrelevance of older women in horror is a by-product of the cultural abjection of older women and of female bodies that no longer express or connote fecundity in a culturally sanctioned manner. These abject barren bodies, while perhaps excluded in this particular iteration, are nonetheless ever-present elsewhere: they are a conceptual and affective extension and a part of every other expression of barrenness or infertility, and thus are another register of a non-normative mode of unfecund femininity that is unable to be fully expelled.

The ageing woman as (American) horror story

In light of the broader absence on women in horror, I finish by suggesting that some of the most interesting and nuanced representations of older women in horror can be found not in film but in television. This is most apparent in *American Horror Story* (2011–present, hereafter *AHS*), an anthology series that offers a different story every season, each set at a different time and in a different archetypal site of horror: a haunted mansion with a history of violent murders in present day Los Angeles; an asylum in 1960s Massachusetts; a coven in present day New Orleans; a travelling freak show in 1950s Florida; a haunted hotel in present day Los Angeles; and the site of the missing 16th-century Roanoke colony in present day North Carolina. The first season, which is set in a so-called 'murder house' that at was once an illicit abortion clinic, is particularly fixated upon issues of gender, sexuality, reproduction, abortion, sexual violence, infidelity, and the relationship between mothers and children, alongside numerous gothic "sexualised hauntings" that trouble the intersections of class, gender, sex and the home (Taylor 2012, 139). Indeed, the first present-day scene in the first episode, "Pilot", features middle-aged Vivian Harmon (Connie Britton) undergoing a gynaecological examination as she discusses menstruation, hormone replacement therapy and her recent miscarriage with a fertility specialist; he impresses upon her the importance of ensuring that her 'house' (her reproductive body) has sound foundations – that is, that it is healthy and appropriately fertile before any treatment, or 'work', starts. These deeply gendered and often female-centric concerns continue throughout the series in various forms, and are perhaps offered more purchase in this serialised form, as opposed to the form of the standalone film, given the show's frequent nods to the narrative and characters excesses of the soap opera. I acknowledge that there are significant formal differences between film and television, but in this instance *American Horror Story* lends itself well to a comparative analysis. It is deeply invested in the history of cinematic modes of deeply gendered horror, and it playfully situates itself, quite obviously, within the same narrative, thematic and aesthetic spaces as cinematic (gynae)horror.

Like other shows by series creators Brad Falchuck and Ryan Murphy, including *Nip/Tuck* (2003–2010), *Glee* (2009–2015), and the comedy horror *Scream Queens* (2015–),[7] *AHS* demonstrates an explicitly camp and queer sensibility, particularly in the manner that it explores issues of sex, gender, taste, identity and the capacities of abject and transgressive bodies. The series also has an effusive attitude towards horror tropes that can be loosely (and cheekily) described as 'throw it all at the wall and see what sticks'. The second season alone includes (but is not limited to) serial killers, alien abductions, wicked nuns, demonic possessions, mutants, a Nazi doctor, racial hate crimes, a rapist in a Santa suit, lobotomies, the forced institutionalisation of a lesbian journalist, and a psychosis-induced musical dream sequence. This madcap semiotic tsunami faces supernatural horrors off against entirely human ones, alternating between outright nastiness and a tongue-in-cheek sense of humour, all of which begs the question as to whether or not it is the inhumanity of people or the bizarre supernatural occurences that are more horrific.

As with film, older women have been consistently underrepresented in American primetime television (Signorelli 2004).[8] Contrary to this broader trend, though, *AHS* offers varied, nuanced and often outlandishly scenery-chewing roles in its large, ensemble casts for a broad variety of women and female-identifying actors. These include critically-acclaimed actors in their 50s and 60s such as Kathy Bates, Frances Conroy and Angela Bassett, whose significant cultural capital adds a degree of heft to the show. The anthologised nature of the show's seasons gives these actors an opportunity, as with their younger female counterparts, to demonstrate range and breadth; for instance, across different seasons Kathy Bates appears as a 19th-century creole socialite and blood-thirsty slave-killer, as a headstrong, earnest and well-respected bearded lady from Baltimore, and as a hotel manager who goes to extreme lengths to feed and tend to the evil that lives there. Angela Bassett appears as Voodoo Queen Marie LeVeau, as a three-breasted intersex freak show performer, and as a glamorous Blaxploitation actress who becomes a vampire. In season six, both women play actors who perform in a televised re-enactment of a violent, real-life haunting, further blurring the registers of representation. These expansive roles express a diversity of embodied female subject positions, and a range of affective capacities, that don't appear on an industrial level, on the surface at least, to be meaningfully available anywhere else, and certainly not for more than one *grande dame* at a time.

Of particular note is the show's repeat headline casting of American actor Jessica Lange throughout the first four seasons. The show celebrates Lange, who came to prominence for her role as the often scantily clad victim-heroine in 1976's *King Kong* and who as of writing is in her mid-60s, as equal parts queer icon, sex symbol and celebrated *grande dame* of prestige television. Each of Lange's storylines draw from the themes, narratives and aethetics of hagsploitation and play with the registers of the abject barren body. They emphasise loss, longing and diverse, intense relationships (and rivalries) between women. They explore, in minute detail, the cruelty that each of her characters have experienced as they have aged, both in terms of their personal lives and more broadly within a society that marks them as increasingly irrelevant and unworthy of status because of their age. They embrace theatricality and fantasy, often drawing from both the heightened, expressionistic visual language of the gothic melodrama, the fantastic excesses of the musical, and the lurid aesthetics of the exploitation film. Importantly, these themes act as blood and marrow to each season. They are never sidelined as less worthy than the concerns and affairs of younger characters, and perhaps indicate that televisual, rather than cinematic space might better facilitate nuanced and diverse expressions of gynaehorror that spread across an entire female lifetime.[9]

Lange's characters express the broad, generative complexity of the abject barren. They are complex, strong-willed and tragic figures who are willing to do terrible things to advance their own interests. Season one's Constance Langdon (*AHS: Murder House*) is a vindictive and self-interested woman whose one-time ambitions to be a Hollywood star were thwarted firstly by her unwillingness to appear naked, secondly by motherhood, and later by outright tragedy. Constance is obsessed with her looks and her social status, and this fixation is exacerbated by her loneliness. Over the course of the season she takes on a role in facilitating a supernatural pregnancy, much like meddling neighbour Minnie Castavet in *Rosemary's Baby.* In season two (*AHS: Asylum*), Lange plays the stern Sister Jude – named for St Jude, that patron saint of lost causes – a strict disciplinarian who displays abject cruelty towards her charges in the asylum she oversees. Her hard line against perceived sinfulness is problematised by her secret history as a promiscuous, alcoholic nightclub singer, her ongoing conflict about her own lustful passions and her anger at the misogyny of the both the church and the world at large. Despite her transgressions and her initial role as a villain, she is offered a positive resolution to her story arc that emphasises compassion and companionship over vindictive punishment. Season four (*AHS: Freak Show*) casts Lange as ageing German singer Elsa Mars, a one-time rival of Marlene Dietrich who now runs a failing travelling freak show that, like Elsa herself, is a relic of a former time. Elsa is herself a secret freak – she had her lower legs violently removed and now wears cunning prostheses – and in her vanity and her obsession with fame and glamour she fearfully tries to present herself as 'normal', often at the expense of the freaks she has promised to care for. Elsa's increasingly grotesque appearance is emphasised during the season's shimmering, sometimes hallucinatory musical numbers, including Elsa's anachronistic performances of David Bowie songs. Her renditions combine the eroticism of Bowie's glam rock personae and Dietrich's gender-bending sensuality, but her haggard, thick stage make-up, and her yearning pathos, directly references the abject decline of Baby Jane Hudson. Like Norma Desmond in *Sunset Boulevard* she desperately tries to remake herself as a star, but like Norma, she is firmly rejected by the system that once supported her.

Lange's storyline in season three, *AHS: Coven,* is the most explicit interrogation of the social and cultural implications of female ageing in an environment where the most powerful woman – the Supreme witch of a coven – is quite literally drained of her life and immense powers. These powers are then transferred to a younger witch as a part of the coven's natural regeneration in a process that is like a spiritual menarche, situating the interplay between barrenness and fecundity as one of many blocks of becoming that are manifest in the broader rhythmic expression of the reproductive. Fiona Goode is the Supreme of the Salem Coven, which is now based out of a girls' school, Miss Robichaux's Academy for Exceptional Young Ladies, in modern day New Orleans. Now in her 60s and horrified at her impending demise, she resorts to extreme measures, including murdering younger witches, in an attempt to retain her status – a status that conflates youth, beauty and desirability with raw power.[10] In the season's opening episode ("Bitchcraft") Fiona – chic, wealthy and elegant, prone to self-indulgence and boozy, drug-fuelled hard living – visits a young scientist she has been funding in an attempt to obtain a serum, only tested on monkeys, which will reverse the deep-set effects of ageing such as organ failure. When the serum fails to work on her immediately, and he tells her that as organic matter we must all rot and die, she seduces him, straddling and kissing him, before quite literally draining the life-force from him. Even this brief injection of vitality doesn't last. As she admires herself in the mirror her skin visibly wrinkles and sags. Later, in a fit of rage and disgust, she smashes the mirrors around her, refusing the visual evidence of her own ambiguous yet dynamic corporeality.

Fiona's furious refusal to accept her fate is bound up with her immense vanity, her taste for drink and drugs, and her inability to consider an existence without the sort of beauty and influence she has curated and leveraged throughout her life. The overlay of her decline and her belligerent performance of youth evokes the sense of zombified sexual subjectivity, or living decay, I refer to earlier. She acts as a crystalline, gynaehorrific and liminal articulation of the toxic veneration of normative female sexuality, although this subject position offers her a lascivious power over those around her that connects her own desirousness and self-serving eroticism to that of the rapacious *vagina dentata*. Over the course of the season her unwillingness to pass on her immense powers to another, and her violent, murderous attempts to avoid the inevitable become increasingly tragic and desperate. In her self-service she refutes the reality that she is not alone, but one of many, and this collection – this coven – form their own empowered feminine ecosystem that exists to serve, and protect, itself from the predations of the outside world; compare this transgressive veneration of female community to the ending of *The Witch*. In the season finale ("The Seven Wonders"), Fiona is shrunken, wizened and nearly hairless, resembling an elderly cancer patient in the end stage of their disease, and she spitefully tells her now all-powerful daughter, the new Supreme, that her very existence (and, perhaps, the living evidence of her own reproductive use-value) has always been a reminder of Fiona's own mortality. The moments before her death are deeply uncomfortable, and like *The Taking of Deborah Logan* connect age-related disease with monstrosity. Given the presence of a diverse range of other older witches, it is emphasised that Fiona's 'ugliness' comes from her selfishness and her inherent cruelty, not from the effects of age. Her life-long unwillingness to firstly lead the coven responsibly and, secondly, to step down 'gracefully', in lieu of indulging herself, is intertwined with her own attempts to retain what she sees as the connection between normative attractiveness, youth and power. She cannot accept, as her daughter puts it, that she is just a woman capable of human feeling, rather than an immortal divine being – a statement that, perhaps, acts as a broader commentary on the immortalisation of women on screen, and the nature of consumption itself.

I suggest that it is here that *AHS* offers a helpful, even provocative site of inquiry regarding the presence (or absence) of horror films that deal with menopause – or, more to the point, the sorts of attitudes towards women and ageing that inform the gendered pathologisation of ageing and also, indirectly, the relative absence of women from the screen. On one hand, the show's repeat casting of Lange, and the concerns outlined above that are addressed within her storylines and by her characters, act as explicit interventions with deeply problematic value judgements that surround older women's bodies, identities and sexualities. However, this discursive construction of the ageing female body is complicated within *AHS*. In *What Ever Happened to Baby*

Jane and other hagsploitation films, we are asked implicitly to marvel and perhaps cringe at the shift – that is, the *decline* – from the actor's youthful elegance and curated beauty to the presentation of the actor as a ghastly, camp, witch-like figure. We are invited, implicitly, to experience disgust and participate in their cultural expulsion. This trajectory crystallises women's cinematic (and societal) value as objects to-be-looked-upon, instead of as agents with sexual desires and lives of their own. Within *AHS,* we certainly bear witness to the abject deterioration of Lange's various characters – in some cases to shocking effect. *AHS* positions itself as a queer, anarchic exploration of all manner of sites of archetypal American horror, and one of those sites, quite clearly, is the body of the older woman. This is not just horror and the ageing body, but the horror *of* the ageing body and the abject barren: an exploration of the effects of a misogynistic representation of women that elevates youthfulness, fecundity and sexual availability, suggesting that only by fulfilling these criteria might individual worth be found or mined.

And yet, unlike some of the *grande dames* of earlier hagsploitation films, there is a disjuncture between these on-screen grotesqueries and Lange's off-screen presentation and celebrity persona. The characters played by Joan Crawford and Bette Davis in films such as *Hush, Hush… Sweet Charlotte, Strait-Jacket* and *What Ever Happened to Baby Jane* are compared, generally unfavourably, to images of the actors' past selves. 'Real life' promotional pictures, film stills and head shots are placed strategically throughout the world of the film, serving as evidence of a glamorous past that no longer correlates to the body of the present, and marking a dissonant slippage between the diegetic and the extradiegetic that marks the female body as always-already socially and corporeally abject, and always on the precipice of decline. In comparison, throughout these first four seasons of *American Horror Story*, we are also asked to compare Lange's own glamorous past with her equally glamorous present, be it on-screen, through the show's promotional material, or in her appearances at awards shows and fan conventions; that is, in terms sexuality and commodity, of intertextuality and history (Dyer 2004, 2–3), Lange is, perhaps, a star in the *present*, not a star of the past. Further, Lange is consistently, explicitly presented to the viewer as unapologetically erotic and sexually active. Even within the context of the emergence of more positive media images and accounts of sexuality and ageing – the figure of the aforementioned 'sexy oldie' (Gott 2005) with its emphasis upon sexual activity and a performance of youthfulness as a part of 'healthy' ageing – Lange's roles are remarkable in their depth and their sensual frankness, let alone the way that they juxtapose the abject with the erotic. Many of Lange's characters are forthright and sensual. They seek out – and find, often easily – sexual pleasure and sexual partners, although how this need plays out depends on the specificities of the season and the character. This re-centres sexuality and pleasure within the space of the conceptually barren.

Most radical and transgressive – in the context of a media environment that usually serves to cover up older women's bodies (Kaplan 2011; Markson

2003) – is the fact that we often see Lange in various stages of undress, or mid- and post-coitus. Her figure is not abjected or otherwise occluded. These are certainly not scenes that are framed in a manner that serves to denigrate her body or present her sexuality as grotesque or inappropriate. Consider the opening episode of *AHS: Asylum* ("Welcome to Briarcliff"), during which Sister Jude prepares to have dinner with her Monsignor, who she secretly lusts after. Interspersed with swiftly edited, frenetic shots of her preparing coq au vin, chopping onions and splashing red wine, we see her dressing herself in anticipation of her meeting. She stands in her room, her nun's coif and veil offset by her slinky red negligee, and she slowly dots herself with perfume and caresses her chest. This scene, which is accompanied by yearning choral music, is strikingly similar in its sense of private pleasurable reverie to that of Carrie washing herself in the shower, especially in its languid tempo. During the dinner Sister Jude fantasises about removing her habit to reveal her red underwear and seamed stockings, shaking out her hair, and straddling the Monsignor – a fantasy that is however swiftly disabused. Her largely suppressed sensual other half, which we later learn relates to her pre-Order career as an alcoholic nightclub singer, offers a powerful juxtaposition throughout the series in its evocation of suppressed desires and its playful engagement with the virgin/whore dichotomy. In the case of season three, *AHS: Coven*, we see as much of Fiona Goode's sex life, if not more, than that of the much younger characters, including the intimacies of her ongoing affair with the ghost of a murderous jazz musician. Throughout the series there is no 'convenient' fade to black, but instead a distinct, unapologetic emphasis upon the sexuality and desires of a sexual and desirous body. Indeed, Jessica Lange is framed through her four seasons not just as attractive but as, specifically, the deserving object of the audience's objectifying, voyeuristic gaze. She gazes back confrontationally, too, as both a queer icon and as a sex symbol who challenges assumptions about female worth and the veneration of the younger body, embracing the slippage and ambiguity that usually marks older bodies to be cast out.

I suggest, then, that *American Horror Story* offers a significant shift in the representation of older women in horror, let alone on screen in general. Throughout this chapter I have asked what it is that horror films about menopause might look like, and I offer that *AHS* gives us something of an answer, for although menopause itself is not a topic per se, the show engages with what we might think of as menopause and the abject barren in a conceptual or thematic sense. By this, I mean that *AHS* interrogates the highly negative social, sexual and cultural myths and discourses that inform Western understandings of the physical and emotional changes that women might undergo as they get older, which reach their institutionalised apotheosis in the biomedical model of menopause-as-disease. Beyond its ongoing exploration (and exploitation) of all manner of archetypal, supernatural and entirely human horrors, *AHS* actively explores the impacts of the marginalisation of the experiences of older women. It highlights the ways that women might be allowed or denied social, cultural and sexual agency. It plumbs some of the awful depths of the discursive construction of female ageing, which marks the older woman's body as unfeminine, unruly, leaky and in need of medical intervention. It simultaneously challenges women's relative invisibility: it offers a range of diverse, nuanced roles for women, including celebrated roles for women in middle-age and beyond, and it centralises and celebrates the subjective experiences of older female characters. It dances with the narrative and aesthetic concerns of hagsploitation, but does not limit itself to its modes of representation, nor does it insist upon the sadistic, even ritualised denigration of its older female leads. It embraces, even exposes, that which is ordinarily abjected, and it situates the older body not as the other to the younger, reproductive body, but as an alternate expression of embodied female subjectivity that is not less-than nor other-to.

This is not to say, though, that this is straightforward, nor unproblematic. *AHS* offers a transgressive and, perhaps, progressive alternative representation of older women onscreen, but this representation in some cases remains planted within broader constraints. It is significant that some of these challenges to normative standards of youth-as-beauty, as evidenced in the centralisation of Jessica Lange's characters and storylines, sit within narrow aesthetic parameters. Lange herself is white, elegant, slender and conventionally attractive. She brings to her current roles, including her presentation in the media, a continuation of her bombshell past to her glamorous present in a manner that, perhaps, serves to maintain the smooth mask of femininity. Her performance of abject grotesquery sits in contrast to what the viewer knows to be her 'real' appearance. Importantly, this challenge occurs within an already ambivalent, niche space, for the horror genre and the show's camp, often queer mode of representation both trade upon and encourage a playful blurring of boundaries that highlights rather than excludes the abject. Might this sexualisation have occurred within a more 'mainstream' text, or with one of the older female actors of *AHS* who conform less to normative standards of beauty?

Nonetheless, perhaps horror is, if anything, the ideal site through which to interrogate and expand the representation of older women. As a genre that is largely deemed to be transgressive and Other, abject and expansive, it offers already potentially marginalised older female actors a degree of freedom that is arguably not available elsewhere, as well as roles of great power and expressive magnitude. Horror's psychobiddies, *grande dames* and harridans certainly articulate, with melodramatic and gothic theatricality, some of the worst, most conservative attitudes towards women and ageing, especially as they sit in seeming opposition to the explosion of power that is associated with menarche. And yet, from a radical perspective, these gynaehorrific performances also serve to highlight how implicitly constructed the categories of normative femininity, youth, beauty and female worth are. They also expose that there are many forms of power. In their refusal to act 'appropriately', and adequately shrink back into a culturally sanctioned docility, abject barren bodies demand to be seen and heard.

Notes

1 Portions of this chapter were first published in Peer Reviewed Proceedings: 6th Annual Conference, Popular Culture Australia, Asia and New Zealand (PopCAANZ), Wellington 29 June–1 July, 2015, pp. 54–62.

2 Significantly, re-usable and more environmentally-friendly menstrual products, such as menstrual cups, are sometimes framed as dirty and messy (see Stewart, Greer and Powell 2009), perhaps because the individual must address the lost blood through emptying and cleaning the cup; similarly, modern reusable cloth pads suffer from an association with a lack of hygiene. That said, reusable and alternative menstrual products are an important part of third-wave feminist menstrual activism, also known as anti-tampon activism, menstrual anarchy or (delightfully) menarchy (Bobel 2006).

3 In her introduction to *The Curse: Confronting the Last Unmentionable Taboo: Menstruation* (2000), which offers a cultural history of menstruation, 'menstrual etiquette', and the messages sold by the sanitary protection industry, Karen Houppert writes, "Blood is kinda like snot. How come it's not treated that way?" (p. 4)

4 The specific visual presentation of this inciting incident is echoed in two later adaptations and remakes of the film, which are perhaps, to a degree, bound by the power, the impact, and the visual language of the original film. In the 2002 remake of *Carrie* she is inside a cubicle, as opposed to an open communal shower, but her sudden menses appears like a river of blood that washes towards a neighbouring girl; the cubicle is an oppressive containment, and Carrie's jeering, baying classmates bang the walls and peer in on her as if she is an animal. In this remake, as with the 2013 version of *Carrie*, the camera lingers voyeuristically on individual parts of Carrie's body. The casting has a further impact: Sissy Spacek's transformation from odd, scrawny, bug-eyed loner to smiling prom queen in the 1976 original plays with then brutally undermines the 'ugly duckling' trope. The same is true, but to a lesser extent, with the casting of Angela Bettis in 2002, who likewise evokes a sense of intensity and awkwardness. The casting of blonde, normatively attractive Chloë Grace Moretz in the 2013 film marks Carrie as a more traditional object of desire from the outset, which perhaps renders her presentation at the beginning of the film as an erotic object, and her transformation into a prom queen, as less complex that the previous films.

5 Kyle Buchanan's article for pop culture website Vulture, "Leading Men Age, But Their Love Interests Don't" (2013), highlights this well in its use of a series of graphs that demonstrate the often pronounced age difference between A-list Hollywood actors (including Denzel Washington, Harrison Ford and Tom Cruise) and their on-screen love interests over time.

6 A segment from the American sketch comedy show *Inside Amy Schumer*, which went viral after its release online, highlights this beautifully. In a sketch from the episode "Last F…able Day" (2015), Schumer comes across celebrated, normatively attractive middle-aged actors Tina Fey, Patricia Arquette and Julia Louis-Dreyfuss having a tea party in the woods, where they are celebrating 54-year-old Louis-Dreyfuss's 'last fuckable day', the event horizon after which female actors aren't considered to be believably 'fuckable'. While the women remark that this signals a shift in their career trajectory that desexualises, stereotypes and side-lines them, and that Louis-Dreyfuss has had a surprisingly good run, the payoff is that they are thrilled that they no longer have to spend excessive amounts of time, energy and money maintaining a degree of normative attractiveness, and can instead guzzle ice-cream, belch, fart and wear their comfy clothes. Men, in contrast, are 'fuckable' forever.

7 *Scream Queens*, which celebrates the slasher genre, makes good use of the intertextual casting of older women, in particular through its use of 1970s and 1980s

scream queen Jamie Lee Curtis in the role of the dean of a college at which a sorority is being terrorised by a serial killer. This self-reflexivity continues throughout the show and reaches its apotheosis during a black and white shot-for-shot recreation of the shower scene from *Psycho*, with Curtis taking the place of her mother, Janet Leigh, who played Marion Crane in the 1960 film. In this latter version, Curtis's character prevails, fighting off not one but three attackers.

8 Outside of terrestrial and cable television this is shifting somewhat; for example, the recent, celebrated Netflix comedy-drama series *Grace and Frankie* (2015–) stars Lily Tomlin and Jane Fonda, both of whom are in their 70s.

9 It is significant that Lange's performances across multiple seasons of *AHS* have garnered extensive critical acclaim, including nominations and awards from the Golden Globe Awards, the Critics' Choice Television Awards, the Primetime Emmy Awards, and the Screen Actors' Guild Awards. This indicates broad-spectrum, mainstream appeal, alongside more niche recognition, as from the Dorian Awards, which are awarded by the Gay and Lesbian Entertainment Critics Association, and the Saturn Awards, which are presented by the Academy of Science Fiction, Fantasy & Horror Films.

10 In the context of the juxtaposition between menopause and menarche, it is significant that the personal power of one of the youngest of the witches is explicitly associated with 'first' blood. Teenager Zoe, one of our key point-of-view characters, is sent to Miss Robichaux's Academy after her power first manifests itself in a particularly gruesome fashion: when she has penetrative sex with her boyfriend for the first time she causes him to haemorrhage violently, killing him. She later uses this 'black widow' power to get revenge on a college student who had stupefied and raped another one of the younger witches.

Bibliography

Badley, L 2009, 'Bringing it all back home: horror cinema and video culture', in I Conrich (ed), *Horror Zone: the Cultural Experience of Contemporary Horror Cinema*, London: I.B. Tauris & Co., pp. 45–64, accessed February 17, 2014, from <http://public.eblib.com/EBLPublic/PublicView.do?ptiID=676670>.

Bazzini, D G, McIntosh, W D, Smith, S M, Cook, S & Harris, C 1997, 'The aging woman in popular film: underrepresented, unattractive, unfriendly, and unintelligent', *Sex Roles*, 36(7–8), pp. 531–543.

Beral, V & Million Women Study Collaborators 2003, 'Breast cancer and hormone-replacement therapy in the Million Women Study', *The Lancet*, 362(9382), pp. 419–427.

Bishop, K W 2010, *American zombie gothic: the rise and fall (and rise) of the walking dead in popular culture*, Jefferson NC: McFarland & Co., accessed December 17, 2016, from <http://public.eblib.com/choice/publicfullrecord.aspx?p=1594824>.

Bobel, C 2006, '"Our revolution has style": contemporary menstrual product activists "doing feminism" in the Third Wave', *Sex Roles*, 54(5–6), pp. 331–345.

Bobel, C 2010, *New blood: third-wave feminism and the politics of menstruation*, New Bruswick, NJ: Rutgers University Press.

Boluk, S & Lenz, W (eds) 2011, 'Introduction: Generation Z, the age of apocalypse', in *Generation zombie: essays on the living dead in modern culture*, Jefferson, NC: McFarland, pp. 1–17.

Braidotti, R 2002, *Metamorphoses: towards a materialist theory of becoming*, Cambridge, UK and Malden, MA: Polity Press in association with Blackwell Publishers.

Briefel, A 2005, 'Monster pains: masochism, menstruation, and identification in the horror film', *Film Quarterly*, 58(3), pp. 16–27.

Buchanan, K 2013, 'Leading men age, but their love interests don't', *Vulture*, accessed September 12, 2016, from <http://www.vulture.com/2013/04/leading-men-age-but-their-love-interests-dont.html>.

Buckley, T & Gottlieb, A 1988, 'A critical appraisal of theories of menstrual symbolism', in T Buckley & A Gottlieb (eds), *Blood magic: the anthropology of menstruation*, Berkeley, CA: University of California Press, pp. 1–50.

Child, B 2015, 'Maggie Gyllenhaal: at 37 I was "too old" for role opposite 55-year-old man', *The Guardian*, accessed July 27, 2015, from <http://www.theguardian.com/film/2015/may/21/maggie-gyllenhaal-too-old-hollywood>.

Comentale, E P & Jaffe, A 2014, 'Introduction: The Zombie Research Centre FAQ', in E P Comentale & A Jaffe (eds), *The year's work at the Zombie Research Center*, The year's work: studies in fan culture and cultural theory, Bloomington, IN: Indiana University Press, pp. 1–58.

Conrich, I 2009, 'Introduction', in I Conrich (ed), *Horror zone: the cultural experience of contemporary horror cinema*, London: I.B. Tauris & Co., pp. 1–8, accessed February 17, 2014, from <http://public.eblib.com/EBLPublic/PublicView.do?ptiID=676670>.

Creed, B 1993, *The monstrous-feminine: film, feminism, psychoanalysis*, London and New York: Routledge.

Datan, N 1995, 'Corpses, lepers, and menstruating women: tradition, transition, and the sociology of knowledge', *Feminism & Psychology*, 5(4), pp. 449–459.

Deleuze, G & Guattari, F 2004, *A thousand plateaus: capitalism and schizophrenia*, London: Continuum.

Dendle, P 2007, 'The zombie as barometer of cultural anxiety', in N Scott (ed), *Monsters and the monstrous: myths and metaphors of enduring evil*, At the interface, probing the boundaries, Amsterdam: Rodopi, pp. 45–57.

Douglas, P M 2013, *Purity and danger: an analysis of concepts of pollution and taboo*, Abingdon and New York: Routledge.

Dyer, R 2004, *Heavenly bodies: film stars and society*, 2nd ed., London and New York: Routledge.

Elliott, C 2003, *Better than well: American medicine meets the American dream*, New York: W.W. Norton.

Fisiak, T 2014, 'Hag horror heroines: kitsch / camp goddesses, tyrannical females, queer icons', in J Stępień (ed), *Redefining kitsch and camp in literature and culture*, Newcastle upon Tyne: Cambridge Scholars Press, pp. 41–52.

Fritz, M A & Speroff, L 2012, *Clinical gynecologic endocrinology and infertility*, Philadelphia, PA: Lippincott Williams & Wilkins.

Fugh-Berman, A 2015, 'The science of marketing: how pharmaceutical companies manipulated medical discourse on menopause', *Women's Reproductive Health*, 2(1), pp. 18–23.

Gannon, L & Stevens, J 1998, 'Portraits of menopause in the mass media', *Women & Health*, 27 (3), pp. 1–15.

Gott, M 2005, *Sexuality, sexual health and ageing*, Maidenhead, UK and New York: Open University Press.

Green, A 2011, 'The French horror film Martyrs and the destruction, defilement, and neutering of the female form', *Journal of Popular Film and Television*, 39(1), pp. 20–28.

Grosz, E 1994, *Volatile bodies: toward a corporeal feminism*, Bloomington, IN: Indiana University Press.

Houck, J A 2003, '"What do these women want?": feminist responses to Feminine Forever, 1963–1980', *Bulletin of the History of Medicine*, 77(1), pp. 103–132.

Houppert, K 2000, *The curse: confronting the last unmentionable taboo: menstruation*, New York: Farrar, Straus and Giroux.

Kaplan, E A 2011, 'Un-fashionable age: clothing and unclothing the older woman's body on screen', in A Munich (ed), *Fashion in film*, New directions in national cinemas, Bloomington, IN: Indiana University Press, pp. 322–344.

Kristeva, J 1982, *Powers of horror: an essay on abjection*, New York: Columbia University Press.

Kwok, W L 1996, 'On menopause and cyborgs: or, towards a feminist cyborg politics of menopause', *Body & Society*, 2(3), pp. 33–52.

Lauzen, M M & Dozier, D M 2005, 'Maintaining the double standard: portrayals of age and gender in popular films', *Sex Roles*, 52(7–8), pp. 437–446.

Lobato, R & Ryan, M D 2011, 'Rethinking genre studies through distribution analysis: issues in international horror movie circuits', *New Review of Film and Television Studies*, 9(2), pp. 188–203.

Lock, M 1993, *Encounters with aging: mythologies of menopause in Japan and North America*, Berkeley, CA: University of California Press.

Lock, M 1998, 'Anomalous ageing: managing the postmenopausal body', *Body & Society*, 4(1), pp. 35–61.

Markson, E W 2003, 'The female aging body through film', in C A Faircloth (ed), *Aging bodies: images and everyday experience*, Walnut Creek, CA: AltaMira Press, pp. 77–102.

Markson, E W & Taylor, C A 2000, 'The mirror has two faces', *Ageing & Society*, 20(2), pp. 137–160.

Martin, E 1987, *The woman in the body: a cultural analysis of reproduction*, Boston, MA: Beacon Press.

Martin, E 1991, 'The egg and the sperm: how science has constructed a romance based on stereotypical male–female roles', *Signs*, 16(3), pp. 485–501.

Mathijs, E & Mendik, X 2008, 'Editorial introduction: what is cult film?', in E Mathijs & X Mendik (eds), *The cult film reader*, Maidenhead, UK: MacGraw-Hill, pp. 1–11.

Miller, A 2005, '"The hair that wasn't there before": demystifying monstrosity and menstruation in "Ginger Snaps" and "Ginger Snaps Unleashed"', *Western Folklore*, 64(3/4), pp. 281–303.

Mulvey, L 2000, 'Visual pleasure and narrative cinema', in E A Kaplan (ed), *Feminism and film*, Oxford readings in feminism, Oxford and New York: Oxford University Press, pp. 34–47.

Powell, A 2005, *Deleuze and horror film*, Edinburgh: Edinburgh University Press.

Russell, L 2004, 'Queering consumption and production in *What Ever Happened to Baby Jane?*', in S Hantke (ed), *Horror film: creating and marketing fear*, Jackson, MS: University Press of Mississippi, pp. 213–226.

Shelley, P 2009, *Grande Dame Guignol cinema: a history of hag horror from Baby Jane to Mother*, Jefferson, NC: McFarland.

Signorielli, N 2004, 'Aging on television: messages relating to gender, race, and occupation in prime time', *Journal of Broadcasting & Electronic Media*, 48(2), pp. 279–301.

Sobchack, V 2000, 'Revenge of "The Leech Woman": on the dread of aging in a low-budget horror film', in K Gelder (ed), *The horror reader*, London and New York: Routledge, pp. 336–346.

Sobchack, V 2009, 'Scary women: cinema, surgery and special effects', in D M Jones & M C Heyes (eds), *Cosmetic surgery: a feminist primer*, Farnham, UK and Burlington, VT: Ashgate, pp. 79–95.

Springer, C 2015, 'Introduction', in C Springer & J Levinson (eds), *Acting*, New Brunswick, NJ: Rutgers University Press, pp. 1–24, accessed from <http://www.jstor.org/stable/j.ctt19jch2h.3>.

Stephens, J 2003, '"I'll never be the same after that summer": from abjection to subjective agency in teen films', in K Mallan & S Pearce (eds), *Youth cultures: texts, images, and identities*, Westport, CT: Praeger, pp. 123–138.

Stewart, K, Powell, M & Greer, R 2009, 'An alternative to conventional sanitary protection: would women use a menstrual cup?', *Journal of Obstetrics and Gynaecology*, 29(1), pp. 49–52.

Takahashi, T A & Johnson, K M 2015, 'Menopause', *Medical Clinics of North America*, 99(3), pp. 521–534.

Taylor, T 2012, 'Who's afraid of the rubber man? Perversions and subversions of sex and class in American Horror Story', *Networking Knowledge: Journal of the MeCCSA-PGN*, 5(2), pp. 135–153.

Tyler, I 2013, *Revolting subjects: social abjection and resistance in neoliberal Britain*, London: Zed Books Ltd., accessed December 17, 2016, from <http://public.eblib.com/choice/publicfullrecord.aspx?p=1160737>.

Ussher, J M 2006, *Managing the monstrous feminine: regulating the reproductive body*, London and New York: Routledge.

Ussher, J M 2011, *The madness of women: myth and experience*, London and New York: Routledge.

Vares, T, Potts, A, Gavey, N & Grace, V M 2007, 'Reconceptualizing cultural narratives of mature women's sexuality in the Viagra era', *Journal of Aging Studies*, 21(2), pp. 153–164.

Walter, B S G 2015, *Our old monsters: witches, werewolves and vampires from medieval theology to horror cinema*, Jefferson, NC: McFarland.

Watson, P 1997, 'There's no accounting for taste: exploitation cinema and the limits of film theory', in D Cartmell (ed), *Trash aesthetics: popular culture and its audience*, London: Pluto Press, pp. 66–83.

Wilson, R A 1966, *Feminine forever*, New York: Evans.

Wilson, R A & Wilson, T A 1963, 'The fate of the nontreated postmenopausal woman: a plea for the maintenance of adequate estrogen from puberty to the grave', *Journal of the American Geriatrics Society*, 11(4), pp. 347–362.

Writing Group for the Women's Health Initiative Investigators 2002, 'Risks and benefits of estrogen plus progestin in healthy postmenopausal women: principal results from the women's health initiative randomized controlled trial', *JAMA*, 288(3), pp. 321–333.

Afterword
Monstrous miscarriages and uncanny births

The ABCs of Death (2012) is an anthology that offers 26 short films, each named for a letter of the alphabet, and each exploring a different way to die. According to the film's opening titles, selected directors from around the world were given a $5000 budget, a letter of the alphabet around which to shape their film, and free range to do as they pleased. As such, the only overt editorialisation of the abecedary comes from the choice of directors made by the film's producers, Tim League and Ant Timpson, both of whom are well-known distributors, festival programmers and independent and genre film producers. The directors themselves represent 15 different countries across Europe, the Americas, Asia, Scandinavia and Australasia. The film's website frames this collection as an international snapshot of the genre as it is today, as presented by some of horror's best and most exciting directors (*The ABCs of Death*).

At the beginning of this book I situated my analysis within my own viewing practice, and in a presentation about female spectatorship and horror cinema at an academic conference I talked about the somewhat unruly experience of watching this film with a female group of fellow horror fans. In particular, I discussed our mounting frustration at the patterns of content that built up over the course of the anthology. While the filmmakers had ostensibly been offered complete artistic freedom, this seemed to result in many of them giving in to the impulse to use the short film format as a vehicle for the cinematic equivalent of quick, dirty punchlines involving toilet humour, ultraviolence and sex. The films vary in tone, content and quality, which is perhaps to be expected for such a collection, but more concerning to me was the overall matrix of misogyny that quickly developed. In the parlance of comedy, many of these films punch down, not up. I suggested that the patterns of representation that build up in the anthology reveal the extent to which a certain set of tastes and expectations were being implicitly catered to, and whose viewing positions, and voices, were being excluded. In particular, the feeling for those of us women watching together was that too many of the cohort of directors were being lazy and playing to a presumed 'ideal' viewer: male, heterosexual, voyeuristic, a little adolescent in their tastes, interested in the shock value of content that could be quickly designated as 'badass'.

Certainly, watching 26 short films in a row can be an addling experience, but as the anthology wore on the tone in the room shifted markedly from excitement to disappointment to irritated disdain.

As the anthology plays out, women's bodies are predominantly presented in ways that are hypersexualised and often misogynistic. This becomes increasingly gauche, such that the originality of darkly comic films about killer spiders (Angela Bettis's "E is for Exterminate"), talking birds and marital infidelity (Banjong Pisanthanakun's "N is for Nuptials") and some endearingly bizarre claymation work about a child's fear of the toilet (Lee Hardcastle's "T is for Toilet") is undermined by image after image of objectification and degradation. Fourteen of the 26 films feature explicitly sexualised content. Thirteen of the films feature women who are partially clothed or naked, compared to six that feature men in this way; of those six, one is a man in an open backed surgical gown – nothing erotic to see here – and the only instance of full-frontal male nudity is in a situation where men are being sexually humiliated, not sexually objectified. Twelve films feature the explicit sexual objectification of women, and others are certainly borderline. Seven – over a quarter – feature sexual assault, rape or other forms of sexual coercion. One (Timo Tjahjanto's "L is for Libido") deals, outright, in sexualised horror. The three examples of female-to-female sexual content are explicitly 'performed' to satisfy a presumably heterosexual male gaze. Only two of the 26 films have a female director, and one of those – "O is for Orgasm", an artful exploration of BDSM and pleasure co-directed by Bruno Forzani & Hélène Cattet – is the only film in which women's sexuality (and consensual sex!) is framed in a positive manner. For the female viewer, this is alienating to say the least.

Even worse, the patterns of gender and power established within the anthology undermine some of the more thoughtful and creative offerings. According to the film's credits, Jorge Michel Grau's short "I is for Ingrown" is intended to act as a serious commentary on rates of domestic violence and femicide in Mexico. When placed alongside these other films its content, which includes gritty footage of a woman bound, gagged and injected with poison by a person we are led to believe is her husband, reads not as plaintive but as exploitative.

One very short film is a brief but telling example of some of the worst, most conservative and reactionary applications of the gynaehorrific, and begs the question as to why it is women in film are framed as they are. It shows a quirkily well-dressed woman trying, and failing, to awkwardly flush something down a toilet. She is clearly flustered. From the perspective of the toilet's bowl we see her leaning in with a plunger, tentatively, and a reverse shot shows a bloody, clotted mess collected in the water. The title card at the end acts as a punchline: "M is for Miscarriage". The short film renders its female lead a cardboard cut-out, without personality or feeling beyond a set of hipster affectations – thick rimmed spectacles, red lipstick, polka-dotted shoes. It frames her reproductive body and its products as abject, leaky, broken and yet – somehow, allegedly – groan-inducingly funny. If this counted as an example of the best of independent horror, then I suggested at the conference that our sneering response *en masse* was a belligerent refusal: I is for 'I Don't Think So'; please try harder.

I offer an account of this film to reiterate the point I have made throughout this book that gynaehorror certainly lends to conservative, even misogynistic accounts of women's sexed, reproductive bodies that reveal as much about deep-seated attitudes towards women as they do about what qualifies as 'horrific'. It is apt, then, that the anthology's sequel offers an outstanding example of gynaehorror as a site of radical, progressive expression that might engage in a nuanced, complex way with issues of women, sex and reproductive bodies. In spite of the claim, again, that its directors were given free reign, *The ABCs of Death 2* (2014) presents a significantly more interesting and diverse set of films – films that do not seem to need to rely on rape, objectification and hypersexualisation to make their point – to the extent that I wonder whether the adolescent excesses of the first were noted and gently marked 'please avoid'. Its final offering, Canadian director Chris Nash's "Z is for Zygote", is deeply provocative.

The film is set in an oneiric rural space that seems to sit out of time: a rustic wooden house sits surrounded by woods, all brown and grey, and the dreamy isolation gives the impression that we are looking into an old photograph. A heavily pregnant woman cries as her disinterested, dismissive husband leaves out into the snow; he promises to return soon, but gives her a large jar of special 'medicine', a dried root that will stave off labour in the meantime. Thirteen years later the woman lies on the floor, surrounded by filth, maggots and the bones of small animals she has hunted to stave off starvation. Her stomach is now an enormous distended sac, home to the unborn thirteen year old, and she is unable to stand; instead, she must drag herself around on the floor. While the image is horrific and the atmosphere unsettling, the tone is unexpectedly light and genial; the woman and her unborn child chat away happily as the woman tries to trap a cat for their dinner, making do as they always have done. The muffled unborn – who voices its hopes that it might be a boy so that 'he' can go hunting with his absent father – wants to be allowed out and is feeling a little cramped, but its mother doesn't want to be left alone, and asks why it doesn't want to spend more time with her.

Terror and violence comes when the woman realises she has finally run out of the labour-stifling root, and she screams, in crippling agony, that she doesn't want the unborn to leave her. In keeping with this request, the unborn forces the mother out of her own body – broken bones, organs, blood and viscera all forced through her distended mouth. It slips into the mother's skin like a hand into a glove before cutting away the immense stomach flap and carefully stitching up the wound; they are now together forever in a new form of symbiosis. Finally, father arrives home to a clean and tidy house and, disappointed that the baby has seemingly been and gone, suggests that the thing to do is to re-impregnate 'mother' and try again. The film ends as mother's dress, unzipped, falls to the floor.

In just under seven minutes, "Z is for Zygote" explores in compelling detail many of the key features of the gynaehorrific, and it does so with both horror and a wry sort of humour. It offers a portrait of a woman abandoned by her uncaring husband, of a mother who cannot give up her intimate, flesh-and-blood alliance-relationship with her child, and of a child who must literally tear itself away from its mother's smothering love. It looks to loss, ageing and the dismissal of female experience, especially as when father re-appears he seems irritated that his 13-year absence has even provoked a reaction, and he certainly doesn't notice that his wife has changed. Its gothic domestic space conflates the emotional and physical entrapment of mother with the corporeal entrapment of the child. It plays with gender and sexuality in the indeterminacy of the unborn and in mother's 'remaking' as a new self in a mother-skin. It looks to the nature of reproduction – the production of children, the reproduction of a certain type of sexed, gendered self, and the reproduction of families and relationships. Its shift from winter to spring marks the reproductive body as cyclical. It positions essential motherhood as something violent and corporeal, but also perhaps as inevitable. Its shocking act of birth – or, rejection – produces not a whole child, but a new mother-self and a torrent of viscera that is summarily, almost cheerfully, dumped in a nearby field. It takes an almost comically pragmatic attitude towards the violence of birth and its dripping by-products, and to the practicalities of the fleshy shift in body and in subjectivity required by pregnancy. Its final, quietly horrific and uncomfortably incestuous moment comes as father tells this new mother that they will just have to put another one 'inside' her, in a reproduction of horror that is inflicted, again and again, specifically *upon* the woman's body, whether she particularly wants it or not.

Importantly, this film shows that the horror genre can, and should, do interesting things with women, sex and reproduction in a manner that enriches, reveals and provokes rather than belittles and reduces. Gynaehorror does not have to be something implicitly misogynistic. Instead, it can be monstrous in its most generative, provocative sense: a zygote that indicates new life, new congruities and new possibilities, rather than the miscarried leavings of a thoughtless representation.

Index

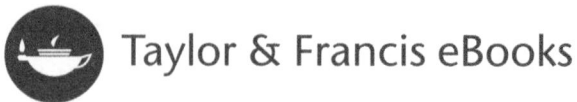
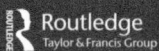